BASIC PATHOPHYSIOLOGY

Modern Stress and the Disease Process

BASIC PATHOPHYSIOLOGY

Modern Stress and the Disease Process

J. M. Ramsey

Professor, Biological Sciences
University of Dayton
Dayton, Ohio

Addison-Wesley Publishing Company
Medical/Nursing Division • Menlo Park, California
Reading, Massachusetts • London • Amsterdam
Don Mills, Ontario • Sydney

Sponsoring Editor: Pat Franklin
Assistant Editor: Thomas Eoyang
Production Coordinators: Karen Bierstedt and Susan Harrington
Book and Cover Design: Judith M. Sager

Library of Congress Cataloging in Publication Data

Ramsey, J. M.
   Basic pathophysiology: modern stress and the disease
process.

   Includes index.
   1. Stress (Physiology) 2. Environmentally induced
diseases. 3. Physiology, Pathological. I. Title.
(DNLM: 1. Stress—Complications. 2. Stress, Psychological
—Complications. 3. Disease—Etiology. QZ 160 R183b)
QP82.2.S8R35   616.07   81-15004
ISBN 0-201-06329-8   AACR2

ISBN 0-201-06329-8
ABCDEFGHIJ-HA-8987654321

The paper in this book meets the guidelines for permanence and durability
of the Committee on Production Guidelines for Book Longevity of the
Council on Library Resources.

The author and publisher have exerted every effort to insure that drug
selection and dosage set forth in this text are in accord with current
recommendations and practice at the time of publication. However in view
of ongoing research, changes in government regulations and the constant
flow of information relating to drug therapy and drug reactions, the reader
is urged to check the package insert for each drug for any change in
indications of dosage and for added warnings and precautions. This is
particularly important where the recommended agent is a new and/or
infrequently employed drug.

Addison-Wesley Publishing Company
Medical/Nursing Division
2725 Sand Hill Road
Menlo Park, California 94025

The requirements of health can be stated simply. Those fortunate enough to be born free of significant congenital disease or disability will remain well if three basic needs are met: they must be adequately fed; they must be protected from a wide range of hazards in the environment; and they must not depart radically from the pattern of personal behavior under which man evolved, for example, by smoking, overeating or sedentary living.—Thomas McKeown

Foreword

I am glad to have been given this opportunity to write a foreword for Professor Ramsey's new textbook, which focuses on the ways the peculiar stresses of modern society lead to disease, and on the more common forms of such derangements. Perhaps it will not be out of place for me to respond with a few comments about how we can in some measure control and prevent the pathogenic process.

The direction of modern stress research reflects a growing awareness of the effects of industrialization on modern human illnesses. In this respect, important work is being conducted concerning the nervous pathways that mediate and condition the stress response. These pathways are operative both if the conditioning factors originate outside the individual, as do family problems, air pollution, and crowding, and if they originate inside the individual, as do genetic predisposition, previous medical interventions, diseases of old age, accidents resulting in irreparable handicaps, and various psychologic factors.

Undoubtedly, in any working environment, as in all stress situations, psychologic conditioning factors cannot be neglected, because whatever a person's position in the hierarchy of command, the stressor effect of one's decision-making depends not only upon what one decides or even what the consequences will be, but also upon the way one reacts to his or her particular position. In essence, this explains the many contradictory ideas about whether being a boss or being bossed is more distressful. Some people are leaders, others followers, in their mental tendencies and habits. In the words of Professor Ramsey, "The degree or severity of psychologic stress is related to the individual's ability to recognize, know, and understand the stress as well as how much control the individual feels he or she has over the situation" (see Chapter 17).

One problem all living beings share is that of surviving as happily as possible in an ever-changing environent. Microbes, plants, and most of the living organisms situated lower on the evolutionary scale achieve this by means of more or less automatic cellular responses or instincts, which have evolved in accordance with "the survival of the fittest." Only the higher organisms, and particularly humans, have acquired brains sufficiently complex to endow them with a sense of logic and ethics, through which they can learn to control, at least in part, their hereditary impulses.

It is a biologic law that humans—like animals—must fight and work for some goal that they consider worthwhile. We must use our innate capacities to enjoy the fulfillment derived from successfully coping with stress. Only through effort, often aggressive egoistic effort, can we maintain our fitness and assure our adaptive equilibrium with the surrounding society and the inanimate world. To achieve this state, our activities must earn lasting results; the fruits of work must be cumulative and must provide a capital gain to meet future needs. To succeed, we have to accept the scientifically established fact that humans have an inescapable natural urge to work selfishly for things that can be stored to strengthen their homeostasis in the unpredictable situations with which life may confront them. These are not tendencies we should combat or try to hide. It is primarily for our own good that we can do nothing about having been built to work. Organs that are not used (muscles, bones, even the brain) undergo atrophy due to inactivity, and every living being looks out first of all for itself. There is no example in nature of a creature guided exclusively by altruism and the desire to help others. In fact, a code of universal altruism may be seen as highly immoral, since we would expect others to look out for us more than for themselves.

"Love thy neighbor as thyself" is a command full of wisdom, but as originally expressed it is incompatible with biologic laws; no one needs to develop an inferiority complex if one cannot spontaneously love all fellow human beings. Neither should we feel guilty because we work for treasures that can be stored to ensure our future homeostasis. Hoarding is a vitally important biologic instinct that we share with other creatures such as ants, bees, squirrels, and beavers.

How can we develop a code of ethics that accepts egoism and working to hoard personal goods as morally correct? That is what I attempted to do in *Stress without Distress*, and here are the basic tenets of the code of behavior I have put forth:

1. Find your own natural stress level, the level at which you can comfortably advance toward your own selected port of destination.

2. Be an altruistic egoist. Do not try to suppress the natural instinct of all living beings to look after themselves first. Yet the wish to be of some use, to do some good for others, is also natural. We are social beings, and everybody wants somehow to earn respect and gratitude. You must be useful to others. This gives you the greatest degree of safety, because no one wishes to destroy a person who is useful.

3. EARN thy neighbor's love. This is a contemporary modification of the maxim "Love thy neighbor as thyself." It recognizes that all neighbors are not lovable and that it is impossible to love on command.

A clear distinction must be made between treatment techniques (for example, biofeedback, relaxation, physical exercise) and a philosophy of life; the latter is, in the long run, much more potent. The greatest challenge to humanity, I believe, is to understand such a philosophy of life, which gives good guidance, not on how to avoid stress (for that cannot be done), but on how to cope with it to achieve health, long life, and happiness.

Hans Selye
April 1980

Preface

Subject and scope

The relationship between disease and our physical environment changes as the stressors of that environment change. The development of today's industrialized society has transformed the environment on a mammoth scale and continues to do so at an ever-increasing rate. *Basic Pathophysiology: Modern Stress and the Disease Process* introduces the reader to the physiologic processes of the body during dysfunction, in the context of our modern environment and the stresses it imposes.

To integrate the disease process with its environmental setting, this text takes a different approach from the traditional one of listing diseases, system by system, in an encyclopedic manner. The book's main focus is on the dynamics of *how the body's normal processes become pathologic,* emphasizing how underlying physiologic stress mechanisms lead to maladaptation. The duality of *stress and adaptation* is thus the conceptual basis throughout the book. Physiologic stress is related to its major pathologic consequences and to the need for preventive measures.

Special effort has been made to explore topics neglected or treated cursorily in more traditional texts on pathophysiology; this effort reflects the intention to focus specifically on the disturbances brought about by the stressors of modern life. Information is presented that is usually contained in works on environmental or applied physiology; the inclusion of this information, however, is essential to the novel approach taken by the text.

Audience

The timely approach of this text will prove especially useful to students of nursing, the life sciences, and allied health because it makes unique connections between concepts of the basic sciences and the physiology of human disease. The material has been prepared for the undergraduate to use as a text or adjunct reference in a one-term course in pathophysiology. It is also appropriate as a supplementary text for a course, such as medical-surgical nursing, where pathophysiology may be an important secondary thread to the main subject.

Organization

The book is organized into five parts. Part One follows a brief introduction and enunciates the conceptual principles underlying the unique perspective of the text. It covers the nature of disease and of physiologic stress, the role that the neuroendocrine system plays in homeostasis, and the relation of physiologic stress to pathology. Discussion of human disease occupies the remainder of the book and is arranged according to the source of stress: physical, chemical, biologic, and cultural. Part Two deals with disease arising from the physical stressors of radiation, temperature change, and sound. Chemical stressors, which are discussed in Parts Three and Four, have been divided into those that occur in the body's natural functioning (Part Three)—oxygenation, physical exertion, and nutrition—and those that occur as a result of human alterations of the body's surroundings (Part Four)—environmental pollution and substance abuse. Part Five discusses biologic and cultural stressors from infection and immune response, psychosocial sources, emotionally induced chemical imbalance, and the effects of biologic time.

Because accounts of various diseases have been arranged according to the sources of stress associated with them, a "disease finder" has been included as Appendix A, identifying the chapters and sections in which principal discussion of each major disease may be found. Appendix B offers the normal adult ranges for clinical laboratory values. A special illustrative feature are the Color Plates, located after Appendix B, showing various dermatologic disorders discussed in the text. A Glossary of important terms precedes the index. Each chapter after Chapter 1 begins with briefly stated student objectives and ends with a summary, chapter glossary, and list of references.

Acknowledgements

I wish to acknowledge the invaluable effort and services provided by several persons without whom this book would not have materialized. Mrs. Ann Feldmann spent countless hours typing and retyping the manuscript and its revisions, and Ms. Barbara J. Banik, Curriculum Coordinator, Department of Baccalaureate Nursing, Austin Peay State University, offered constructive suggestions upon critically reading and rereading the manuscript. In addition, the following people critically reviewed the manuscript and made valuable suggestions: Dr. Margaret Mullins of the Wright State University School of Medicine; Dr. June C. Abbey, Professor and Director of Nursing Research, University of Pittsburgh School of Nursing, and formerly Director of Physiological Nursing Programs, University of

Utah School of Nursing; and Professor Jane Taylor, College of Nursing, University of Delaware.

Appreciation is expressed also to Dr. Hans Selye for graciously consenting to write the Foreword, and gratitude is expressed to the many investigators, authors, and publishers who have granted permission for the various citations and adaptations.

Finally, I wish to extend a word of appreciation to my publisher, Addison-Wesley, and especially to editor Pat Franklin, to Karen Bierstedt and Susan Harrington for production coordination, and to assistant editor Thomas Eoyang.

J. M. Ramsey

Contents

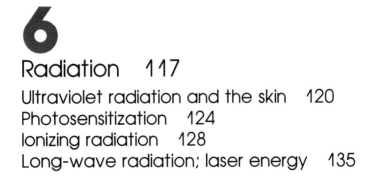

10

Stress from Physical Exertion   227

11

Malnutritive Stress and Disease   255

12

Caloric Imbalance and Food Intolerance   287

PART IV. STRESS AND DISEASE FROM MAN-MADE CHEMICAL STRESSORS   317

Health Effects of Environmental Pollution   319

Tobacco, Alcohol, and Drugs   343

BASIC PATHOPHYSIOLOGY

Modern Stress and the Disease Process

1

Introduction

A fundamental principle in biologic sciences is that an organism must be able to adapt to its environment to survive and remain healthy. Inability to adapt invites disease and risks premature death. Adaptability may be especially problematic for the human species because most of us inhabit a somewhat artificial environment that is becoming more complex and poses novel demands. In addition to natural physical, chemical, and biologic forces, many more environmental conditions have been developed by humans themselves.

There has been a dramatic shift in the major causes of death in all industrialized regions of the globe since 1900. For the most part, the current medical problems in all technological societies are not the illnesses familiar to past generations. As the noted medical historian Rene Dubos has stated, "Each civilization has its own kind of pestilence and can control it only by reforming itself . . . just as the great epidemics of the nineteenth century were precipitated by environmental factors which favored the activities of pathogenic microorganisms, so many of the diseases characteristic of our times have their origin in some faulty factor of the modern environment. . . ."[1]

It is true that today infectious and contagious diseases have been replaced largely by cardiovascular disease, hypertension, malignant neoplasms, arthritis, diabetes, emphysema, gastrointestinal disorders, mental illness, allergic disease, and other chronic conditions. Undoubtedly the increased frequency of some of these illnesses is due in part to extension of the average life span, which in turn has stemmed from the conquering of infectious disease. However, numerous clinical specialists are beginning to realize that the health problems characteristic of our times are somehow linked with the way we live in our modern environment. They contend that the difficulties involved in adapting to today's world constitute an important component of the etiology.

Many of us these days do suffer from the onslaught of the

[1]R. Dubos. 1959. *Mirage of health*. New York: Harper & Bros. p. 164.

multiple stresses of the modern urban jungle with its overcrowding, competition, rush, noise, dirt, chemicals, bright lights, excitement, polluted air, rich and salty foods, temperature changes, disease, and threat of bodily harm. Moreover, those of us who tolerate these stresses poorly sometimes resort sooner or later to the crutches of alcohol, drugs, and endless varieties of medications, which in many instances merely contribute additional stress and heighten the risks of serious pathology.

In recent years there appears to be a growing awareness of the role of the environment in promoting disease; accordingly, the health care professions are showing more consideration for the whole patient. More attention is being paid to the significance of our habits, where we live, where we work, and our personal problems. Along with these developments there has been an increasing interest in preventive medicine. The recognition of health threats from the environment and the need to understand the nature of the stresses they impose warrant educational emphasis on the relation of stress to disease, particularly if preventive medicine is to be soundly and effectively pursued. Our modern environment has become much more physically, chemically, socially, and psychologically complex.

There will be physiologic stress and consequent disease as long as there is human existence. However, various stressors tend to become more or less formidable with time. In ancient times people were often subjected to severe stress, although they were not confronted with as many different stressors as are their modern counterparts. Thermal stress, infectious disease, and malnutritive stress occasionally got the better of them, but they were spared the din of incessant vibratory energy, and they were free from the compulsive rapid pace of living and the bombardment of manufactured chemicals that plague us today.

Although evidence of improvement in the effective control of today's stressors is generally meager, there are a few encouraging indicators. For example, male deaths from heart attacks during middle age are occurring less frequently than was the case fifteen years ago. Whether this is a transient or a genuine trend of longer range remains to be seen. On the other hand, cancer is being detected more frequently than ever before. Moreover, there appears to be no appreciable reduction in the incidence of alcoholism, mental illness, hypertension, emphysema, diabetes, obesity, liver damage, toxic blood disorders, kidney disease, arthritis, allergic diseases, and hearing impairment. Since the body is being accosted by a large assortment of chemicals to which it was never exposed throughout most of human existence, there is little wonder that there are increasing incidences of some of these disorders.

In regard to the physiologic stress-disease relationship, clear-cut conclusions and indisputable points are not easily established despite numerous investigations of the consequences of exposure of laboratory animals and humans to various stressors. Though many concepts have been introduced, a surprising number of points remain equivocal and unresolved. This is especially true with respect to utility of the knowledge. As a result, people are frequently confused, especially by popular reports in the media which often are the principal sources of information available to the public on matters of health. Should one eat this, or avoid that? Will transcendental meditation relieve one's hypertension?

Why do reports, even technical ones in professional journals, occasionally contradict each other? There are good reasons. Living organisms, and especially mammals, are fantastically complex machines. The chemical and physical variables seem endless. The permutational potential of nucleic acids (genes) and proteins is the basis for the likelihood that no two individuals will respond in the same way to the same conditions. By the same principle, each investigator is a different human being with a different background who cannot help but view matters from a unique angle. Hence, the possibility of different results from different laboratories always exists, and it must be conceded that medical science is not exact.

A few points of caution are in order here. Of necessity, a considerable amount of controlled research pertaining to stress and its relation to disease is done with laboratory animals, and it is risky to extrapolate interpretation of data from animals to humans. Also, the student of any science must learn to discriminate between theory and fact. When controversial points are addressed, it must be realized that we are born into a world of people; thus, we normally become attuned to a social and psychologic reality that by nature is steeped in subjectivity. It is not easy to make the mental transition to a more objective, less personalized *physical* reality that is so important in the pursuit of science.

With these introductory remarks in mind, let us begin by examining the nature of disease.

PART ONE
GENERAL PRINCIPLES

This section introduces the concepts of disease and physiologic stress, followed by a background of neuroendocrine control mechanisms. The section concludes with an insight into the stress-disease relationship, with special focus on cardiovascular pathology and cancer.

2

The Nature of Disease

Functional and Organic Disorders
Tissue Damage
    Inflammation
    Degenerative Damage
    Regressive Injury
    Cellular Chemical Stress
Tissue Repair
Classification of Pathology-Producing
Disturbances
Diagnosis and Treatment
Pathology Today

|| Objectives: Upon completing this chapter you should:

1. Understand the concept of disease as a dynamic process.
2. Be able to distinguish between functional and organic disorders.
3. Be acquainted with the physiologic and cellular bases of disease.
4. Be able to categorize the types of body disturbances associated with pathologic development.

What is disease? More to the point, how does it come about? The word itself literally means lack of ease. That doesn't tell us much. There are various synonyms, among them illness, absence of health, sickness, abnormality. As practical as these words are in common usage, concepts based upon them alone are unavoidably superficial. Many reputable works on pathology define disease as deviation beyond the limits of normal. What are these limits? Does this mean that an individual who has lost a hand in an accident is suffering from a disease? Is a color-blind person diseased? Since normalcy is essentially a statistical concept and therefore quite relative, does this mean that everyone is diseased? Obviously the distinction between what is normal and what is pathologic is somewhat arbitrary. The two conditions occur as related points along the same continuous spectrum.

Diseases traditionally are given specific names and descriptions which may lead us to the naive idea that they are static, well-defined entities. Disease is a complex, dynamic process. The potential for developing disease is ever present to varying degrees in all of us. Disease is latent within the adaptive mechanisms of our bodies. It is sometimes manifested as a finely graded series of stages, many of which are not clearly recognizable. With proper measures, disease often can be arrested, reversed, or both in all but the later stages.

Perhaps the most realistic concept of disease regards it as a *distinct inability to maintain the proper chemical and physical balances throughout the body, not only within the cells themselves, but among their various interactions as well*. In health we are in reasonable balance with the antagonistic forces of our environment. In disease the balance becomes disturbed. If uncorrected the imbalance leads to specific functional and structural alterations in the cells, tissues, and organs. Environmental changes and their demands on the body require continual physiologic adaptation to maintain physical and chemical balances within our tissues. When these balances are disturbed to the point that they stress our adaptive mechanisms, we may be risking the initiation of a vicious cycle in which less effective

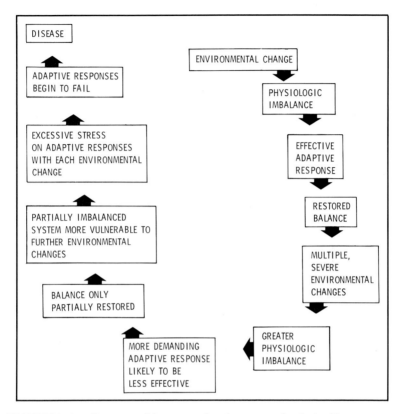

FIGURE 2-1   **Concept of how unrelenting stress leads to disease.**

adaptability is followed by further imbalance which in turn leads to further strain on adaptive mechanisms (Figure 2-1).

When adaptive responses to stresses become faulty and ineffective, disease begins to be recognizable. Hence, one must fully understand the nature of physiologic stress to adequately comprehend the disease process. Both stress and disease can be conceived as related points along the same continuum. (Physiologic stress is defined in Chapter 3.)

The appearance of disease depends upon the interaction of two factors. One is the variation in the original chemical nature of our cells that is determined at fertilization; in other words, our heredity, about which we can do very little at the present time. Lifelong environmental confrontations with physical forces, chemical agents, parasitic microbes, and psychosocial interactions constitute the second factor. These are the so-called stressors that continually challenge the capacity of our cells, tissues, organs, and systems to counteract disturbances prompted by environmental change. Unlike the genetic factor, we can do something about our exposure to stressors. Indeed, an awareness of the role of stress in pathogenesis offers possibilities for preventing disease and prolonging life.

In certain diseases the genetic factor is by far the more significant. The occurrence of hemophilia and sickle-cell anemia, for example, depends almost exclusively on gene determination. On the other hand, there is no special underlying genetic predisposition to syphilis. In most of our serious, major diseases such as hypertensive cardiovascular disease, cancer, arthritis, and diabetes, both heredity and environmental stress are significant contributors in varying degrees. However, the actual precipitation of a recognized disorder and when in a lifetime it appears often depend upon the intensity and chronicity of stress on a particular system.

FUNCTIONAL AND ORGANIC DISORDERS

A disorder that is produced by functional disturbances or changes in chemical composition in the absence of a lesion is distinguished as *functional impairment*, whereas structural alterations make up what is known as *organic disease*. In reality it is not always possible to separate the two, and in most diseases, especially those that have progressed, a composite effect is usually present.

In the earlier days of the study of pathology, structural changes received the most consideration. However, over time functional, or biochemical disorder as it is sometimes called, began to gain much more attention and assume greater importance for two reasons. First, functional imbalance became better understood than formerly, and second, it has become apparent that structural change in tissue is usually caused and preceded by chronic biochemical disturbances. Since derangements of biochemical systems are often gradual and tend to result from multiple stressor effects over periods of time, and since we are particularly concerned with how disease comes about, our attention is especially directed toward chronic, functional forms of pathology.

Functional disorders are considered to be reversible. They may be initiated by psychophysiologic factors, and they often involve the autonomic nervous system (ANS). Although no lesions can be demonstrated in these disorders, recent methods are revealing significant biochemical changes with respect to neurotransmitting substances, hormones, and other chemical mediators. Immune reactions also may become altered in functional disease.

TABLE 2-1

Some Frequently Encountered Disorders Considered Functional in Nature

Migraine

Colitis

Indigestion

Labile forms of hypertension

Insomnia

Depression

Hypersensitivity reactions

Constipation

Diarrhea

Reactive hypoglycemia

Some forms of dermatitis

Cardiac arrhythmia and palpitations

Menstrual discomfort

Impotence

In many instances of progressive, chronic disease, the typical sequence of events often begins with a weakening of adaptive responses due to overstressing an already predisposed constitution. The consequence is the chemical imbalance that characterizes functional disorder. If functional impairment is allowed to remain uncorrected, structural alterations in cells will follow sooner or later. A list of some of the more frequently encountered disorders that are usually considered to be functional is provided in Table 2-1.

Despite our emphasis on functional derangement, it must be acknowledged that all pathology is not chronic in nature. There are disorders in which organic changes may occur first. Acute disease is a consequence of such stressors as trauma, shock, and various forms of infection.

The detectable morphologic changes that characterize organic disease are termed *lesions*. They are most often revealed by microscopic examination of tissue, although inspection of gross morphologic features may show advanced stages of organic pathology. Electron microscopy is required to detect earlier structural alterations. Lesions detected by routine light microscopy are usually a late manifestation of the disease process.

Since most uncorrected disease processes sooner or later reach the point of recognizable structural alterations, it behooves us to learn more about tissue damage in general.

TISSUE DAMAGE

Stress that is applied directly to cellular material can result in alterations that are generally designated as damage or injury. Injury may be defined as any adverse influence that deranges the cell's ability to maintain a steady, adaptive homeostasis. Physical stressors such as mechanical trauma, radiation, and temperature change are capable of adverse influences. Damage also is produced by chemical stressors and infectious agents. If cells are restricted in the necessary supply of molecular materials such as oxygen and nutrients, or if noxious chemical agents such as irritants, toxins, infiltrating lipid, and antigen-antibody complexes are present, then disturbances in membrane integrity, enzyme activity, energy production, and osmotic regulation may occur, leading to disorganization within the cells. Much of the disorganization is reversible and the damage repairable, although in time this regenerative capability tends to diminish, particularly when the injury occurs again and again.

Ischemia (diminished blood supply) is the foremost factor underlying cellular injury in mammalian systems. It is a pathway that may allow other injurious agents to become effective. Indeed, hypoxia (insufficient oxygen) is probably the most common cause of cell injury. When the mitochondrial system of aerobic respiration is impaired, the integrity of cell membrane transport is compromised, leading to a disturbance of ionic and osmotic homeostasis that can become destructive.

Tissue damage has been classified as inflammatory, degenerative, infiltrative, and regressive. However, these conditions are variously interrelated and more than one may be present simultaneously.

Inflammation

Inflammation is defined as a localized reaction of vascularized tissue to nonspecific injury. Thus it is more of a tissue response to damage than an actual injury in itself. Inflammation is characterized by prominent microvascular changes around the cells. It serves a defensive purpose since these changes attempt to neutralize and destroy noxious agents at the site of injury and prevent their dissemination elsewhere. Inflammation can accomplish this defense largely through available blood supply. Despite the useful purposes it serves, inflammation itself can be potentially harmful and debilitating.

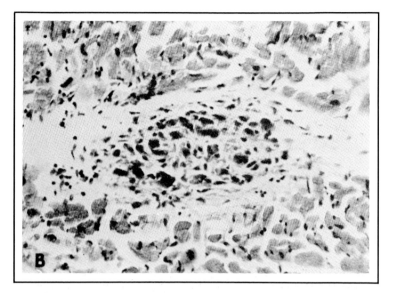

FIGURE 2-2   A histological section of connective tissue in which there is granulomatous inflammation. Note the edematous separation of the cells. The dark inclusions are Aschoff bodies. Section taken from a patient with acute rheumatic fever. (From R. Perez-Tamayo, *Mechanisms of disease—an introduction to pathology.* Philadelphia: W. B. Saunders Co., 1961.)

Heat, redness, swelling, and pain are the cardinal signs and symptoms of inflammation. Heat and redness result from an abnormal accumulation of blood due to localized vasodilation, which may reach a maximum in 10 minutes and is mediated by histamine and prostaglandins. A delayed phase, requiring one to several hours, culminates in the infiltration of tissue with leucocytes, followed by stasis and local hemorrhage. Neutrophils are the first leucocytes to appear. They begin to adhere to the inner surface of blood vessel endothelium, in a process known as *chemotaxis.* Monocytes follow, and once present in the damaged tissue they are transformed into macrophages which become effective phagocytes. A histological section of inflamed tissue is shown in Figure 2-2.

Inflammatory vasodilation is associated with increased capillary permeability, resulting in a leaking of plasma proteins, which produces a shift in osmotic balance. Water follows the protein, leading to much fluid congestion around the cells, which then become edematous (swollen) with fluid infiltration. The accumulation of fluid and cellular matter is called *exudate.* In some instances, exudate consists primarily of fluid and solutes with very few leucocytes, whereas in other cases neutrophils are predominant, producing

TABLE 2-2
Mediators of Inflammation

Vasodilation	Histamine
	Prostaglandins
Increased vascular permeability	Histamine
	Bradykinin
Fever	Pyrogens
	Prostaglandins
Chemotaxis	Neutrophils
	Monocytes
Pain	Bradykinin
	Prostaglandins
Tissue damage	Lysosomal enzymes (from
	neutrophils and macrophages)

what is known as *purulent* or *suppurative* exudate (pus). Suppuration occurring within connective tissue is called an *abscess*.

In inflammation a sustained mobilization of leucocytes and macrophages together with a release of lysosomal enzymes can be damaging to tissue, and the state may be perpetuated by additional release of vasoactive mediators. Pain is believed to be due to localized pressure caused by the swelling, as well as to stimulating action on the nerves by bradykinin and prostaglandins. A list of mediators associated with inflammation is provided in Table 2-2.

Acute inflammatory damage is typically reversible, but there are chronic forms associated with autoimmune processes, and there may be systemic manifestations of the localized reactions. Systemic effects include fever and increases in the sedimentation rate of red blood cells. The stressors most notably associated with inflammatory response include infection, antigen-antibody reactions, and radiation. Further attention is given to inflammatory reactions in the chapters devoted specifically to these stressors (Chapters 6 and 15).

Degenerative Damage

Degenerative injury is usually more chronic than acute. It is characterized by a progressive loss of biochemical organization within the cell cytoplasm, and it is usually associated with disturbances in cell energy metabolism. Degenerative change is typified by an accumulation of water within the cytoplasm. Impairment of cell membrane transport stemming from diminished energy metabolism interferes with the cell's normal ability to pump out sodium ions.

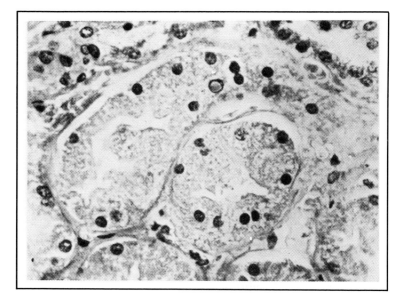

FIGURE 2-3   An example of cellular swelling in renal tubular cells.
The cytoplasm is swollen, finely granular, and its staining becomes less
defined. On the other hand, the nuclei stain more intensely, but appear
small. (From R. Perez-Tamayo, *Mechanisms of disease—an introduction to
pathology.*)

An increase in intracellular sodium alters osmotic balance and draws
water into the cell. Damage of this type is often described by histolo-
gists as *cellular* or *cloudy swelling.* The mitochondria also may swell. If
the influx of water becomes severe enough, the cytoplasm may become vacuolated. This state is designated *vacuolar degeneration.*

Degenerative changes are often associated with *fatty accumulation,* although significant increases in intracellular lipid can occur
without degenerative change. Accumulation of lipid may occur in
the kidney, heart, and especially the liver. The cell cytoplasm may
appear vacuolated, but in this case the vacuole content is lipid, not
water. The degeneration associated with fatty accumulation is usually chronic. Overeating stresses the liver, and hypoxia tends to enhance a build-up of lipid by restricting the cellular production of
energy. An agent most notable for producing fatty changes of the
liver is ethanol, or alcohol.

Many degenerative changes are reversible, at least in principle. In actuality, many of them slowly progress to greater degrees of
degeneration because the metabolic irregularities underlying them
are sustained. For example, the mitochondrial enspherulation in cel-

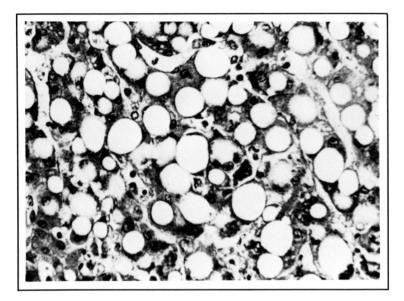

FIGURE 2-4   Fatty deposition in liver cells. The spherical bodies, light in color, are droplets of lipid. (From S. L. Robbins and R. S. Cotran, *Pathologic basis of disease*, 2d ed. Philadelphia: W. B. Saunders Co., 1979.)

lular swelling is related to an impairment in the organization and function of the respiratory chain within the cell. Since this type of change is associated with interference of respiratory mechanisms, essentially it is a nonspecific degeneration and therefore can be found in many organs such as the myocardium, kidney, liver, pancreas, and blood vessels. The histological appearance of cellular swelling is shown in Figure 2-3. Fatty accumulation and vacuolar degeneration, respectively, are depicted in Figure 2-4 and Figure 2-5.

Degenerative change tends to progress with age, particularly after the fifth decade, even without the recognized presence of specific disease. This form of tissue alteration is the principal type of lesion underlying atherosclerosis and consequent cardiovascular disease.

In respect to infiltrative injury, fluid infiltration that accompanies both inflammation and degenerative damage already has been mentioned. In addition, injured cells may be characterized by an increase in mucin and other colloidal materials, which, if they are mesenchymal or epithelial in origin, indicate that they are infiltrations. Examples of fluid infiltration may be found in such conditions as nasal catarrh and gastritis, where infiltration often accompanies inflammation.

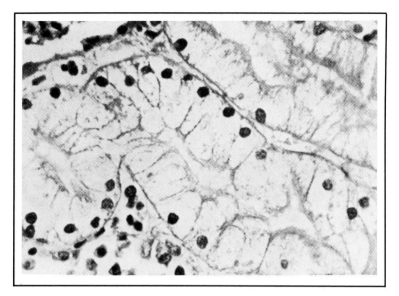

FIGURE 2-5   An example of vacuolar degeneration in renal tubular cells. Cell limits are discernible but the cytoplasm itself is primarily vacuole space and appears mostly empty. (From R. Perez-Tamayo, *Mechanisms of disease—an introduction to pathology.*)

Regressive Injury

Regressive tissue damage is irreversible. Examples include damage resulting in the specific hyaline structures in cells, such as those of the pancreatic beta cells, which consequently no longer secrete insulin, and *necrosis*, which represents the actual death of localized tissue. In these cases, changes are apparent in the cell nuclei. In some instances the necrotic cells disintegrate, as in tuberculosis. Such disintegration is termed *caseous* necrosis. When necrotic cells maintain their outlined appearance, despite shrunken, damaged nuclei, we describe the necrosis as *coagulative* (see Figure 2-6). Coagulative necrosis is usually the result of a severe restriction in blood supply (ischemia). Coagulative necrosis of a localized area, whether due to occluded arterial supply or venous drainage, is termed an *infarct*. The development of *gangrene,* or tissue death, usually follows, and saprophytic bacteria multiply in the dying tissue.

Cellular Chemical Stress

Most cellular injury is initiated by chemical stressors. Cell hypoxia has been mentioned already as a foremost factor leading to an over-

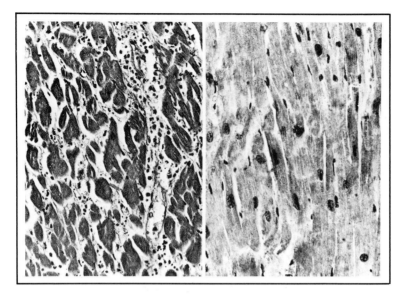

FIGURE 2-6   An example of coagulative necrosis in heart muscle.
Left, observe the necrotic cardiac muscle cells with well-preserved outlines.
The cytoplasm is coagulative and granular, and the nuclei have
disappeared. Compare with the normal cardiac muscle, *right*. (From S. L.
Robbins and R. S. Cotran, *Pathologic basis of disease.*)

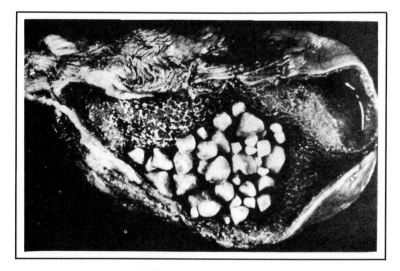

FIGURE 2-7   A group of gallstones within a diseased gall bladder.
Calculi of these dimensions block the common bile duct thereby
obstructing the flow of bile. (From S. A. Price and L. M. Wilson,
Pathophysiology—clinical concepts of disease processes. Copyright © 1978 by
McGraw-Hill, Inc. Used with permission of McGraw-Hill Book Co.)

all biochemical derangement within cells. On the other hand, as strange as it may appear, there also can be damage associated with the presence of oxygen. Oxidative reactions can lead to the formation of what are known as *free radicals* within cells. Free radicals are groups of atoms such as superoxides and hydroxyls that have electron orbitals with unpaired electrons, making these substances highly reactive and capable of entering into many chemical-bond formations. Much biochemical derangement can result from the oxidizing potential of free radicals. Since polyunsaturated lipids are prime targets of free radicals, and since such lipids form essential portions of cell membranes, then damage to cell membranes can result from this type of disturbance. The subject of lipid peroxidation and damage from free radicals will reappear from time to time throughout subsequent chapters, particularly Chapters 6, 9, and 18.

In certain pathologic changes in tissue, there is a deposition of insoluble calcium salts from the bloodstream. Such calcification occurs in tuberculosis and arteriosclerosis. Sometimes the calcium forms particles called *calculi* within ducts of major organs. Calculi (gallstones) tend to form around cholesterol globules in the biliary tract (Figure 2-7). Noncholesterol calculi also may be found in the urinary system, where they are called *kidney stones.*

TISSUE REPAIR

The human body possesses a remarkable ability to recover from injury and reconstruct damaged cells. Two distinct processes are involved, though they are often combined. The first is *regeneration,* in which there is proliferation of new *parenchymal* tissue identical to that lost. Regeneration constitutes a replacement by the same kind of cells, which are usually the essential or functional elements of an organ. However, an underlying framework or supporting *stroma* for the parenchymal cells must remain intact to permit this form of healing. Regenerative replacement also occurs normally. For example, the epithelial surfaces of the body are continually being replaced. The majority of the body's tissues can be regenerated, nerve cells being the most notable exception. Once damaged, all nervous system tissue, including that of the brain, cannot be restored.

A second type of repair process usually predominates. It involves the proliferation of connective tissue. We call the ground substance or framework of an organ the stroma, meaning the connective and fibrous tissue that supports the functioning cells (parenchyma). The proliferation of stroma-type cells in the repair

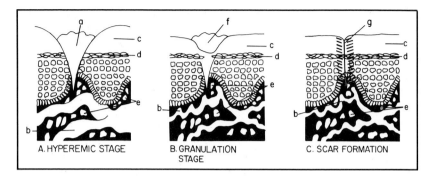

FIGURE 2-8   Steps in the healing of a wound. A. The swelling and vascular dilation stimulate the proliferation of stromal cells. B. (granulation) and new epidermis. C. The fibrosis proceeds outward resulting in scarring. a = fibrin formation induced by bleeding; b = capillary loop; c = superficial swelling of outer epidermis from infiltration of plasma; d = advancing layer of multiplying epithelial cells (parenchymal); e = dermal connective tissue cells which become granulation tissue impregnated with collagen; f = scab formation; g = contracted scar formation.

process leads to *fibrosis*, or scarring. Ingrowth from this process consists of proliferating fibroblasts and capillary sprouts. Actively growing, highly vascularized connective tissue is referred to as *granulation* tissue. As time goes on, more and more collagen is deposited in granulation tissue, which progressively matures into a scar. A diagrammatic account of wound healing is presented in Figure 2-8.

If healing of damaged tissue is accomplished entirely by regeneration, a near perfect reconstruction of the original tissue will result. However, repair that primarily involves connective tissue leads to fibrosis, which does not restore the original function as effectively. Indeed, heavy scarring can seriously impair function. This distinction has clinical significance. For example, injury to such organs as the liver and skin are repaired primarily by regeneration. Unfortunately, the healing of tissue in the heart, lung, and kidney involves scarring. Regardless of the type of repair, adequate nutrition and a normal blood supply are essential for the healing process.

CLASSIFICATION OF PATHOLOGY- PRODUCING DISTURBANCES

There are many strategies for classifying diseases. Each plan has its own rationale and individual appeal. Among clinical specialists, diseases traditionally are grouped according to the organ or part of the body affected. This scheme may mislead one into thinking that disease is restricted to compartments within the body, when in actuality a disturbance in one organ tends to provoke imbalances elsewhere. Furthermore, despite their origin in the same organ, diseases like tuberculosis, emphysema, asthma, pneumonia, and bronchial carcinoma are distinctly different pathologies with different causes.

In addition to organ classification, patterns of disease may also be classified according to their association with the following types of disturbances:

1. circulatory
2. infective or immune
3. nutritive or metabolic
4. toxic
5. neurohormonal
6. traumatic (physical)
7. growth (neoplasm)

There are numerous interrelationships among the seven groups, a point that cannot be overemphasized. For example, the inhalation of carbon monoxide (toxic) disturbs blood transport of oxygen (circulatory), which in turn impairs function of the nervous system (neurohormonal) and alters tissue metabolism (metabolic) in a manner that favors lipid deposition, which in time can produce arterial disease (circulatory). In many instances the disturbances themselves are synonymous with specific diseases, the presence of which enhances the probability of further disease development. For example, a disturbance in glucose metabolism (diabetes mellitus) often leads to vascular disease. Developments of additional disturbances from preexisting pathology are known as *complications.*

Much of the remainder of this book is devoted to discussions of the seven general types of physiologic disturbance listed in this section and their stress-pathology relationships.

DIAGNOSIS AND TREATMENT

Physical examination, measurements in the clinical laboratory, and reported symptoms constitute the basis for arriving at a diagnosis of disease. Laboratory data and clinical signs are considered to be objective, while symptoms by nature are largely subjective data. This does not mean that symptoms are unimportant and laboratory findings infallible. Negative laboratory results do not always rule out the pos-

TABLE 2-3

Examinations Demonstrating Organic Lesions

FORM OF EXAMINATION	EXAMPLE
Tissue sections (from surgery and autopsy)	Microscopic examination of excised lung tissue
Biopsy (small bit of tissue removed in vivo)	Portion of lymph node for microscopic examination
Exfoliative cytology (cells sloughed from surface)	Pap test
Radiography (x-ray and fluoroscopy)	Pyelography (kidney)

sibility of disease. Biochemical alterations that are rather subtle can produce symptoms, and the earlier stages of many forms of pathology may be undetected by ordinary methods. The earlier manifestations of disease are called *subclinical* stages, and they often progress to clinical disease. Once the presence of disease is clearly established, predicting its course and outcome is known as the *prognosis*, which of course can be favorable or unfavorable.

Once diagnosis is reasonably established, a course of treatment is chosen. Thus diagnosis and treatment constitute the procedural tandem that is the essence of clinical practice. Proper treatment depends upon the accuracy of diagnosis, which in itself can prove to be elusive. Each individual is unique and may not fit the usual pattern described in textbooks. Moreover, human beings are not constructed exactly like pieces of machinery. Consequently, identifying defects and correcting them is sometimes not always a simple matter. The dynamic nature of disease must be kept in mind, especially when dealing with chronic ailments. In this light, the patient as a whole organism represents a unique history of attempting to adapt his or her inborn predispositions to the vicissitudes and capriciousness of the physical, chemical, biologic, and psychologic components of today's environment.

A disease can be diagnosed and treated without knowledge of its cause, or pathogenesis. Indeed, the etiology of many ailments is not clearly understood. This matter traditionally resides in the domain of the researcher. However, if preventive programs are to flourish, medicine will have to become more concerned with etiology.

The modern clinical laboratory has assumed a dominant role in the diagnosis of pathology. Since most diseases are dynamic processes that sooner or later produce lesions, various methods for examining cells, tissues, and organs have been developed. A list of

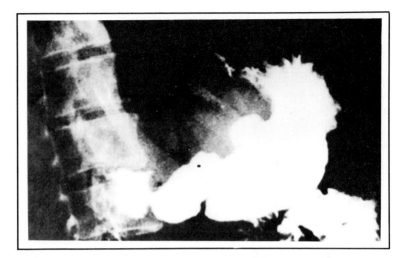

FIGURE 2-9   A barium x-ray of the stomach. Note the nodule along the stomach wall opposite the side with curvature. This is indicative of a gastric ulcer. (From S. A. Price and L. M. Wilson, *Pathophysiology—clinical concepts of disease processes.* Copyright © 1978 by McGraw-Hill, Inc. Used with permission of McGraw-Hill Book Co.)

several of these types of examinations appears in Table 2-3. One of the best known examples is the use of x-ray (Figure 2-9). Examinations that show electrical changes and chemical alterations are examples of methods for demonstrating functional disorders. Some of these methods are listed in Table 2-4.

Modern medical treatment of disease consists largely of surgery and the administration of drugs; both modalities are sometimes thought to be overused. Indeed, we now speak of *iatrogenic* disease, which is disease resulting from medical treatment.

PATHOLOGY TODAY

In the Introduction it was stated that the diseases most frequently found in modern technological societies were not as well known three-quarters of a century ago. For the most part, degenerative types of pathology that run a chronic course have replaced infectious diseases, which typically are acute in effect. Emphysema was a rarity at the turn of the century. Arthritis, hypertension, liver and kidney disease, heart disease, adult-onset diabetes, cancer, depression, suicide, hearing impairment, addiction to alcohol and drugs,

TABLE 2-4

Examinations Demonstrating Electrical and Chemical Changes

Electrocardiography (ECG)

Electroencephalography (EEG)

Blood chemical analysis

Urinalysis

Analysis of cerebrospinal fluid

Chemical analysis of sputum, exudates, and transudates

and various forms of allergic disease all have shown dramatic increases during the past 50 years. More and more birth defects are appearing. Likewise, there has been a phenomenal increase in behavioral deviations and functional irregularities of the nervous system among children born since World War II. It can be argued that the observed increases in so many of these conditions are due to more extensive programs of screening and detection. This may explain some of the dramatic shift. However, truly pernicious maladies such as cancer, arthritis, and emphysema are not likely to progress into later stages undetected.

There are two ways of looking at the prevalence of the various illnesses that plague us today. On one hand the mere frequency of the condition is to be considered, regardless of its seriousness. The ten leading reasons given for consulting physicians are listed in order in Table 2-5. Primarily these are symptoms or complaints, not diseases per se. Although the underlying causes could be serious, this is not likely. Scrutiny of the list suggests the possibility that either psychosomatic or allergic factors may be responsible for the symptoms in some instances.

On the other hand, when a disease has a known probability of becoming terminal, or of greatly limiting one's powers, it must be considered serious. To obtain some idea of the frequency of these illnesses, all we need to do is examine a list of the leading causes of death. The ten leading causes of death in the United States are presented in order in Table 2-6. It is immediately apparent that either cardiovascular disease or cancer is the form of pathology that will terminate most of us. Both pathologies have shown an amazing increase in incidence since the turn of the century, and neither condition develops overnight. Some think that our present way of living in our modern environment is a significant factor in the etiology of each illness.

TABLE 2-5

The Ten Most Frequent Reasons Given for Consulting a Physician

Upper respiratory distress (infections, allergy, etc.)

Rheumatic pain and discomfort (includes headache)

Weight problems

Gastrointestinal distress

Bronchial congestion

Fatigue

Nervousness

Insomnia

Urinary disturbances

Female problems

Source: Personal communications to the author.

In this chapter it has been implied that various forms of environmental stress are highly significant components in the development of disease processes. Therefore, before we proceed in respect to the stress-disease relationship and its many individual examples, let us explore in the following chapter exactly what stress means to a physiologist.

‖ SUMMARY

Disease is a dynamic process characterized by an inability to maintain the proper chemical and physical balance within the tissues and integrative functions of the body. The interaction of genetic predisposition with the effects on the body produced by unrelenting environmental stresses leads to this inability.

Disorders produced by chemical disturbances in which lesions are not apparent constitute functional disease, whereas the recognition of structural abnormalities indicates organic disease.

In organic disease there are characteristic forms of tissue damage. Inflammation is a common vascular response to cellular injury. It features vasodilation, increased capillary permeability, and an infiltration of fluid and white blood cells, leading to localized redness, heat, swelling, and pain. Degenerative damage, which involves the cell cytoplasm, leads to fluid infiltration, lipid accumulation, vacuolation, and disorganization of the respiratory chain within the mitochondria. Many forms of tissue injury are potentially

TABLE 2-6

Leading Causes of Death in the United States

CAUSE OF DEATH	APPROXIMATE NO. PER 100,000 POP.
Heart disease	735
Cancer	340
Stroke	218
Accidents	109
Pneumonia	58
Diabetes	39
Cirrhosis of the liver	34
Suicide	25
Emphysema	23
Homicide	20

Source: National Center for Health Statistics, 1980.

repairable. Repair is accomplished by the regeneration of new, functional cells and/or by the proliferation of cells from the connective tissue framework, or stroma, resulting in nonfunctional scar tissue.

The development of most diseases involves disturbances related to circulation, nutrition, metabolism, growth, infections, toxins, physical trauma, and functional abnormalities of the neurohormonal and immune systems. These disturbances are interrelated, one promoting the occurrence of others.

Diagnosis of disease is based upon physical examination, symptomatology, and clinical laboratory findings, whereas treatment often involves either the administration of drugs or surgery.

The major diseases confronting us today are chronic, degenerative types of pathology that were much less frequent at the turn of the century.

Chapter Glossary

acute   a condition developing rapidly and running a short course

chronic   a slowly developing condition running a prolonged course

collagen   a fibrous protein necessary for support in connective tissue

degenerative   involving progressive loss of cellular organization

etiology   the causes, precipitating factors, and methods of introducing disease

hypoxia   a reduction in the required supply of oxygen

ischemia   insufficient blood supply
lesion   a morbid change in the structure of cells, tissues, or organs
stasis   retardation or stoppage of normal flow or movement

For Further Reading

Anderson, W. A. D., and Kissane, J. M., eds. 1977. *Pathology.* 7th ed. Vol. 1. St. Louis: C. V. Mosby Co.

Anderson, W. A. D., and Scott, T. M. 1976. *Synopsis of pathology.* 9th ed. St. Louis: C. V. Mosby Co.

Boyd, W., and Sheldon, H. 1977. *An introduction to the study of disease.* 7th ed. Philadelphia: Lea & Febiger.

Buehlmann, A. A., and Froesch, E. R. 1979. *Pathophysiology.* New York: Springer-Verlag.

Dannenberg, A. M., Jr. 1975. Macrophages in inflammation and infection. *N. Eng. J. Med.* 293:489.

Frohlich, E. D., ed. 1976. *Pathophysiology: Altered regulatory mechanisms in disease.* 2d ed. Philadelphia: J. B. Lippincott Co.

Green, J. H. 1978. *Basic clinical physiology.* 3d ed. New York: Oxford University Press.

Houck, J. C. 1976. *Inflammation: a quarter century of progress.* Jour. Invest. Dermatol. 67:124.

Price, S. A., and Wilson, L. M. 1978. *Pathophysiology—clinical concepts of disease processes.* New York: McGraw-Hill Book Co.

Robbins, S. L., and Cotran, R. S. 1979. *Pathologic basis of disease.* 2d ed. Philadelphia: W. B. Saunders Co.

Roddie, I. C., and Wallace, W. F. M. 1975. *The physiology of disease.* Chicago: Year Book Medical Publishers.

Selye, H. 1976. *Stress in health and disease.* Boston: Butterworths.

Sodeman, W. A., and Sodeman, W. A., Jr. 1974. *Pathologic physiology: Mechanisms of disease.* Philadelphia: W. B. Saunders Co.

Young, C. G., and Barger, J. D. 1977. *Introduction to medical science.* 3d ed. St. Louis: C. V. Mosby Co.

Zweifach, B. W.; Grant, L.; and McCluskey, R. T., eds. 1974. *The inflammatory process.* 2d ed. Vol. 2. New York: Academic Press.

3

The Nature of Physiologic Stress

Internal Environment and Homeostasis
A Multiplicity of Stressors
Control Systems and Chemical Mediators
Physiologic Reserve
Manifestations and Assessment of Stress

|| **Objectives:** Upon completing this chapter you should:

1. Have a broad concept of physiologic stress.
2. Understand the role of the internal environment in maintaining homeostasis.
3. Be acquainted with the operative principle of control systems in counteracting stress disturbances.
4. Appreciate that stress stimuli exist in great variety.
5. Perceive the importance of the variation in the body's capacity to respond to stress.

What does the word *stress* mean to you? Is it worrying about an impending exam? Playing a competitive tennis match on a hot, humid day? Driving in congested, noisy traffic in heavily polluted city air? In themselves these are not considered to be stresses, but technically are referred to as *stressors*—factors that activate specific physiologic mechanisms in the body.

Although the word stress is formalized in science to mean any change within a system induced by an external force, it generally has an indefinite meaning and symbolizes different things to people of different disciplines. Psychologists, as well as nonprofessionals, usually employ the term stress to denote emotional tension emanating from psychologic demands. Physicists and engineers define stress as the force per unit area that tends to distort an object. The physiologist, however, utilizes a broad concept, implying that something in some way is disturbing the chemical or physical balance somewhere within an organism. Yet, even physiologists are not unanimous in defining stress. Some have stated simply that stress is a physiologic response to aversive stimuli. Those following the concept of Hans Selye view stress as a nonspecific response of the body to any demand, with emphasis on nonspecific. Physiologic stress may be defined as *a chemical or physical disturbance in the cells or tissue fluid produced by a change occurring either in the external environment or within the body itself that requires a response to counteract the disturbance.* According to this definition, stress comprises three components: (a) the exogenous or endogenous stressor initiating the disturbance; (b) the chemical or physical disturbance produced by the stressor, which can be conceived as the stress itself; and (c) the body's counteracting response to the disturbance. It should be pointed out that some physiologists do not separate the first and second components, and many investigators consider the counteracting response to be the essential part of stress, considering a response as evidence for the presence of stress.

Even though stress, like disease, can be either localized or widespread in the body, responses to it often involve some degree of systemic mobilization. Indeed, at the very outset it is important to distinguish a localized, specific stress disturbance from its more generalized manifestation by use of an example. When one burns a finger, there is an immediate, localized disturbance from the heat. At the same time, this localized disturbance is detected by a system of nervous and hormonal mediators which mobilize responses via the circulation. When the neurohormonal system becomes involved, the response is widespread throughout the body. Neuroendocrine responsiveness to stress is sometimes looked upon as a *generalized stress syndrome*.

Obviously we are experiencing some degree of stress all the time. In fact, just remaining alive implies physiologic stress. Much attention has been given to the idea that stress is an important factor in promoting chronic disease and shortened lives, and in general this seems to be true. On the other hand, without stress there is no responsiveness, and we must concede that stress can be constructive and desirable as well as destructive and undesirable. For example, it has been shown that stress contributes to the learning process. Moreover, eating, sexual excitement, participating in sports, socializing, and striving for professional achievement, while pleasurable and rewarding, can also be quite stressful. Regardless of how personally desirable the habit or activity may be, there may be risks of maladaptive stress responses when exposure to stressors becomes especially severe or is sustained for too long a time. This emphasizes the point that *it is not so much the stress itself but the body's capability in responding to it that constitutes the significant variable*, especially in regard to our interest in disease. As long as our bodies can cope with the changes, then the stress effect can be overcome.

INTERNAL ENVIRONMENT AND HOMEOSTASIS

As implied in the previous section, an important aspect of stress is the body's ability to counteract the disturbances produced by stressors, otherwise the system rapidly becomes disorganized. According to the second law of thermodynamics, all systems tend to become random (disorganized), stable, and probable. Living systems represent an extreme in organization, instability, and improbability. Therefore, we can expect them to be maintained for relatively brief periods only. The fact that such systems remain living for as long as

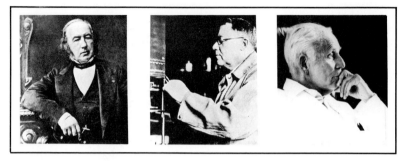

FIGURE 3-1   **Pioneers in stress physiology.** *Left to right:* Claude Bernard (1813–1878), Walter B. Cannon (1871–1945), and Hans Selye (1907–).

they do can be attributed to the many regulatory mechanisms that serve to restrict chemical and physical alterations within the cells. To maintain intracellular balance, the specialized cell aggregations constituting the mammalian form must be provided with an intimate fluid environment. Cells of the most primitive simple organisms are thought to have been exposed directly to a stable fluid of the external environment: the ocean. Most cells of complex, multicellular forms inhabiting land are not directly exposed to the external environment. Claude Bernard (Figure 3-1), a nineteenth-century French physiologist, first introduced the concept of the *internal environment.* This concept implies that each cell of a complex multicellular organism is bathed by fluid called *extracellular fluid* which constitutes the immediate environment of the cells. Extracellular fluid is the medium of exchange with the cell for oxygen, carbon dioxide, nutrients, wastes, ions, and numerous other molecular species. Obviously this fluid must provide the correct physicochemical composition for stable cell function.

Of course, fluid occurs within cells (intracellular fluid) as well as without. Extracellular fluid, however, is the internal environment of the body and constitutes approximately 20% of body weight, while intracellular fluid amounts to about twice that much. In actuality extracellular fluid has two compartments. About 80% of it is directly dispersed around and among the cells and is known as *interstitial fluid.* The remaining 20% is confined within blood and lymph vessels and constitutes the fluid portion (plasma) of the blood. Circulation of the blood represents the dynamic component of extracellular fluid. This component responds physically and chemically to changes in the external environment. In turn the physical and chemical conditions of interstitial fluid depend upon the conditions of the blood. Thus, changes in the external environment can affect

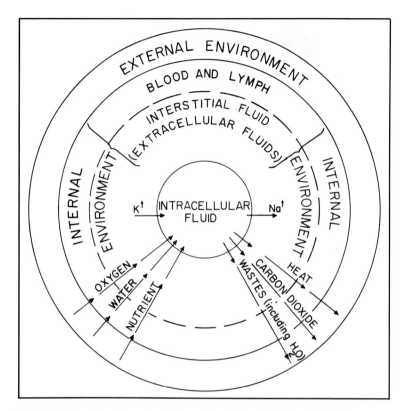

FIGURE 3-2   Functional relationship of the three body fluids.
Blood, lymph, and the interstitial fluid directly bathing cells make up the
internal environment of tissues and serve as the regulators of the
intracellular fluid under changing conditions of the external environment.

conditions within the cells, first through changes in the circulating
body fluids, followed in turn by appropriate alterations in the interstitial fluid. All three fluids are interchangeable to a degree; in fact,
capillary exchanges between plasma and interstitial fluid result in
solute concentrations in the two that are virtually identical except
for protein, which is normally confined to the plasma. A diagrammatic illustration of the three fluids and their relation to each other
and the external environment appears in Figure 3-2.

Bernard considered that all physiologic mechanisms, however varied, have one adaptive consequence, that of preserving the
conditions in the internal environment. This concept was further
advanced by Walter B. Cannon (Figure 3-1), an American physiologist, who coined the term *homeostasis*. He postulated that tissues and
organs must be regulated and integrated with each other in such a

way that any change in the internal environment initiates a reaction to counteract or at least minimize the change. The result is maintenance of a steady state (homeostasis) within the tissues. Some homeostatic mechanisms regulate the balance of physical parameters such as heat and pressure, but most regulations are concerned with chemical balance.

The constancy of the internal environment is maintained in respect to innumerable variables such as acid-base equilibrium, temperature, osmotic pressure, gas pressures, and solute concentrations. The constancy is not absolute: slight variations occur under normal conditions. However, if the stresses imposed upon the system become too great, the composition of the internal environment may alter significantly, sometimes with disastrous effects. Thus a change in plasma pH value from 7.4 to 7.0, or a change in serum calcium level from 10 to 6 mg/dl, or a change in blood glucose level from 90 to 35 mg/dl,[1] all can produce an immediate danger to the functioning of the central nervous system, which is especially sensitive to chemical change.

A MULTIPLICITY OF STRESSORS

What types of changes in the external environment or in the body itself elicit responses to demands for adaptation? In Parts II through V of this book the effects from an array of stressors that commonly confront us and pose risks of developing disease are discussed in some detail. Prolonged exertion, noise, infection, exposure to cold and heat, shock, fatigue, decreased oxygen supply, pain, malnutrition, radiation, obesity, anger, fear, old age, excitement, anxiety, pregnancy, injuries, drugs, disease, medical treatment, and surgery account for most of the stressors with which the physiologist is concerned. Even though the body's response to low temperatures is something quite different in specific ways from response to anxiety, it has been shown that one aspect of the response is the same in either case. Apparently most stresses share a common reaction in the body, regardless of the distinctions among individual stressors. Hans Selye (Figure 3-1), a Canadian physiologist, first introduced the concept that in responses to various stressors the adrenal cortex is activated and there is an increase in cortisol secretion. In fact,

---

[1]The unit mg/dl is milligrams per deciliter of blood. It is equivalent to milligrams per 100 milliliters, or mg%.

some physiologists conceive of stress as being any event resulting in an increase in cortisol secretion. Selye exposed rats to extreme cold, intense sound, and physical restraint for periods of 48 hours. In each instance there was a prominent elevation of secretions from the adrenal cortex and a characteristic triad of tissue changes: hypertrophy of the adrenal cortex, atrophy of lymphatic organs, and ulceration of the stomach and duodenum. Selye termed these responses the *general adaptation syndrome*. He postulated that animals go through three distinct stages in their response to stressful situations. First, there is an alarm reaction in which the hypothalamic action systems are aroused and the body's defensive forces are mobilized. This leads to a stage of adaptation. However, unrelenting stress may introduce a third stage in which there is a progressive loss of acquired adaptation that can lead to exhaustion and the breakdown of homeostatic mechanisms. Such breakdowns represent impairments that we equate with disease or more specifically, disease of adaptation.

Selye has a special talent for incorporating many facts into a unified generalization, which led to his concentration on the common denominators in stress reactions. However, in addition to response from the adrenal cortex, there may be other effects provoked by stressors that can be specific and may vary according to the nature of the individual stressor. An example is erythema and damage to skin from ultraviolet radiation. Nevertheless, Selye's discoveries justify his acknowledged position as the preeminent pioneer in establishing the stress concept, and his investigations were instrumental in developing the groundwork that led to the recognition of the hypothalamic-pituitary-adrenal cortex involvement in responses to stress. As pointed out earlier, regardless of the specific nature of the stress, there tends to be a generalized responsiveness of neurohormonal components. It was the generalized stress syndrome involving pituitary-adrenal activation that occupied Selye's attention.

Selye also proposed that diseases may be the result of faulty adaptation by the body. Indeed, a number of pathologic changes have been induced in laboratory animals upon their being subjected to such stressors as intense noise and electric shocks. Hypertension, gastrointestinal ulcers, and nephrosclerosis were a few of the pathologic consequences. More attention is given to this important topic in Chapter 5.

In reality we are seldom confronted with a single stressor at a time. For example, in a heated tennis match on a hot day, we can expect heat stress, exercise stress, and psychologic pressure all at the same time. It has been shown that the response to one stressor can automatically alter responses to other, simultaneous stressors. Usually this results in a less effective response to any one stressor. Multiple stresses rather than single ones are more likely to initiate breakdowns in homeostatic mechanisms.

CONTROL SYSTEMS AND CHEMICAL MEDIATORS

To maintain physical and chemical balance within the tissues and the internal environment, a series of integrated components serving as a system of control must be operative. One can appreciate the characteristics of a control system by referring to a simplified, non-biologic example. To maintain the temperature of a room at 20°C during cold seasons, homes and other buildings are equipped with automatic heat controls. As the room begins to lose heat to the outside air, the temperature inside drops below 20°C, the figure at which the heat control system (thermostat) is set. This change activates the first component of the system, a temperature-sensitive material (sensor) that generates electric current which ignites the furnace fuel jets from a pilot light and starts a fan motor. As hot air accumulates in the room the temperature returns to 20°C and even exceeds it slightly for a moment. The sensor then initiates a breaking of the current to the burners and fan and they stop. The action in which an increase in output (heat) results in a decrease of input (current to burners and fan) is known in principle as *negative feedback.* It stabilizes the system and is a common feature of biologic control systems. However, biologic control systems are usually much more complex than the example just described.

In physiologic terms a detectable change in the environment (external or internal) is designated as a *stimulus.* Changes in blood pressure and serum glucose concentration would be examples. The component detecting the change (the sensor in our previous example) is termed a *receptor.* The receptor communicates information to an intergrating component which relays it to the last component of the system, termed an *effector* (the burners and fans in our previous example). As already stated, the effector's response can abolish or at least diminish the receptor activity and its input (negative feedback).

There also can be *positive feedback* in a system. In such instances the effector's response intensifies receptor activity, reinforcing and increasing the response from effector components. Positive feedback leads to instability and tends to disrupt balance and destroy control. This principle is popularly described as a vicious cycle.

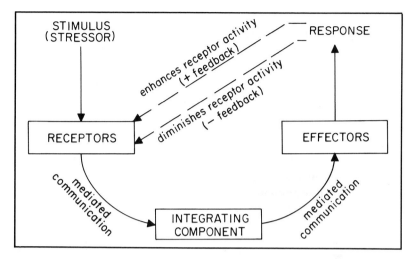

FIGURE 3-3   Simplified model of the physiologic control principle.
Observe that the response can either diminish (negative feedback) or
enhance (positive feedback) further action throughout the system.

With few exceptions, positive feedback in the body tends to promote
disease. (One exception that can be beneficial to the body is blood-
clotting.)

Reflection upon the operation of a control system in response
to stress reveals that the stimulus is the stressor, and the effector
action represents the counteracting response. A simplified diagrammatic model of a physiologic control system is shown in Figure 3-3.

Control systems in physiology often involve neural pathways
and hormonal secretions. However, a control system can be localized without hormones or nerves being involved. An example is
the release of carbon dioxide from exercising muscle into extracellular fluid, where the gas promotes dilatation of the local blood vessels, enhancing perfusion of the muscle with blood.

A great deal of the integrating action in homeostasis is based
upon the capacity of one cell to alter the activity of another. For the
most part these alterations are mediated chemically, and there are
many different molecules that serve as mediators. Specific mediators
that alter cell activity some distance from their source and are conveyed by the bloodstream are usually classified as *hormones.* Neural
pathways also function through chemical mediation, one neuron altering the activity of the next neuron by releasing a chemical *transmitter.* In still other instances chemical mediators are operative that
are not traditionally classified as hormones or neural transmitters.
The stimulation of the breathing center in the medulla oblongata of
the brain by hydrogen ions is an example.

TABLE 3-1

Maximum Reserve Capacities in Young Men

PHYSIOLOGIC PARAMETER	MEASUREMENT
Vital capacity (pulmonary)	5 liters
Cardiac output*	20–25 liters/min
Maximum oxygen consumption*	3 liters/min
Adrenocorticotropin (ACTH) (pituitary response to stress)	70 pg/ml of plasma
Hemoglobin (oxygen-carrying capacity)	18 g/100 ml of blood
Heat production	960 kcal/hr
Sweat production	3–4 liters/hr

*Untrained.

PHYSIOLOGIC RESERVE

Persistent stressing obviously presents a challenge to control mechanisms. Furthermore, homeostatic capacity varies considerably from individual to individual and from time to time in the same individual. In addition, one control mechanism in an individual may perform capably, whereas another mechanism may be impaired. The potential capacity of a systemic mechanism to respond beyond its ordinary functional requirement is termed *physiologic reserve.* Thus we speak of cardiac reserve, pulmonary reserve, insulin reserve, and renal reserve. A list of some of the maximum reserve capacities for several physiologic parameters in young, healthy, adult males is provided in Table 3-1.

In aging and disease, physiologic reserve is compromised. For example, a 60-year-old man in reasonably good health can expect to have lost more than one-fourth of his pulmonary and renal reserves due to age. The development of habits that tend to maintain substantial reserve in homeostatic mechanisms should promote good health and longevity. However, agreement on how this is achieved is somewhat divided. Some professionals and nonprofessionals alike take the view that as much avoidance of stressors as possible offers the best means of preserving physiologic reserve and preventing chronic, degenerative disease. Much can be said in favor of such a policy although stressful conditions cannot be circumvented in many instances. Moreover, obsession with such a regime could very well result in a dull life. It would seem sensible to avoid certain stressors such as long-term inhalation of tobacco smoke, which has been shown to stress the pulmonary and cardiovascular systems with serious pathologic consequences.

Another school of thought contends that the best way to insure optimum physiologic reserve is to challenge the response, regularly and prominently, so that through the system's habitual acclimation, it progressively develops more reserve. There is no doubt that such a policy is effective in improving certain reserves. For example, exercise will build up reserves for the pulmonary and cardiovascular systems. However, it is doubtful if long-term stressing of the liver and insulin response with an excessive intake of concentrated sweets will do those systems any good. Thus, it would appear that certain responses may benefit from habitual challenge much more than others. In any case, age and general health must be considered in respect to the advisability of so-called stress conditioning. Nor should the individual lose sight of the significance of genetic predisposition in regard to physiologic reserve. Inherited genes constitute a major variable in determining reserve capacity, though this is a factor that we can do little about.

MANIFESTATIONS AND ASSESSMENT OF STRESS

How do we know if stress is occurring? Since the idea of stress denotes a degree of subjective abstractness, can we expect to demonstrate its presence objectively? Can it be measured? If physiologic stress is a disturbance in chemical and physical balance within the organism, then theoretically it should be detectable and measurable. However, in practice the matter is not so simple. First of all, what do we look for? Do we measure the stressor? Certain stressors such as temperature, radiation, sound, and oxygen deficiency are quite measurable. Others such as psychosocial stimuli do not lend themselves well to measurement. However, the measurement of stressors is necessary in quantifying the degree of a stress response to a given magnitude of the stressor.

Because certain parts of the body are not accessible for in vivo study, certain stress-induced disturbances are not readily assessable. For example, a number of important morphologic changes, such as atherosclerotic plaques of arterial walls, or malignant cell growth in lung parenchyma, are not usually detectable during their early development. Likewise, many important functional changes in the hypothalamus cannot be directly observed. Therefore, a number of stress manifestations are not accountable with traditional clinical tests. In other instances, results of laboratory evaluations are merely suggestive of disturbance in the body without providing specific information as to the nature or location.

It is the counteracting response to a stress that constitutes the most fertile ground for quantitative study. The detection and measurement of such responses provide the most practical evidence that stress is occurring or has just occurred. No one would dispute that an increase in ventilation rate or cardiac output is a valid indication of the presence of one or more stressors.

The assessment of stress in the body may be approached by observing deviations in body chemical composition, morphology, and function. Clinical chemists have developed capabilities for measuring an extensive number of metabolites, hormones, and other chemical mediators from blood, urine, and tissue. Microscopic morphology and diagnostic radiology have been the domain of the pathologist for some time. Changes in tissue, both reversible and irreversible, reflect the impact of stressors; and deviations in functional parameters are studied regularly by stress physiologists.

In view of the fact that the concept of stress in general has been associated with activity of the adrenal glands, one of the most frequently employed methods for assessing stress has been the measurements of catecholamines and adrenal steroids in the blood and urine. It is shown in subsequent chapters that these measurements can be of value in studying the generalized responses that typify emotional stress, thermal stress, and exertion. However, we shall see that there are specific responses to individual stressors in which these determinations may not be as important.

We must remember that stress in some degree is going on all the time with its characteristic, normal fluctuations in body chemistry. Accordingly, practical distinctions must be made between these changes and the more significant deviations that warrant the label of abnormality. This distinction is not always clear, indeed it is quite arbitrary in many instances. Certainly disease can be a manifestation of stress, and the relationship is significant enough to justify a special treatment in Chapter 5.

SUMMARY

Physiologic stress is a chemical or physical disturbance within tissues or their immediate environment, initiated by a change either in the external environment or from within the body itself. The disturbance prompts a counteracting response.

The role of the internal environment is to provide exchange with the tissues thus enabling them to maintain a steady physicochemical state. The internal environment comprises extracellular fluid, which is divided into circulating fluid (blood), and interstitial fluid, which directly bathes the cells.

Homeostasis is the term employed to denote the body's ability to maintain a narrow range of chemical and physical variation within the tissues and the internal environment.

Many diverse conditions singly and in combination are capable of initiating physiologic stress disturbances. Even though the response to each individual stressor may have its own specific involvements, most stressors provoke the release of hormones from the adrenal cortex, leading to what is known as the generalized stress syndrome.

Common components of homeostatic control systems are receptors that detect changes, and effectors that produce responses to the changes. A frequent control operation is negative feedback in which the effector action suppresses input from receptors. The mediation of the necessary integration in control systems is essentially chemical in nature.

The ability to counteract stress disturbances varies according to genetic factors, age, health status, and the particular homeostatic mechanism in question. The degree of this capacity is known as physiologic reserve.

Though the manifestations of stress are not always directly discernible in the living body, assessment of some responses can be performed by observing changes in body chemistry, morphology, and function.

Chapter Glossary

adrenal steroids   hormones, such as cortisol, secreted by the adrenal cortex

atrophy   a shrinkage or wasting away of tissues or organs

catecholamines   hormones, such as epinephrine, secreted by the adrenal medulla

hypertrophy   an enlargement of tissues or organs

in vivo (in life)   refers to investigations involving the intact, living body

metabolites   compounds degraded from key chemical substances in the body

nephrosclerosis   disease of the renal arteries, in which the vessels harden

psychosocial   pertains to psychologic reactions prompted by social interactions

For Further Reading

Archer, J. 1979. *Animals under stress.* Baltimore: University Park Press.

Bernard, C. 1957. *An introduction to the study of experimental medicine.* New York: Dover.

Burke, S. R. 1976. *The composition and function of body fluids.* St. Louis: C. V. Mosby Co.

Cannon, W. B. 1939. *The wisdom of the body.* New York: W. W. Norton & Co.

Hardy, R. N. 1976. *Homeostasis.* Baltimore: University Park Press.

Keale, C. A., and Neil, E. 1971. *Wright's applied physiology.* 12th ed. New York: Oxford University Press. Chapt. 2.

Langley, L. L. 1973. *Homeostasis: Origin of the concept.* Stroudsburg, Pa.: Dowden, Hutchinson, & Ross, Inc.

McQuade, W., and Aikman, A. 1974. *Stress.* New York: E. P. Dutton & Co.

Milhorn, H. T., Jr. 1966. *The application of control theory to physiological systems.* Philadelphia: W. B. Saunders Co.

Robin, E. D., ed. 1979. *Claude Bernard and the internal environment. A memorial symposium.* New York: Marcel Dekker, Inc.

Selye, H. 1974. *Stress without distress.* New York: J. B. Lippincott Co.

———. 1976a. *The stress of life.* New York: McGraw-Hill Book Co.

———. 1976b. *Stress in health and disease.* Boston: Butterworths.

Vander, A. J.; Sherman, J. H.; and Luciano, D. S. 1980. *Human physiology: The mechanisms of body function.* 3d ed. New York: McGraw-Hill Book Co. Chapts. 7, 17.

The Role of the Neuroendocrine System in Homeostasis

|| **Objectives:** Upon completing this chapter you should:

1. Be informed of the basic neural and hormonal interactions involved in reactions to stressors.
2. Understand the roles of the sympathetic and parasympathetic divisions of the autonomic nervous system (ANS) in maintaining homeostasis.
3. Know how stress activates the adrenal glands.
4. Recognize the key role of the hypothalamus in regulating the ANS and the pituitary-adrenal system.
5. Be acquainted with some of the major disorders of the endocrine system.

It stands to reason that the primary systems of communication in the body play the foremost roles in homeostatic control. These are the neural and hormonal systems. Since both systems employ chemical mediators and in many respects interact as one functional continuum, we may speak of the combination as the neuroendocrine system. This system plays a paramount role in stress and susceptibility to disease. In fact, it is generally acknowledged that many manifestations of stress stem directly from actions of the autonomic nervous system and certain portions of the hormonal system. Neuroendocrine regulation is often complex, and it may involve a number of feedback loops. Moreover, there is much yet to be elucidated in respect to this area of physiology.

In view of our interest in stress and disease, there are certain priorities to be emphasized in a discussion of the neuroendocrine involvements. Therefore, this chapter reviews the functional interactions that are known to exist among such components as the two divisions of the autonomic nervous system, the pituitary and adrenal glands, and the hypothalamus. As a starting point, let us inspect autonomic regulation.

AUTONOMIC NERVOUS SYSTEM

The autonomic nervous system (ANS) is often termed the *visceral* nervous system as opposed to the *somatic*, or voluntary, nervous system. In actuality a clear-cut division between the two systems can be made only with respect to the efferent fibers. Nerves that innervate skeletal muscle are somatic, and those that innervate smooth muscle, cardiac muscle, and glands are visceral.

Because of its effects on smooth muscle and glands, as well as its influence on reticuloendothelial and lymphoid tissues, the ANS has an extremely widespread and important role in the homeostatic control of the internal environment. The ANS has two divisions, *sympathetic* and *parasympathetic*, each concerned with the regulation of visceral activities. Generally speaking, the sympathetic division acts in response to sudden demands or threats, usually from the external environment. Parasympathetic activity is generally more responsive to an internal need for restoration and conservation. This division also promotes elimination of wastes and other noxious materials. The individual who manages to survive some sort of unexpected emergency, then later becomes weak and faints (vasovagal syncope), exemplifies how stress can produce a shift in autonomic balance between the two divisions. Sympathetic activity tends to sustain us during a crisis, but after it has subsided, we may be left with a strong parasympathetic response that can result in pronounced hypotension.

Characteristically, sympathetic response shows a composite of activities, the division tending to respond as a whole with multiple, widespread effects. On the other hand, parasympathetic activity is more discrete because of the limited distribution of its efferent fibers, there being stimulation of only one organ at a time in some instances. Each division of the ANS is capable of causing excitatory effects in some organs but inhibitory effects in others, and, taken as a whole, neither division can be classed as excitatory or inhibitory. However, most visceral effectors have a dual innervation system composed of an efferent pathway from each division, and it is generally true that a given organ which is excited by one division is inhibited by the other. Yet there are several visceral effectors that are supplied with efferent fibers from only one division. The sweat glands, pilomotor muscles, and smooth muscle of certain blood vessels have sympathetic innervation only. The innervation of the body with efferent pathways from both the sympathetic and parasympathetic divisions is illustrated in Figure 4-1.

In discussions of ANS function, it is primarily the efferent fibers that are emphasized. However, there are afferent fibers originating from visceral receptors which transmit impulses to centers in the spinal cord and brain stem. These fibers are located in the cranial and spinal nerves. Visceral receptors are sensitive to such things as effector action, organic sensation, and pain.

Acetylcholine is the neurotransmitter released from postganglionic efferent fibers in the parasympathetic division of the ANS; hence the term *cholinergic* is used in expressing parasympathetic ac-

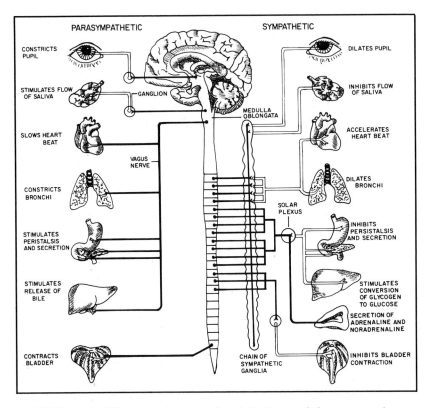

FIGURE 4-1   Efferent pathways of each division of the autonomic nervous system. Relation to the autonomic centers of the brain and cord, and specific actions on the various organs are indicated. Heavy lines represent preganglionic neurons, and light lines are postganglionic neurons.

tion. Most postganglionic fibers of the sympathetic division secrete norepinephrine, and their action is described as *adrenergic*. Visceral effectors may be sensitive also to other chemical mediators. Smooth muscle responds to various *prostaglandins* and to certain amines such as *histamine* and *5-hydroxytryptamine* (serotonin). (Reference is made to histamine and prostaglandins in regard to inflammation discussed in Chapter 2.) There are at least 14 different prostaglandins along with a number of related materials known as *thromboxanes*, all of which are synthesized from arachidonic acid, an unsaturated fatty acid. Prostaglandins are released in response to a wide variety of stress stimuli.

    Dopamine and *gamma-aminobutyric acid* (GABA) are two neurotransmitters of importance in brain physiology, and many additional brain neurotransmitters and neuromodulators are discussed in Chapter 17.

Systemic Effects of the ANS

It has been implied already that sympathetic activity is often characterized by widespread systemic effects. Thus a mass sympathetic discharge results in a stimulation and increased activity of many functions in the body: the major ones include cardiac output, arterial blood pressure, blood perfusion of skeletal muscle, blood glucose concentration, rate of cellular metabolism, rate of blood coagulation, lipolysis, and mental arousal. Walter B. Cannon (see Chapter 3) termed this battery of responses the *stress reaction.* It is true that many stressors are capable of eliciting sympathetic responses, and it is obvious that the sum of these effects permits the individual to perform strenuous physical activity far more effectively than would otherwise be possible. Yet sympathetic activity is not always manifested as a mass discharge. In heat stress, for example, the sympathetic impulses can regulate sweating and blood flow in the skin without action from other effectors innervated with sympathetic fibers.

Though we do not commonly consider parasympathetic activity to show widespread systemic effects, nevertheless there often is an allied association among parasympathetic actions. For example, salivary secretion, gastric secretion, and pancreatic secretion normally occur together in association with gastrointestinal motility. For a list of autonomic effects on individual organs, see Table 4-1.

Stress and Autonomic Balance

Although we tend to associate stress with sympathetic activity, it is often overlooked that the parasympathetic division also responds to stressors. In actuality both systems may respond to stress at the same time. However, there may be a predominance in activity of one or the other of the divisions; which one depends upon a number of variables. It must be realized that both divisions are continually active even in the absence of externally applied stimuli. Such basal rates of activity are respectively called sympathetic and parasympathetic *tone,* which is maintained chiefly through the action of the autonomic centers, particularly those of the medulla oblongata and the hypothalamus. For example, sympathetic tone keeps blood vessels constricted to about one half of their maximum diameter. Sympathetic stimulation constricts these vessels even more. However, inhibition of the normal tone dilates the vessels. In this way the modulation of impulses in the ANS can result in *both* vasoconstriction and vasodilation, not just vasoconstriction alone.

TABLE 4-1

Effects of Autonomic Nervous System on Various Organs

ORGAN	PARASYMPATHETIC STIMULATION	SYMPATHETIC STIMULATION
Eye (pupil)	Contracts	Dilatates
Salivary glands	Thin, copious secretion	Scanty, thick secretion
Stomach	Promotes motility and secretion	Inhibits motility and secretion
Pancreas	Promotes secretion	Inhibits secretion
Gall bladder	Promotes secretion	Inhibits secretion
Colon and rectum	Increases motility	Inhibits motility
Liver	No effect	Stimulates glucose release
Basal metabolism	No effect	Greatly increases
Eccrine glands	No effect	Copious secretion
Apocrine glands	No effect	Thick secretion
Heart muscle (contraction)	Decrease in rate and force	Increase in rate and force
Bronchial airways	Constricted	Dilatated
Blood vessels to muscle	No effect	May constrict or dilatate
Blood vessels to skin	Dilatates	May constrict or dilatate
Other blood vessels	No effect	Constricts
Blood glucose	No effect	Increases
Blood lipids	No effect	Increases
Blood coagulation	No effect	Increases
Skeletal muscle	No effect	Increases glycogenolysis
Adrenal cortical secretion	No effect	Increases
Secretion from adrenal medullae	No effect	Increases
Kidney	No effect	Decreases output
Urinary bladder	May stimulate or inhibit	May stimulate or inhibit
Piloerector muscles	No effect	Stimulates
Mental activity	No effect	Stimulates

In the absence of strong stimuli we may expect some degree of *autonomic balance* between actions of the two divisions, keeping in mind that they tend to produce opposing effects on the viscera. When a stressor is applied, there is usually a predominance of effector response from one or the other division, at least for a time. Generally speaking, sympathetic predominance is more likely. However, activity of the ANS can vary considerably in response to stress.

Hereditary predisposition, past experience, state of health, age, sex, the nature of the stressors, and drug intake are several important variables underlying potential imbalance in the overall responsiveness of the ANS.

Stress in certain animals such as rats and dogs tends to elicit a predominance of sympathetic activity, yet other animals such as rabbits and sheep are often disposed to a predominance of parasympathetic discharges. In a like manner there are humans who appear to manifest parasympathetic predominance much of the time, with consequent complaints of weakness, hypersensitivity, bronchial constriction (asthma), and gastrointestinal disturbances (ulcers and colitis). On the other hand, those with sympathetic predominance are more likely to be candidates for hypertension, elevated blood lipids and glucose, and thrombus formation, all of which dispose the individual to cardiovascular disease.

In some instances sympathetic influence on one organ may be accented along with a predominance of parasympathetic action on another organ at the same time. Hence, with chronic stress, it would not be unreasonable to find hypertension and duodenal ulcers in the same individual. Moreover, the autonomic response to a given stimulus may at one time be predominatly sympathetic and at another time parasympathetic. Evidently the system can be set so that one or the other division becomes more responsive, thereby facilitating impulses along particular pathways. Ernst Gellhorn, an eminent neurophysiologist, termed such changes in reactivity *autonomic tuning*. Apparently tuning reflects the state of neural activity in the autonomic centers of the hypothalamus. These centers in turn can be influenced by mental states.

A number of studies support the concept of autonomic imbalance and its relation to stress and disease. Wenger studied the resting autonomic patterns of thousands of young, healthy, Air Force cadets during World War II. Autonomic measurements in cadets who began to develop psychosomatic disorders indicated that the majority showed sympathetic predominance in the resting state. The sympathetic tone of these persons was being maintained at a higher level. Moreover, a follow-up study of the medical histories of these individuals in later life indicated a preponderance of hypertension, heart disease, and a greater than average susceptibility to such conditions as hyperlipidemia, hyperglycemia, and kidney problems.

Of special interest were a few cases in which there appeared to be alternating periods of sympathetic and parasympathetic predominance. Under mental demands characterized by a sense of urgency combined with exposures to cold, these individuals exhibited an inability to relax that became associated with a significant elevation in blood pressure and serum lipids. Six months later in a warm, humid, tropical environment the same persons became lethargic and developed lower than average blood pressures. In addition they complained of numerous symptoms of allergic and gastrointestinal nature.

ANS in Relation to Other Areas of the Central Nervous System

Since efferent autonomic impulses emanate from centers in the brain and spinal cord, we would conclude that there must be associations of some sort between autonomic function and central nervous system (CNS) pathways. Most of the autonomic centers are located in the hypothalamus and medulla oblongata of the brain. These centers receive afferent input from many sources, including visceral and peripheral receptors. In addition there are descending afferent pathways from the cerebrum and limbic system of the brain. Furthermore, the nuclei making up the autonomic centers themselves function as chemoreceptors or thermoreceptors.

There are specific hypothalamic nuclei that control respectively the sympathetic and parasympathetic divisions of the ANS. These nuclei in turn can be stimulated by input from the cerebral cortex via the limbic system. In fact, recent studies have shown that animals and humans can learn visceral responses in the same way that they learn skeletal responses. (More attention is devoted to these intriguing possibilities in Chapter 16.) The hypothalamus is of such monumental importance that a later section of this chapter is devoted exclusively to it.

HORMONAL REGULATION AND INTERACTION

Though all endocrine activity in a strict sense has some relation to stress, the sites of primary significance are the *adrenal glands* and the *pituitary gland.* In fact, the adrenal glands are often referred to as the stress glands. An adrenal gland is actually a double gland. Each portion has a different embryonic origin, and synthesizes distinctly different types of hormones which evoke different effects. The outer tissue, or *cortex,* synthesizes a variety of *steroid* hormones, whereas

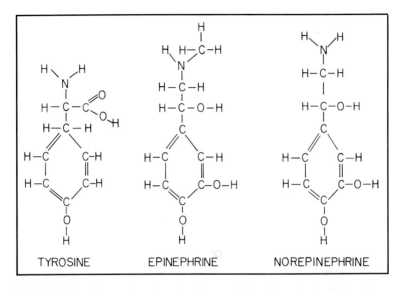

FIGURE 4-2   The molecular structure of the adrenal catecholamines.
Note the similarity of epinephrine to norepinephrine. Both are derived
from the amino acid tyrosine, *left*. The action of these amines is believed to
be associated primarily with the O-H groups.

the inner tissue, or *medulla,* is composed of chromaffin cells which
synthesize two separate *catecholamines.* Both portions of the gland
indirectly respond to most stressors.

The Adrenal Medullae

The adrenal medullae are stimulated by preganglionic sympathetic
nerves to secrete the catecholamine hormones *epinephrine* and *norepinephrine.* On the average about 75% of the total secretion is epinephrine. Adrenal catecholamines are derived from the amino acid
tyrosine. Their molecular structure is shown in Figure 4-2.

The circulating catecholamines have essentially the same effects on the viscera as those caused by direct sympathetic stimulation, except that the effect may persist almost ten times as long
because the hormone is not rapidly degraded and removed from the
blood. Hence, secretions from the adrenal medullae reinforce and
prolong sympathetic effects in the body. Norepinephrine is the primary constrictor of smooth muscle in all the blood vessels. In addition it can inhibit gastrointestinal activity and dilate the pupil of the
eye.

Although epinephrine causes some of the same effects as norepinephrine, it has a greater influence on cardiac action, and it is the principal catecholamine involved in metabolic regulations. It is capable of increasing the metabolic rate 100% above normal. Associated with this effect is the ability of the hormone to stimulate the activity of hepatic phosphorylase, which promotes the conversion of liver glycogen to glucose. Thus epinephrine causes transient hyperglycemia. Epinephrine also suppresses release of insulin from the beta cells of the pancreatic islets while stimulating release of glucagon from the alpha cells. In addition it stimulates lipolysis and the mobilization of triglycerides and free fatty acids from fat stores. Moreover, epinephrine stimulates cholesterol synthesis from acetate, while at the same time it inhibits the degradation of cholesterol to bile acids.

There is a synergistic relationship between the action of epinephrine and thyroid hormones. Thyroxin can increase the number of epinephrine receptors in the heart, and epinephrine increases the release of fatty acids from adipose tissue only in the presence of thyroid hormone. Thus each hormone enhances the action of the other.

Other well-known effects of catecholamines include increased coagulability of the blood, increased skeletal muscle contractility and decreased fatigue, dilatation of bronchial passageways, increased arousal of the CNS, and stimulation of activity in the hypothalamic-pituitary-adrenocortical axis. The overall effects of adrenal catecholamines are summarized in Table 4-2.

The sympathoadrenomedullary system is a potent reactor in many stresses, notably exercise, thermal changes, and acute emotional states. Chronic overdrive in this system is a significant factor in the development of cardiovascular pathology, whereas underactivity is associated with asthma, other allergies, and many functional gastrointestinal disorders. The neural input to this system is most directly from specific hypothalamic nuclei which in turn receive afferent impulses from numerous sites of the body and brain.

The Adrenal Cortex

In the preceding chapter reference was made to the pioneer work of Hans Selye in which activity of the adrenal cortex was shown to be a major component in response to many stressors. Indeed, it is well documented that the adrenalectomized animal cannot resist even minor stresses of various sorts. The adrenal cortex secretes steroid hormones, and these are usually divided into three functional groups, the *mineralocorticoids*, the *glucocorticoids*, and the *androgens*. Our interest here is primarily in the glucocorticoids, although some

TABLE 4-2

Physiologic Effects of Adrenal Catecholamines

EFFECT	PRINCIPAL HORMONE
Vasoconstriction	Norepinephrine
Inhibition of gastrointestinal action	Norepinephrine
Pupil dilation	Norepinephrine
Rate of cardiac contraction	Epinephrine
Force of cardiac contraction	Epinephrine
Stimulates metabolic rate	Epinephrine
Stimulates conversion of glycogen to glucose	Epinephrine
Suppresses secretion of insulin	Epinephrine
Stimulates secretion of glucagon	Epinephrine
Stimulates lipolysis	Epinephrine
Stimulates cholesterol synthesis	Epinephrine
Inhibits cholesterol degradation	Epinephrine
Dilates bronchial airways	Both epinephrine and norepinephrine
Stimulates secretion of ACTH	Norepinephrine
Promotes skeletal muscle contractility	Epinephrine
Increases rate of blood coagulability	Epinephrine
Arouses central nervous system activity	Norepinephrine

attention is given to the mineralocorticoids. While the adrenal steroids have remarkably similar molecular structures, their physiologic actions may be quite diverse. There is evidence that they regulate specific intracellular enzymes through the mediation of gene transcription. They are capable also of altering cell membrane permeability and active transport mechanisms. The structures of the two major adrenal steroids in humans are shown in Figure 4-3.

At least 95% of the mineralocorticoid activity of adrenocortical secretion is due to *aldosterone*. The primary effect of this steroid is an increased renal tubular resorption of sodium and increased renal excretion of potassium. Through osmotic force water tends to follow sodium; therefore, excessive resorption of sodium results in an increased extracellular fluid volume which in turn elevates blood pressure. Aldosterone secretion is normally stimulated by a decreased extracellular fluid volume as well as by the renin-angiotensin mechanism, which responds to diminished blood flow to the kidneys.

About 95% of the glucocorticoid activity of adrenocortical secretion is due to *cortisol*, also known as *hydrocortisone*. One of the primary effects of cortisol is the stimulation of gluconeogenesis in the liver. Cortisol action may increase the rate of conversion of amino acids to keto acids to glucose by as much as six to ten times. In addition there is evidence that the presence of cortisol enhances the

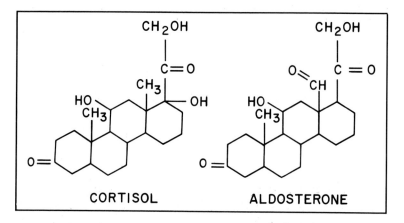

FIGURE 4-3 **The two major steroids secreted from the human adrenal cortex.** Cortisol (hydrocortisone) is a glucocorticoid, and aldosterone is a mineralocorticoid. Like all steroid hormones there are four carbon rings. Most of their action is thought to be associated with the side groupings, such as O-H radicals and double-bonded oxygens.

elevation in blood glucose promoted by other hormones such as epinephrine, glucagon, and somatotrophic growth hormone (STH); thus cortisol is said to be permissive to the action of these hormones. Cortisol also inhibits the uptake and oxidation of glucose by many body cells. For example, it inhibits the activity of hexokinase, the first enzyme involved in glycolysis. It is apparent that the overall action of cortisol in respect to carbohydrate metabolism results in an elevation of plasma levels of glucose, thus constituting a strong insulin antagonism.

Cortisol has a prominent effect on protein metabolism also. It promotes a negative nitrogen balance, both through a stimulation of protein catabolism and a suppression of protein synthesis. The steroid mobilizes body protein, which increases the concentration of amino acids in the blood. There is evidence also that cortisol depresses transport of amino acids into muscle cells, while enhancing their uptake into the liver, where they are converted to glucose. Moreover, cortisol can be responsible for lipid mobilization, resulting in an increase of free fatty acids and cholesterol in the blood.

In addition to its metabolic effects, cortisol exhibits some very interesting influences on vascular reactivity, immune competence, tissue inflammation, and gastric secretion. In ways not thoroughly understood, cortisol activity exerts a counteraction of the vasodilation, capillary permeability, cellular edema, and phagocytosis associated with tissue inflammation. In certain stresses the release of mediators such as histamine and bradykinin promotes vasodilation, capillary leakage, and fluid exudation into cells. The arteriolar dilatation may proceed despite sympathetic discharges. It has been postulated that cortisol is permissive to allow the norepinephrine to be effective in counteracting vasodilation. It does this by influencing the steady-state levels of a rate-limiting enzyme in the synthesis of norepinephrine. In this way cortisol is able to modulate the action at norepinephrine-mediated synapses.

Cortisol also has an immunosuppressive action. Its suppression of protein synthesis includes a diminished production of immunoglobulin. Moreover, cortisol activity results in decreased numbers of eosinophiles, lymphocytes, and macrophages. Substantial dosages of cortisol are known to promote atrophy of lymphoid tissue in the thymus, spleen, and lymph nodes.

Some of the anti-inflammatory action of cortisol may be related to its immunosuppressive effects, although there appear to be other mechanisms as well. For example, cortisol activity is known to stabilize the membranes of cellular lysosomes, thereby inhibiting their tendency to rupture. This prevents cellular damage caused by lysosomal enzymes. In addition the action of cortisol decreases permeability of capillary membranes and inhibits the formation of bradykinin. Finally, the glucocorticoids are noted for promoting gastric secretion, thus reinforcing parasympathetic activity in this regard. Indeed, excessive cortisol may produce ulceration of the gastric mucosa. The known cellular and biochemical effects of the glucocorticoids are listed in Table 4-3.

Exposure to a wide variety of nonspecific stimuli results in marked increases in glucocorticoid secretion. Yet it is not entirely clear just why this response to stress is of benefit. It has been postulated that the pooling of amino acids from labile proteins serves to provide an adequate supply for protein synthesis in certain needy cells. This would amount to a redistribution of protein to sites where replacement is critical. Such would be the case with tissue damage, or where cells undergo temporary depletion of certain proteins. The gluconeogenesis promoted by cortisol is considered to be an adaptation for insuring an adequate source of energy for body tissues, nerve cells in particular. The anti-inflammatory action of glucocorticoids would appear to prevent damage to tissue from the hydrolytic enzymes of cellular lysosomes, or at least the steroid activity would reestablish the membrane stability so important for the repair process. Although these explanations are based somewhat on supposition, the regularity of cortisol secretion in response to stress strongly implies homeostatic value of some sort.

TABLE 4-3

Major Physiologic Actions of Adrenal Glucocorticoids

Carbohydrate and Lipid Metabolism	Diminishes peripheral uptake and utilization of glucose
	Promotes gluconeogenesis in liver cells
	Enhances the gluconeogenic response to other hormones
	Promotes lipolysis in adipose tissue
Protein Metabolism	Stimulates degradation of body protein
	Depresses protein synthesis (including immunoglobulin)
	Increases plasma level of amino acids
	Stimulates deamination in the liver
Membrane Permeability	Suppresses membrane permeability of all cells and organelles, but particularly those of lysosomes, and capillary endothelium
	Inhibits the formation and release of histamine and bradykinin
	Permissive for vasoconstrictive action of norepinephrine
Immune Reserve	Decreases the tissue mass of all lymphatic tissues
	Promotes rapid decrease in circulating lymphocytes, eosinophiles, basophiles, and macrophages
Other Effects	Promotes gastric secretion
	Enhances urinary excretion
	Decreases proliferation of fibroblasts in connective tissue

Adrenal reserve of glucocorticoids varies considerably among individuals and at different times in the same individual. The reserve may temporarily approach exhaustion in those confronted continually with multiple stressors, foremost of which are mental strain, thermal change, noise, and inadequate rest. Fatigue, gastrointestinal upset, irritability, allergic symptoms, hypoglycemia, and unusual sensitivity to temperature change are common manifestations of diminished adrenal reserve. On slightest exertion the individual may experience tremor and feel weak from hypotension. Adequate rest and avoidance of stress are necessary to restore normal adrenal responses. Otherwise there may be risk of eventual tissue damage.

Regulation of Cortisol Secretion

It has been repeatedly confirmed that various forms of stress not only increase the output of adrenal glucocorticoids, but they also increase circulating levels of a peptide hormone, adrenocorticotropin (ACTH), from the anterior lobe of the pituitary gland (adenohypophysis).[1] Increases in levels of ACTH always precede the

1There is recent evidence that the secretion of beta-endorphin, another pituitary peptide, often accompanies secretion of ACTH. Beta-endorphin is discussed at length in Chapter 17.

elevation of glucocorticoids. Moreover, injections of ACTH are followed by an increase in adrenal glucocorticoids. Small quantities of ACTH are secreted continually by the adenohypophysis. In the presence of physiologic stress, however, ACTH secretion can be increased by as much as 20-fold within a few minutes. Therefore, the elevation of cortisol levels in stress depends upon elevations of ACTH. Furthermore, the primary regulator of ACTH secretion is the central nervous system, more specifically a secretion from certain hypothalamic nuclei. It is well established that the secretion of all hormones from the anterior pituitary is controlled by the hypothalamus. Thus, in response to various changes in the external or internal environment, the output of the appropriate pituitary hormone may be selectively altered. Therefore it is apparent that cortisol response to stress is mediated first through the nervous system and then through the pituitary. These components compose what has been designated as the *hypothalamic-hypophyseal-adrenal axis,* which is functional to various degrees in the nonspecific responses to most stressors.

Control of ACTH secretion is exercised also by the output of the target tissue of cortisol, illustrating the principle of negative feedback. When *corticotropic releasing factor* (CRF) from the hypothalamus stimulates release of ACTH, which in turn stimulates an increase in blood levels of cortisol, the effects of the cortisol in some way act upon the anterior pituitary and the hypothalamic nuclei to inhibit secretion of ACTH, thus diminishing the cortisol output and restoring hormonal balance. Does this imply that elevated levels of cortisol are always transient and do not persist? Ordinarily this might appear to be the case; however, there is evidence that in pronounced, unrelenting stress, release of ACTH may persist independently of existing plasma levels of cortisol, particularly under strong stimulation from the hypothalamic nuclei. Hence, the negative feedback system can be overridden. Moreover, animal studies have suggested that when the stress is sustained, the feedback loop tends to function from a higher set point, with a much greater than usual steroid level being necessary to achieve operation.

Thus, it would appear that in some stresses, ACTH secretion is not always subject to feedback inhibition in the usual manner by customary levels of cortisol. This loss of control would mean that excessive levels of cortisol would persist, a condition that could enhance susceptibility to infectious disease and other immune irregularities. A diagram of potential interactions that can occur among the adrenal gland, pituitary, hypothalamus, and the ANS in response to a stressor appears in Figure 4-4.

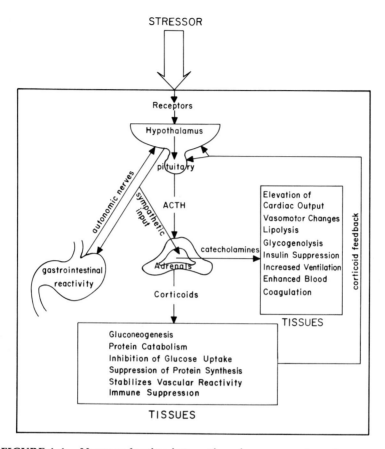

FIGURE 4-4 **Neuroendocrine interactions in response to a stressor.**
Receptors respond to the stressor stimulus and relay the information to the
hypothalamus, which controls both the pituitary (adrenal cortex) and the
ANS (sympathetic pathways). Most of the stress reaction throughout the
body is then mediated by secretions of catecholamines and cortical steroids.

Stress and Other Hormones

A number of other endocrine secretions may become elevated in the
blood when the individual is confronted with physiologic stress.
The mineralocorticoid, aldosterone, often increases, and *antidiuretic
hormone* (ADH), released from the posterior lobe (neurohypophysis)
of the pituitary, likewise may show increased levels in the plasma,
although the evidence in regard to this hormone in stress has been
somewhat contradictory. ADH is antidiuretic in action; therefore, together with aldosterone these two hormones would promote retention of water and sodium in the plasma, resulting in a greater

extracellular fluid volume. Such hormonal mechanisms would counteract hypovolemic and hypotensive tendencies as occur in shock, for example.

Certain types of stress via a hypothalamic releaser stimulate secretions of *growth hormone* or *somatotropin* (STH) from the adenohypophysis. Exertion, exposure to cold, trauma, hypoglycemia, and emotional arousal are examples of stresses known to elevate STH. The action of this hormone reinforces the insulin antagonism of cortisol and the lipolytic action of epinephrine. The result is an elevation of glucose and lipids in the blood. STH also blocks synthesis of triglycerides from glucose. This is one of its mechanisms responsible for blood glucose elevation. *Glucagon* from alpha cells of the pancreatic islets also is released in response to hypoglycemia and numerous other stresses. Glucagon promotes an elevation in blood glucose. Exercise, exposure to cold, and acute anxiety can result in dramatic rises in glucagon output.

A few stressors, among which are temperature reduction, exercise, infections, and acute anxiety, operate through a hypothalamic releasing factor to stimulate production of *thyrotropic hormone* (TSH) from the anterior pituitary. TSH in turn stimulates the thyroid gland to release its hormones, *thyroxin* (T_4) and *triiodothyronine* (T_3). However, in some stresses the output of thyroid hormones is diminished. Indeed, some studies have led to the idea that there may be an inverse relationship between thyroid output and adrenal cortex activity. According to this idea, since stresses activate the adrenal cortex, thyroid secretions would be expected to decrease. The generally accepted concept is that thyroid output may increase in response to severe, acute stress, but may decrease with chronic forms of stress.

The discovery of a hypothalamic peptide hormone, called *somatostatin*, that inhibits secretion of both pituitary growth hormone and TSH, has stimulated considerable interest since it has been shown that it also acts directly on the pancreas to suppress output of both insulin and glucagon. Many forms of stress such as fatigue, mental strain, and infections tend to inhibit secretion of somatostatin. The resulting excess of glucagon can elevate blood glucose and stress the insulin response mechanism. For this reason there has been speculation concerning the role of somatostatin regulation in diabetes mellitus.

There is also a decrease of certain other hormones during stress. For example, the pituitary gonadotropins, follicle stimulating hormone (FSH) and luteinizing hormone (LH), as well as the gonadal steroids that respond to them are all somewhat diminished in the stressed organism. In addition, plasma levels of insulin may be reduced, which is largely due to the action of catecholamines. However, in a stressed individual who responds with parasympathetic predominance, the cholinergic mediator acetylcholine is known to stimulate insulin release.

It is noteworthy that catecholamines, glucocorticoids, growth hormone, thyroxin, and glucagon (the stress hormones) all have a predominantly catabolic effect on the body.

THE SIGNIFICANCE OF THE HYPOTHALAMUS

Though the direct response to many stressors is through the activity of the ANS and adrenal glands, it is apparent from the foregoing discussions that the major component directing these actions is the hypothalamus. Indeed, the hypothalamus is the primary integrator in sorting out afferent input and relaying it to the appropriate efferent output for both the ANS and the pituitary-adrenocortical system. Thus the hypothalamus is the single most important control area for regulating the internal environment.

The hypothalamus lies at the base of the brain behind the optic chiasm, just above the pituitary. It is sometimes considered a part of the *limbic system,* along with the hippocampus, amygdala, and thalamus—structures which from the standpoint of evolution are older regions of the brain. The general structural relationship of the hypothalamus to the rest of the brain is illustrated in Figure 4-5. It is truly remarkable that this small region with a volume of only 5 to 6 cubic centimeters, weighing only 4 grams, is the principal director of the neuroendocrine system.

In addition to its control of the ANS and the pituitary, the hypothalamus comprises a number of distinct centers or nuclei that operate the neural pathways involved in body temperature regulation, hunger, thirst, satiety, water regulation, sleep, waking, pain, instinctive sexual reflexes, and emotional states such as fear, rage, and hostility. All of these expressions emanate from a compact conglomeration of nuclei, some of which are only half a millimeter apart.

ANS Regulation

The hypothalamus controls the responses of the parasympathetic division of the ANS through several nuclei in its anterior and medial regions. Stimulation of these regions, which include the *preoptic, supraoptic,* and *dorsomedial* nuclei, produces a decrease in heart rate and blood pressure, a dilatation of blood vessels, an increase in gastroin-

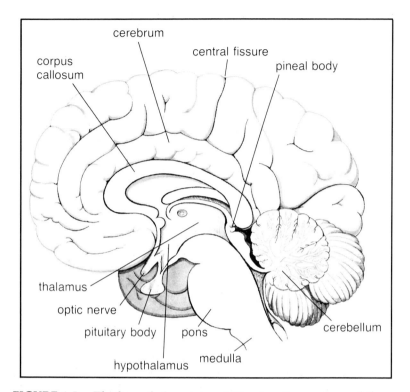

FIGURE 4-5   The hypothalamus in relation to other regions of the brain (sagittal section). Observe its intermediate position between the thalamus and the pituitary.

testinal motility and secretion, bronchial constriction, and increased sweating. Most of these effects are known to result from direct vagal impulses.

The hypothalamus excites sympathetic pathways of the ANS through several nuclei located in its posterior and lateral regions. Stimulation of these regions, which include the posterior and *mammillary* nuclei, produces an increase in heart rate and blood pressure, a constriction of blood vessels, a decrease in gastrointestinal activity, bronchial dilatation, shivering, and a release of catecholamines from the adrenal medullae. Some of the various hypothalamic nuclei and their regulatory capabilities are shown in Figure 4-6.

It is apparent that the hypothalamus may evoke changes in autonomic activity in response to its afferent input. This afferent input in turn can be modified by efferent autonomic activity. Not only does the hypothalamus direct the activity of visceral effectors, but this activity itself can stimulate visceral receptors which relay information back to the hypothalamus. Therefore, autonomic function re-

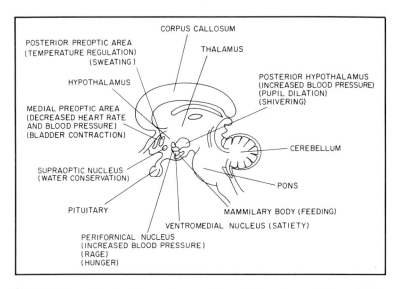

FIGURE 4-6   The location of several hypothalamic nuclei (sagittal section). The particular body regulation of each is indicated.

flects the variable state of activity occurring among the various centers of the hypothalamus.

Earlier in this chapter mention was made of autonomic tuning, in which neural activity of specific autonomic nuclei becomes facilitated, resulting in a disposition for one division of the ANS to show a functional predominance over the other when certain stressors are applied. Evidence from experiments with animals supports this idea. For example, it would appear that afferent input from higher centers in the brain can effect tuning through the facilitation of certain pathways as a result of conditioning. This may explain why mental distress in one instance may produce a predominance of sympathetic activity (elevation of heart rate and blood pressure, and tensing of the muscles); whereas in another instance the same stimulus may elicit a predominance of parasympathetic activity (trembling and diarrhea). Leastwise, the nature of the overall autonomic action is dependent upon the particular way in which the various hypothalamic nuclei are functionally disposed at a given time in a given individual.

Pituitary Regulation

Almost all secretion from the pituitary gland is controlled by signals transmitted from the hypothalamus. Secretion from the posterior lobe of the pituitary is regulated by nerve fibers originating in the

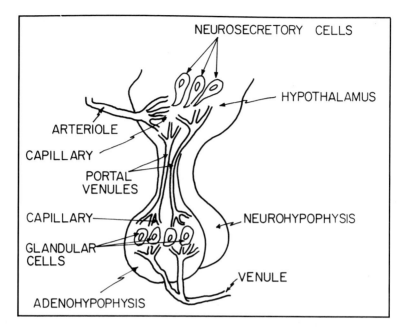

FIGURE 4-7   The hypothalamic-hypophyseal portal system.
Neurosecretory cells of the hypothalamus release peptides that are
conveyed to the anterior pituitary (adenohypophysis) by two portal
venules. The hypothalamic releasers then stimulate the glandular cells of
the anterior pituitary to release their specific hormones into the
bloodstream.

hypothalamus. Hormones such as ADH that are released from this
region are synthesized in the supraoptic and *paraventricular* nuclei of
the hypothalamus itself. In respect to control of the anterior lobe,
both releasing and inhibiting factors are synthesized by hypothalamic neurons, and moved by way of axons to the *median eminence,*
whence they are released into portal capillaries, and then transported to the anterior pituitary. These neurosecretions are peptides
whose target cells lie in specific regions of the adenohypophysis, a
highly vascularized lobe with extensive blood sinuses around the
cells. The neurosecretions are conveyed through what is termed the
hypothalamic-hypophyseal portal system, which consists of a hypothalamic capillary bed drained by two portal venules which form a second capillary network among the sinuses of the adenohypophysis.
This structural arrangement is shown in Figure 4-7.

   Apparently there is a different hypothalamic releasing factor
for each of the tropic hormones of the anterior pituitary. In view of
our concern with stress, the major hypothalamic releaser is corticotropic releasing factor (CRF), which stimulates the release of

ACTH from the anterior pituitary. As has been mentioned, STH and thyrotropic hormone are other secretions from the adenohypophysis that may respond to stress.

The hypothalamus governs much of the endocrine system through its control of pituitary secretions. In many functional disorders characterized by an imbalance of pituitary hormones, the malfunction is usually hypothalamic rather than a problem stemming directly from the pituitary itself.

In addition to effects mediated through the pituitary, the hypothalamus is involved in governing other endocrine tissues in a more direct manner. For example, direct nerve connections have been demonstrated to the islet cells of the pancreas, which produce insulin and glucagon. In addition, it has been shown that lymphatic tissues such as the thymus are influenced by the hypothalamus. Thus this important part of the brain must also govern immune phenomena in some way.

Afferent Input

The hypothalamus receives neural and hormonal input, both facilitory and inhibitory, from all areas of the body. As previously mentioned, this includes input from visceral receptors, peripheral receptors, and higher centers in the brain. Moreover, these are two-way pathways with reciprocal connections. Therefore, practically all body changes are made known to the hypothalamic centers, which in turn can respond with the appropriate efferent output.

There are numerous pathways connecting the hypothalamus with many centers of the cerebrum and brain stem. Indeed, the hypothalamus receives a large part of its neural influx by way of the limbic forebrain structures that consist of some of the more primitive cortical and subcortical regions. It is well established that the cerebral hemispheres as a whole, and the frontal lobes in particular, are capable of exerting considerable inhibitory action on the hypothalamus. Obviously the functional association between the cerebral cortex and the hypothalamus underlies the role played by the mind in physiologic stress. Mental conflict is such an important and ever-present stressor that it is discussed at considerable length in Chapters 16 and 17.

Certainly the hypothalamus is by far the most important region of the nervous system in regulating somatic balances throughout the body, and many functional types of disorders are rooted in the inability of the hypothalamus to adequately regulate homeostasis. When we see a happy, well-controlled individual who is free of chronic disease throughout a long life, we may well conclude, "There goes a master of his hypothalamus."

ENDOCRINE DISORDERS

When neurohormonal response mechanisms become overloaded with demands from stressors, functional hormonal imbalances may develop. Eventually the imbalances may be alleviated by the subsiding of stress or by medical intervention. On the other hand they can progress to greater severity and become persistent. Long-term hormonal disorder leads to tissue damage. In other instances endocrine disorder is a consequence of direct localized stress on the glandular cells themselves from infective agents, immune reactions, or abnormal growths. However, it cannot be overemphasized that endocrine disorders are often generated through alteration of hypothalamic activity stemming from stress, particularly emotional upsets and chronic anxiety.

Many endocrine problems are associated with either deficient or excessive hormone production. However, the amount of circulating hormone alone is not always a reliable indicator of the normalcy of its effective action. There also may be some sort of chemical antagonism to the hormone, or it may fail to bind effectively to receptor sites on cell membranes. Hormonal balance depends upon complex interactions and feedbacks among the various secretions as well as upon the integrating influence of the nervous system. Not only can stress lead to endocrine disorder, but, once disease is present, it may itself constitute further stress on the body. The most frequently encountered endocrine disorders involve the pancreas, thyroid, adrenal glands, and pituitary gland.

The Pancreas

Diabetes mellitus is the most common endocrine-related disturbance. Despite its prevalence and incidence it is yet to be completely understood. The essential problem is a relative ineffectiveness in metabolizing glucose, the utilization of which is associated with the action of *insulin* from the beta cells of the pancreatic islets. *Glucagon* from the alpha cells of the islets is antagonistic to the action of insulin.

When blood levels of glucose remain elevated, especially to the point that they exceed the kidney threshold, the diagnosis of diabetes is unequivocal. However, the degree of glucose intolerance varies enormously, and the entire matter affords an excellent example of the principle of graded, progressive stages in the development of pathology. Thus the terms *prediabetes* and *latent* or *chemical* diabetes are used to designate a predisposition, which can be revealed by unusual elevations in blood glucose during times of stress.

There are at least several underlying causes of glucose intolerance despite the traditional notion that it is simply a matter of insufficient insulin from the beta cells. Thus diabetes is not just one disease. Most cases can be divided into two distinct forms, each with a different underlying etiology and set of circumstances. Genetic predisposition has been cited in both forms, but this factor may be overemphasized. In studies of several sets of identical twins, in which one has developed glucose intolerance, the other does not always become diabetic. In the severe form of diabetes with juvenile onset, there is damage to the beta cells and a consequent deficiency of insulin production leading to a dependency on exogenous insulin. Recent evidence suggests that a viral infection of glandular tissue combined with a specific type of immune response initiates the damage in predisposed individuals. This mechanism is pursued further in Chapter 15.

In the milder form of glucose intolerance that typically does not appear until middle age, exogenous insulin is not usually required. Adult-onset diabetes is discussed at length in Chapter 12, and there is reference to the vascular complications of diabetes in Chapter 5. Distinctions between the two clinical types of diabetes are summarized in Table 4-4.[2]

The Thyroid

Excessive thyroid secretion (hyperthyroidism) is usually more frequent in young adults, whereas hypothyroidism (*myxedema*) is more commonly found in those of middle age and older, although occasionally thyroid deficiency has been detected in neonates, a serious matter in view of potential cretinism arising from defective thyroid output. Thyroid disturbances occur more often in women and in individuals inhabiting regions with seasonal temperature change. The most common form of hyperthyroidism is *Graves disease,* charac-

2Quite recently, juvenile-onset diabetes has been distinguished as Type I diabetes and the adult-onset form as Type II diabetes. This reference is realistic in that Type I patients are not exclusively juvenile, and Type II patients are not always adults.

TABLE 4-4

Comparison of Adult-Onset and Juvenile-Onset Diabetes

ADULT-ONSET	JUVENILE-ONSET
Insidious development	Develops suddenly
Symptoms usually vague, or absent	Always symptomatic (polyuria, polydipsia, fatigue, weight loss)
Occurs in adulthood; often after age 40	Occurs in childhood or adolescence
Patient usually overweight	Patient often underweight or at least of normal weight
Hyperglycemia mild to moderate	Hyperglycemia severe
Patient not susceptible to ketosis	Uncontrolled patient develops ketosis
Blood glucose fluctuations relatively stable	Blood glucose fluctuations brittle
Blood insulin levels not deficient, but usually excessive	Blood insulin levels deficient
Treatment consists of weight loss, dietary restrictions, and sulfonylurea drugs	Treatment consists of exogenous insulin and dietary restrictions
Vascular complications can occur, but their development may take longer and are not as severe	Vascular complications occur earlier and may be more severe
Postprandial hypoglycemia common	Postprandial hypoglycemia absent

terized by symptoms that would be expected from an elevated metabolic rate: tremor, insomnia, tachycardia, weight loss, increased appetite, profuse sweating, and heat intolerance. *Exophthalmia* (bulging eyes) often accompanies Graves disease, and it may persist for a time after the condition is under control. In hyperthyroidism the gland may show an enlargement, referred to as goiter, which infrequently may be tumorous.

There is a strong likelihood that multiple stresses in predisposed young adults may be involved in some cases of hyperthyroidism. It is of interest that the onset is usually during winter, and it tends to occur in high-strung individuals known to be under mental strain. It is suspected that the problem is related to the pituitary regulation of the thyroid. The pituitary, of course, responds to hypothalamic direction.

In adult hypothyroidism there is a diminished rate of metabolism, resulting in fatigue, apathy, drowsiness, cold intolerance, and sometimes a gain in weight. The skin is dry and puffy (Figure 4-8). There may also be constipation, depression, hyperlipidemia, and hoarseness. Several causes of hypothyroidism have been cited. In some cases the pituitary regulation may be involved. In other in-

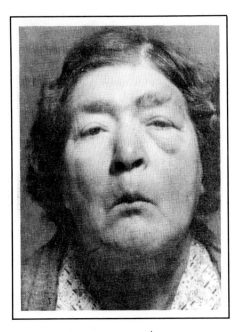

FIGURE 4-8   A person with myxedema (hypothyroidism). Note the
puffiness beneath the eyes, the scaly appearance of the skin and eyebrows,
and the apathetic countenance. (From B. A. Schottelius and D. D.
Schottelius, *Textbook of physiology*, 18th ed. St. Louis: C. V. Mosby Co., 1978.)

stances the fault is a deficiency in dietary iodine, which can lead to a
progressive enlargement of the gland. Iodine-deficiency goiters are
more common than those associated with Graves disease. *Hashimoto
disease* is a form of hypothyroidism of autoimmune etiology.

The Adrenal Cortex

A marked, persistent elevation of blood glucocorticoids produces a
group of metabolic disturbances known as *Cushing syndrome*. The
condition is characterized by hyperglycemia, a characteristic thickening of the trunk, and a wasting effect in the extremities from extreme protein catabolism. There is an increased susceptibility to
infection and a heightened risk of gastric ulcer formation. Mental
depression and irritability sometimes develop. The disease is caused
either by long-term administration of glucocorticoids for such conditions as arthritis, asthma, and autoimmune disturbance, or by an imbalance in function of the hypothalamic-pituitary-adrenal system. In
some cases excessive secretion of ACTH from the pituitary is responsible.

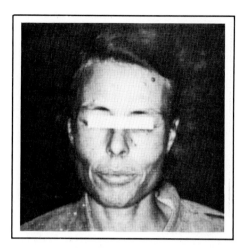

FIGURE 4-9   A case of Addison disease. Observe the dark, bronzed cast to the skin, as well as the dehydrated, wasted appearance of the neck and face. (From J. R. McClintic, *Physiology of the human body.* Copyright © 1975 by John Wiley & Sons, Inc. Reprinted by permission of John Wiley & Sons, Inc.)

When there is an excessive secretion of aldosterone, the mineralocorticoid from the adrenal cortex, a persistent increase in the retention of sodium and water occurs. This maintains an expanded blood volume that results in chronic hypertension. The condition is called *aldosteronism.* It can be a result of chronic stimulation of the renin-angiotensin system, which is discussed in the subsection on hypertension in Chapter 5.

A relative deficiency in secretions from the adrenal cortex is known as *Addison disease.* Levels of both glucocorticoids and mineralocorticoids are diminished. Glucocorticoid deficiency is responsible for low concentrations of blood glucose, and the patient is especially sensitive and vulnerable to such ordinary stresses as temperature change, exertion, and trauma, both physical and psychic. Since the action of *melanocyte-stimulating hormone* (MSH) is inhibited by glucocorticoids, the victim of Addison disease may show greater MSH activity than usual, resulting in hyperpigmentation (Figure 4-9).

Insufficient aldosterone in Addison disease leads to hypotension, which is particularly noticeable when the individual assumes an upright posture. Infections, such as tuberculosis, can damage the adrenal cortex and thereby produce Addison disease. However, the leading cause of the disease is considered to be an autoimmune reaction.

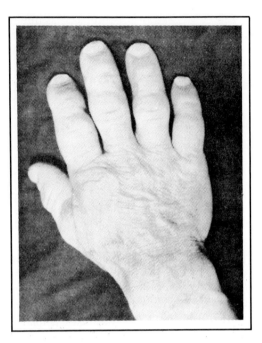

FIGURE 4-10 An acromegalic hand. Note the thickened, clublike fingers. (From B. A. Schottelius and D. D. Schottelius, *Textbook of physiology*.)

Disorders of the adrenal medulla are less frequent than those of the cortex. The pathologic condition found most often is *pheochromocytoma,* a tumor of the chromaffin tissue responsible for intermittent elevations of catecholamines in the blood. The elevations result in sporadic increases in blood pressure and heart rate.

The Pituitary

Pituitary deficiency inevitably affects all the glands controlled by the adenohypophysis. This includes the thyroid, adrenal cortex, and the gonads. Although the pituitary gland itself can be diseased from disturbances involving autoimmune processes, tumorous growths, and ischemia of the pituitary region, the majority of pituitary irregularities are associated with functional disturbances in the hypothalamus.

An insufficiency of growth hormone in adulthood brings about a prominent reduction in fasting blood glucose and a considerable sensitivity to the action of insulin. This is due to the fact that STH is an insulin antagonist. Excessive secretion of STH in adults is known as *acromegaly* (Figure 4-10). In this condition there is a thickening of bones and soft tissue in the hands, feet, and portions of the face. Pituitary tumors are often responsible for acromegaly.

‖ SUMMARY

The neural and hormonal systems play a major role in homeostatic regulation, and much of the control exercised in response to stressors stems directly from activity of the autonomic nervous system and adrenal glands.

Sympathetic impulses produce widespread systemic effects which serve to adapt the body's physiology to changes in the external environment, whereas the parasympathetic division responds to internal, restorative needs. Though stress is often characterized by a predominance of sympathetic activity, parasympathetic responses occur as well. Hypothalamic-induced imbalances among actions of the two divisions often lead to functional disorders.

Sympathetic activity provokes release of catecholamines from the medullae of the adrenal glands, whereas ACTH from the anterior pituitary stimulates release of glucocorticoids from the adrenal cortex. The catecholamines produce effects similar to those of sympathetic stimulation itself, except that the action is prolonged. The glucocorticoids stimulate gluconeogenesis, suppress protein anabolism and immune reactions, and stabilize the vascular reactivity and permeability associated with tissue damage.

The hypothalamus receives neural and hormonal input, both facilitory and inhibitory, from all areas of the body, including the higher brain centers. A distinct group of hypothalamic nuclei regulates respectively the sympathetic and parasympathetic divisions of the ANS. In addition, afferent input to specific hypothalamic nuclei promotes release of hypothalamic hormones, which move through portal veins to the anterior pituitary where they stimulate release of pituitary hormones. The most significant of these hormones in stress is ACTH.

Persistent stress and localized lesions lead to disorder in endocrine function. Among the more frequently encountered endocrine diseases are diabetes mellitus, Graves disease, myxedema, Cushing syndrome, aldosteronism, and Addison disease.

Chapter Glossary

adenohypophysis   the anterior lobe of the pituitary

afferent   refers to nerve impulses that are conducted inward to centers from receptors

efferent   refers to nerve impulses that are conducted outward from centers to effectors

gluconeogenesis   metabolic production of glucose by the liver

hyperglycemia   excessive levels of glucose in the blood

hyperlipidemia   excessive levels of cholesterol and triglycerides in the blood

hypervolemia   excessive extracellular fluid volume

innervation   a supply of functional nerve fibers

lipolysis   a breakdown of lipid stores; the converse of lipogenesis

pilomotor (piloerector)   refers to the smooth muscle action responsible for erecting the hair or producing "goose bumps" on the skin

postganglionic   the final efferent fiber of an ANS pathway, running from a ganglion to an organ

reticuloendothelial   refers to connective tissue derivatives involved with blood cell production and the immune system

shock   a rapid, pronounced decrease in cardiac output and pressure of circulating blood associated with a weak, rapid pulse, and cold, clammy skin

visceral   refers to internal organs or structures suspended in the body cavity as opposed to the skeleton and skeletal muscles

For Further Reading

Archer, J. 1979. *Animals under stress.* Baltimore: University Park Press.

Brothers, M. J. 1976. *Diabetes: The new approach.* New York: Grosset & Dunlap.

Burn, J. 1975. *The autonomic nervous system: For students of physiology and of pharmacology.* 5th ed. London: Blackwell Scientific Publications, Ltd.

Camerini-Davalos, R. A., and Hanover, B., eds. 1979. Treatment of early diabetes. In *Advances in experimental medicine and biology.* Vol. 119. New York: Plenum Press.

Cryer, P. E. 1979. *Diagnostic endocrinology.* 2d ed. New York: Oxford University Press.

DiCara, L. 1975. *Limbic and autonomic nervous systems research.* New York: Plenum Publishing Corp.

Gellhorn, E. 1957. *Autonomic imbalance and the hypothalamus.* Minneapolis: University of Minnesota Press.

Guyton, A. C. 1977. *Basic human physiology: Normal function and mechanisms of disease.* 2d ed. Philadelphia: W. B. Saunders Co.

Jeffcoate, S. L., and Hutchinson, J. S. M., eds. 1978. *The endocrine hypothalamus.* New York: Academic Press.

Johnson, R. H., and Spalding, J. M. K. 1974. *Disorders of the autonomic nervous system.* London: Blackwell Scientific Publications, Ltd.

Loraine, J. A., and Bell, E. T. 1971. *Hormone assays and their clinical application.* 3d ed. Baltimore: Williams and Wilkins Co.

Makara, G. B.; Palkovits, M.; and Szentagothai, J. 1980. The endocrine hypothalamus and the hormonal response to stress. In H. Selye, ed., *Selye's guide to stress research.* Vol. 1. New York: Van Nostrand Reinhold Co.

McQuillan, M. T. 1977. *Somatostatin.* Vol. 1. Annual Research Reviews. Montreal: Eden Press Inc.

Martini, L., and Ganong, W. F. 1976. *Frontiers in neuroendocrinology.* New York: Raven Press.

Martini, L., and Besser, G. M., eds. 1977. *Clinical neuroendocrinology.* New York: Academic Press.

Noback, C. R., and Demarest, R. J. 1972. *The nervous system: Introduction and review.* New York: McGraw-Hill Book Co.

Reichlin, S.; Baldessarini, R. J.; and Martin, J. D. 1978. *The hypothalamus.* New York: Raven Press.

Ryan, W. G. 1979. *Endocrine disorders.* Chicago: Year Book Medical Publishers, Times Mirror.

Unger, R. H.; Dobbs, R. E.; and Orci, L. 1978. Insulin, glucagon, and somatostatin secretion in the regulation of metabolism. *Annu Rev Physiol* 40:307.

Vander, A. J.; Sherman, J. H.; and Luciano, D. S. 1980. *Human physiology: The mechanisms of body function.* 3d ed. New York: McGraw-Hill Book Co. Chapts. 8, 9.

Wenger, M. A. 1966. Studies of autonomic balance: A summary. *Psychophysiology.* 2:173.

Wenger, M. A., and Cullen, T. D. 1973. Studies of autonomic balance in children and adults. In N. S. Greenfield and R. A. Sternbach, eds., *Handbook of psychophysiology.* New York: Holt, Rinehart & Winston.

Williams, R. H. 1974. *Textbook of endocrinology.* Philadelphia: W. B. Saunders Co.

5

The Relation of Physiologic Stress to Pathology

|| **Objectives:** Upon completing this chapter you should:

1. Be able to perceive the role of stress in weakening homeostatic mechanisms, thereby promoting disease development.
2. Be fully informed about the nature and causes of hypertensive cardiovascular disease.
3. Be informed about the nature and causes of cancer.
4. Recognize the relationship of physiologic stresses to the development of cardiovascular disease and cancer.

Practical considerations of physiologic stress inevitably center around its potential relationship to disease. Do stresses produce disease? We already have defined both disease and physiologic stress, and certain parallels are apparent. In each case there are disturbances in the chemical and physical balance within the tissues or their immediate environment. However, the distinction between physiologic stress and the beginnings of disease rests largely upon the degree and duration of the imbalance and *how effectively it continues to be counteracted by the adaptive responses of the organism.* Unless stress-induced alterations are effectively corrected, further disorder may ensue, which then leads to a loss of steady-state control. Widespread failure among a number of control systems can lead to less and less reversibility of unsteady states until life itself becomes threatened.

Stress begins to manifest itself as a disease process when homeostatic response mechanisms become faulty and cannot cope with continued stress. What prompts the failure of the mechanisms? Within their operations designed to achieve states of physical and chemical equilibriums, control systems tend to slightly overshoot or undershoot a precise point of balance, oscillating rather than achieving an exact equilibration. A progressive increase in the degree of such oscillations, due to cumulative and overloaded stressor effects, indicates that the control system is becoming maladjusted, leading to a pendulum effect that threatens the integrity of steady-state maintenance. At this point relief from stressors becomes imperative. Otherwise, the control systems tend to become overwhelmed with demands, and a recovery of balance becomes less likely. If counteracting responses are forced to operate too hard or too fast for too long a time, errors in sensing stimuli or in interpreting signals may ensue. When any of these events transpires, the control system is no longer effective in maintaining stability. This failure leads to progressive biochemical imbalance and may eventually induce cellular damage considered truly pathologic. A major concern of medical and nursing practice is the identification of whatever function is out of control, and the application of measures necessary to repair the damage and restore a normal operation of the system.

Mention is made in Chapter 3 of pathologic changes in laboratory animals that have been induced by subjecting them to various stressors. Hypertension, gastrointestinal ulcers, and nephrosclerosis were among these changes. Experimental results of this nature have prompted Hans Selye and others in his school of thought to proclaim that stresses do produce disease. Caution is advised in extrapolating experimental results of this sort to the ordinary, everyday stressing in human beings. The stressors employed in the animal studies were applied persistently for several days and with extreme intensity, and after all, we are not rats. On the other hand, experimental data of this kind cannot be dismissed, and we must acknowledge that *chronic* exposure to *multiple* stressors carries a strong risk of developing disease, particularly in certain individuals. Also, it must be recognized that there is a reciprocal cause and effect relationship between stress and disease; in other words, not only may stress promote disease; but disease in turn constitutes a stress.

STRESS DISEASES

It has become commonplace to regard certain ailments such as gastrointestinal ulcers, hypertension, migraine headaches, spastic colitis, certain skin problems, and some forms of heart disorders as stress diseases. In these instances, the stressor is usually presumed to be emotional strain, and the ailment is categorized as psychosomatic. Indeed, most people conceive of stress as being synonymous with emotional tension. In reality, however, all diseases are stress diseases, in that stress, as it is broadly conceived in physiology, is inevitably a contributing factor in pathogenesis. Moreover, stress worsens conditions that already are considered pathologic.

Yet, there are certain diseases that warrant priority in consideration of their relation to stress because of their incidence in the population and their probability of becoming terminal. Upon examining Table 2-6, one will note that heart disease and stroke, the first and third causes of death, are closely related and can be considered together as cardiovascular impairment. Diabetes might be so classified as well, since the vascular complications of this disease usually precipitate death. When these three conditions are considered together, over half the deaths in the United States are related in some way to disease of the heart and blood vessels. These facts call for a special look at this form of pathology and its stress relationships.

CARDIOVASCULAR PATHOLOGY

In parts of the world where there is little industrialization and affluence, the incidence of cardiovascular disease is notably low, at least among the middle-aged. Epidemiologic evidence of this sort strongly suggests that the difference in habits of life must be a significant variable underlying the difference in the incidence of cardiovascular pathology. What causes damage to the heart, and what promotes degeneration of blood vessels? How are stresses related to pathology? Apparently the process is inevitable, and anyone who lives long enough will certainly die of arterial degeneration. Yet, why does it appear so much earlier in some than in others?

Heart Disease

Over 90% of all cardiac pathology develops either from coronary artery disease or from pathologic changes in the heart valves. Of these two developments, the occurrence of coronary artery disease outnumbers the cases of valvular pathology by nearly 85 to 1. Thus the term heart disease is sometimes considered synonymous with coronary artery disease.

The prevalence of valvular disease is by far the highest in the mitral valve, and the major cause of the damage is acute rheumatic inflammation with subsequent healing or scar formation. The rheumatic complications are sequels to bacterial infections most commonly experienced in childhood. Characteristic nodular lesions, called *Aschoff bodies*, may appear in the cardiac walls, providing evidence of active rheumatic inflammation (see Figure 2-2). In *mitral stenosis* there is a restriction of blood flow from the left atrium to the left ventricle during diastole. This eventually can lead to hypertrophy of the left atrial muscle, and both the elevated pressure and volume of blood in the atrium are reflected backward into the pulmonary vessels. When the diameter of the valve orifice has been reduced by nearly 50% of normal, dyspnea and tachycardia become apparent, particularly with modest exertion. A diastolic heart murmer is often detectable even before the stenosis has advanced to a symptomatic stage.

As implied above, most pathologic changes in the heart develop in the cardiac muscle as a consequence of biochemical alterations brought about by an insufficient perfusion of the myocardium with blood from the coronary arteries. When the coronary arteries are becoming diseased or are subject to neuromuscular spasms, various degrees of transient ischemia cause reversible changes at the tissue level, depressing myocardial contractility. The critical substance is oxygen; an insufficiency forces the myocardium to shift to anaerobic metabolism. Thus the production of high-energy phosphate is reduced, and the end product of anaerobiosis, lactic acid, reduces cellular pH. Hence the consequences of myocardial hypoxia are less available energy and an acidosis, both of which can greatly impair ventricular contractility and recovery.

The consequent depression of left ventricular function from less available contraction energy and reduced pH reduces the stroke volume, thereby lowering cardiac output. In addition, the slowness in systolic emptying increases ventricular blood volumes, thereby imposing an increase in pressure in the left side of the heart. This elevation in ventricular pressure is compounded by changes in wall distensibility brought on by the ischemia. Thus the myocardial stress originated by coronary ischemia is compounded by added strain on the ventricular wall due to intraventricular pressure.

Myocardial ischemia usually is associated with two noticeable changes in the electrocardiogram (ECG). A normal ECG is shown in Figure 5-1. In Figure 5-2, in which myocardial ischemia is present, note the inversion of the T wave, and the depression of the S-T segment. When unusual concentrations of metabolites, such as lactic acid, begin to accumulate as a result of myocardial ischemia, pain receptors may be stimulated, and it is these that are responsible for the classic symptom, *angina pectoris*. Any additional myocardial demand for oxygen, as in exertion or emotion, can provoke this symptom in those with ischemia from coronary artery disease.

When myocardial ischemia is sustained beyond 45 minutes, cellular changes in the muscle fibers tend to become irreversible, and the permanent damage leads to localized necrosis. As pointed out in Chapter 2, this condition is termed *infarction*. Its seriousness depends upon the size and specific location of the infarct. When the infarction is massive (> 40% of the left ventricle), the resulting cardiogenic shock is fatal in 90% of the cases. Coronary care units are equipped to monitor ECGs so that an impending infarction may be detected and the severity perhaps diminished (Figure 5-3).

The most common mechanical complication following myocardial infarction is *congestive heart failure*, due to the inability of the

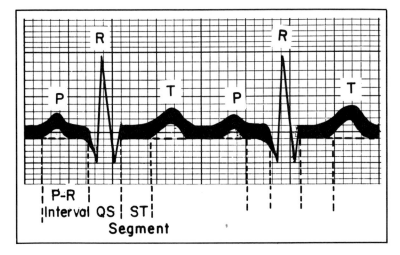

FIGURE 5-1   A normal electrocardiogram (ECG). The ECG measures
electrical changes (in millivolts) occurring in the heart muscle during the
cardiac cycle. The depolarization associated with contraction of the atria is
represented by the P wave, whereas the QRS components express
ventricular depolarization, R indicating the brief contractile peak of the
ventricles. The T wave is produced by repolarization (recovery) of the
ventricles. At rest the R wave spike is about 1 to 2 mv in magnitude, and
one full cycle (P to P) requires about 0.7 to 1.0 seconds.

left ventricle to empty during systole. This coupled with increased
diastolic filling produces high left ventricular blood volume and
pressure, which pushes blood backwards through the left atrium
and into the pulmonary system, resulting in much pulmonary congestion. The occurrence of congestive heart failure is not limited to
cases of myocardial infarction, however. In pathology of the lower
respiratory tract, such as acute respiratory infection, the heart may
become congested.

Another common disturbance during myocardial infarction is
arrhythmia, in which the electrophysiologic timing of the cardiac cycle becomes distorted. The most severe arrhythmia is *ventricular
fibrillation:* in this case the ventricles lose control of regulated contraction and merely quiver in an uncoordinated manner (Figure 5-4).

One must recall that all of these serious and often fatal
changes are a consequence of blood supply that is insufficient for the
demands of the myocardium. Although this insufficiency is often a
consequence of a progressive narrowing that can develop in any artery, there are some cases in which spasm of the coronary arteries is
the basis for the ischemia leading to angina, and even heart attacks.
Coronary artery spasms are the result of nervous stimulation of the

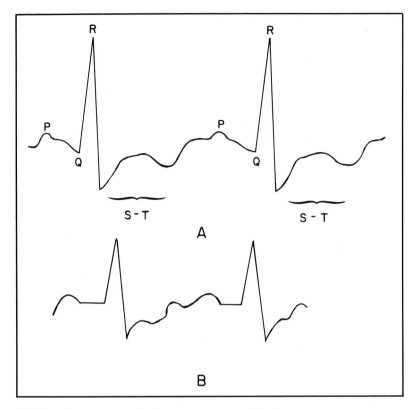

FIGURE 5-2   A. An ECG with inversion of the T wave. A common finding in myocardial ischemia. When the heart muscle is insufficiently supplied with oxygen, normal ventricular recovery is impossible. B. Depression of the S-T segment. Another ECG change in myocardial ischemia.

alpha adrenergic receptors in the vessel wall. Even though spasms may occur in coronary arteries that are not atherosclerotic, diseased arteries are more susceptible to spasms than normal ones. It is apparent, then, that spasms or no spasms, most serious cardiovascular impairment appears to be derived from degenerative changes in the artery wall. For this reason an investigation of what happens to the arteries, and how physiologic stresses contribute to the disease process is in order here.

Arterial Degeneration

Most cardiovascular pathology is based upon progressive degenerative changes in the arterial walls. The changes are characterized by a thickening of the tissues of the wall with lipid deposition and

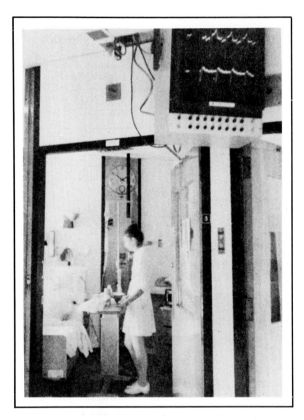

FIGURE 5-3   **A coronary intensive care unit.** Cardiac electrical activity of victims of heart attacks is displayed continuously. (Courtesy of John Withee, The S. A. Levine Cardiac Center of the Peter Bent Brigham Hospital in Boston.)

fibrous accumulation. The thickening narrows the vessels and increases resistance to blood flow, requiring a greater pressure for delivery of blood. Two terms are employed in describing this general form of arterial pathology. *Arteriosclerosis* refers to a well-established thickening or hardening of arteries regardless of the type of lesion. It becomes localized primarily in the middle of the three layers of the artery wall—the *tunica media*. The vessels lose much of their elasticity, becoming rigid, weakened, and easily ruptured. Once well established, the condition is not reversible. An angiogram showing artery disease that has produced an *aneurysm* is illustrated in Figure 5-5.

 Atherosclerosis refers to the major type of arterial change leading to, and accounting for, most instances of arteriosclerosis. The

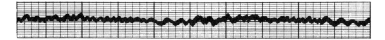

FIGURE 5-4   An ECG record showing ventricular fibrillation.
Observe the complete absence of any semblance to the normal pattern.
Contraction regulation is completely lost.

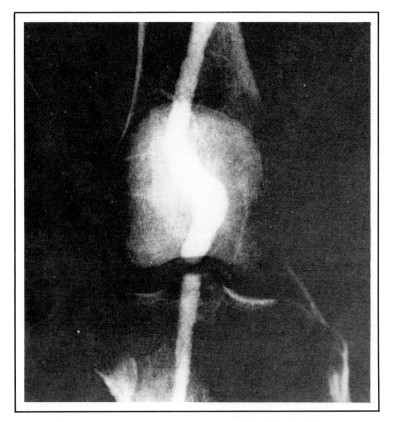

**FIGURE 5-5   An x-ray photograph of a blood vessel injected with a
radiopaque dye.** This particular angiogram shows an aneurysm, an
abnormally dilated segment of an artery due to atherosclerotic weakening
of the arterial wall. (Courtesy of Dr. Irwin Bluth, Brookdale Hospital
Medical Center, Brooklyn, N.Y.)

condition is characterized by hardened, plate-like lipid deposits
called *plaques*, which make their initial appearance in the inner wall
of arteries, the *tunica intima*. The development of atherosclerotic lesions is associated with an intimal proliferation of smooth muscle
cells, accumulation of large amounts of connective tissue matrix, and

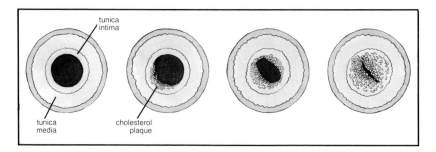

FIGURE 5-6   **Progressive atherosclerotic change in an artery.** *Far left,* the artery cross-section illustrates a disease-free vessel. *Second from left,* following damage to the endothelial layer of the tunica intima, plaques of LDL cholesterol begin to appear. *Third from left,* as more cholesterol is deposited, the plaques, reinforced by production of connective tissue matrix, thicken, resulting in a partial obstruction of blood flow, which enhances the hypoxia of the tissue. *Far right,* the process further expands both outward, invading the tunica media, and inward, resulting in near occlusion of the artery.

deposits of intracellular and extracellular lipid. Hypertension is known to be involved with increases in arterial collagen synthesis. Hyperlipidemia and tissue hypoxia also contribute to the overall atherosclerotic process.

As the lipid-containing plaques enlarge, they tend to protrude into the lumen of the artery. The rough inner surface of the arterial wall then may promote the formation of a *thrombus* (clot). A thrombus may partially or completely occlude a vessel; or it can break loose in the bloodstream and be carried to another location where occlusions may develop. If these conditions develop in a coronary artery, a heart attack (*coronary thrombosis*) occurs. If a vessel is occluded in the brain, the result is a stroke or *cerebral vascular accident.* The structure of an arterial wall and the progressive atherosclerotic changes in it are depicted in Figure 5-6. Photomicrographs comparing healthy with atherosclerotic arteries in humans are shown in Figures 5-7 and 5-8.

Two explanations have been offered concerning the genesis of the atherosclerotic process. One is that the plaques originate from tumorous growth of arterial smooth muscle. However, there is very little support for this theory. The preponderance of evidence favors the second idea, which considers the pathology to be initiated by injury to the endothelial cells lining the artery wall. Even slight damage may reduce the threshold of endothelial stability so that local hemodynamic factors can produce focal endothelial desquamation, thereby exposing the subendothelial connective tissue. The endothelial injury is followed by the aggregation of blood platelets

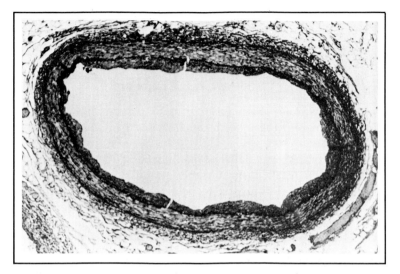

FIGURE 5-7   Photomicrograph of a normal human coronary artery (cross-section). The picture is enlarged about 18 diameters. (Courtesy of Dr. David M. Spain, Director, Department of Pathology, Brookdale Hospital Medical Center, Brooklyn, N.Y.)

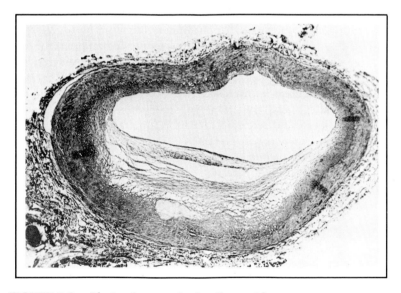

FIGURE 5-8   Photomicrograph of a diseased human coronary artery (cross-section). Compare with Figure 5-7 and note the partially occluded channel brought about by the atherosclerotic process. Much of the thickening is fibrous scar tissue. The clear areas within the thickening are fatty deposits. (Courtesy of Dr. David M. Spain, Director, Department of Pathology, Brookdale Hospital Medical Center, Brooklyn, N.Y.)

at the site of desquamation and the release of their constituents at this site. Throughout the process certain plasma solutes such as low density lipoproteins and mucopolysaccharide complexes pass into the underlying artery wall. Eventually there is an excessive accumulation of intracellular lipid followed by a degenerative formation of connective tissue matrix by the smooth muscle cells. It is the lipid that constitutes the major portion of plaques, but the platelet activity is thought to enhance plaque formation once endothelial injury is initiated.

Everyone is potentially susceptible to endothelial damage as a result of mechanical, chemical, and immunologic assault on the blood vessels. There is reason to believe that the major process is mechanical. In support of this belief, a correlation has been demonstrated between endothelial injury and sites of maximum shear from blood flow forces. It is these sites that are most susceptible to atherosclerosis (see Figure 5-9). The shearing stress of flowing blood produces additional endothelial desquamation once a lowered threshold of endothelial stability has been initiated. Knowledge of this kind has generated much concern over the role of elevated blood pressure (hypertension) in both initiating and perpetuating atherosclerotic pathology.

Studies of cerebral arteriolar damage in cats with acute hypertension indicate that the tissue abnormality is caused by free oxygen radicals generated as a result of increased prostaglandin synthesis. Biosynthesis of prostaglandins from their precursor, arachidonic acid, is reputed to produce free oxygen radicals. The role of free radicals in tissue damage is discussed in Chapter 2.

Hypoxic stress, hypertension, metabolic imbalances associated with dietary indiscretions, and hormonal actions arising from emotional tensions sooner or later culminate in the pathology of atherosclerosis. Typically these stressors operate through time against a background of genetic predisposition. There is evidence from animal studies as well as some suggestion from clinical data that atherosclerotic changes can be delayed and even reversed to some extent. Thus, according to some researchers, cholesterol plaques can be thought of as naturally resorbable foreign material just as one expects resorption of hematomas and unfertilized ova.

Once atherosclerosis has progressed to the point of clinical detection, and the patient complains of symptoms stemming from coronary insufficiency, the therapy of choice is *coronary bypass surgery*. Approximately 100,000 patients undergo this procedure each year. However, a much simpler treatment is beginning to be used. The treatment consists of inserting a balloon into a blocked coronary

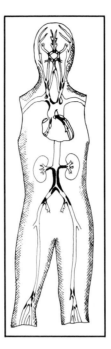

FIGURE 5-9   Arterial sites most susceptible to atherosclerosis. These sites are indicated by the blackened areas. Observe that they occur at or near points where the arteries branch. It is here that flow is more turbulent than laminar, resulting in mechanical stress on the arterial endothelium.

artery and inflating the balloon, which squashes the atherosclerotic plaques against the artery wall. The balloon is then deflated and removed. The method is effective in cases in which there are only one or two plaques that have not yet become calcified.

Hypertension

Most clinicians consider that in the average adult a systolic blood pressure exceeding 140 torr[1] at the lower end of the brachial artery, and diastolic pressure exceeding 90 torr, constitutes a pressure that may be damaging should it remain elevated. On this basis it is estimated that nearly 60 million people in the United States are hypertensive, making this by far the most common of the chronic diseases. High blood pressure is recognized as a significant factor in 68% of all first heart attacks and 75% of all first strokes.

[1]A torr is equivalent to the pressure needed to support a millimeter of mercury (mmHg), and is the standard measurement of blood pressure.

There is evidence that hypertension is actually a complex of diseases in which different defects produce the same result. In a few instances the cause is clearly understood, as, for example, for pheochromocytoma or toxemia of pregnancy. Yet approximately 85% of all instances have been termed essential hypertension, which implies that the cause has not been clearly elucidated. However, recent search has shown some success in identifying some of the underlying factors. Hypertension is generally distinguished as benign or malignant. In the benign form the disease progresses quite slowly, while in malignant hypertension there is a rapid acceleration of the course, often resulting in severe organ damage that especially involves the kidneys and heart.

Aside from the heart stroke force, there are two main variables determining the pressure of blood in the arteries. One is the vasomotor regulation of the vessel diameter, and the other is the volume of fluid in the vessels. In most cases of well-established hypertension, the major abnormality is believed to be increased peripheral blood flow resistance due to arteriole diameters that remain abnormally reduced. Sympathetic stimulation and catecholamine action are powerful vasoconstrictors.

Renin, an enzyme produced by the kidney, and another enzyme catalyze a reaction with a plasma protein that results in the formation of a substance called *angiotensin II*. Angiotensin II reinforces sympathetic action in constricting arterioles. Angiotensin II also stimulates the adrenal cortex to secrete aldosterone, and this hormone promotes resorption of sodium from renal tubules, resulting in an increase in fluid volume of the blood. About 82% of patients with essential hypertension have elevated concentrations of renin in their blood, and it is believed that an increase in renin activity may be the first deviant finding as hypertension begins to develop. A reduction in renal blood flow is one stimulus prompting release of renin, whereas an increase in renal blood perfusion generally acts as a feedback stimulus for inhibiting the release of renin. Therefore, an elevation in blood pressure from this mechanism should be temporary. However, if the feedback operation loses some of its effectiveness, this could lead to chronic hypertension. One factor capable of interfering with the feedback is a persistence of sympathetic discharges, which have been shown to maintain or even increase the release of renin.

Irregularities in kidney function also can disturb the feedback. Many cases of essential hypertension are characterized by various degrees of renal vascular damage and *glomerulonephritis*, conditions in which there may be inflammation and a thickening of

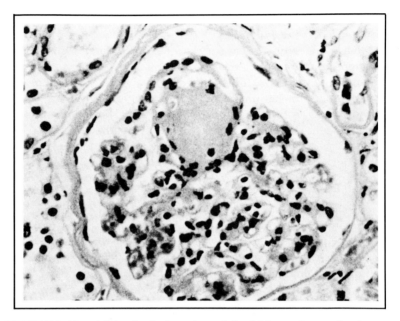

FIGURE 5-10   A histological section of the kidney glomerulus in diabetes mellitus. Within the gomerular capsule is the knotted mass of capillary. Note the rather structureless nodular material in the upper portion of the capillary mass, indicative of the progressive intercapillary glomerulosclerosis that typifies long-standing cases of diabetes. Also, the basement membrane throughout the capillary is diffusely thickened. (From J. R. Anderson, W. W. Buchanan, and R. B. Goudie, *Autoimmunity—clinical and experimental*, 1967. Courtesy of Charles C Thomas, Publisher, Springfield, Ill.)

glomerular basement membranes as well as a narrowing of arteries in the kidneys. This can result in renal blood perfusion that perpetually is recognized by the kidney-renin mechanism as being low. Consequently, high levels of renin are maintained. In addition, irregularities in renal function may be associated with retention of sodium in the blood. Indeed, much evidence points to excessive sodium intake and retention within the body as a common denominator in many cases of renal hypertension. Retention of sodium contributes to chronic hypertension by increasing the blood volume.

The principle of positive feedback can be recognized in the relationship of kidney disease to hypertension: glomerulonephritis contributes to hypertension, which in turn can itself further damage the renal vasculature. It is well established that diabetes mellitus and autoimmunity are two conditions that favor development of chronic glomerulonephritis (Figure 5-10).

Some investigators view many instances of hypertension as being related to increased activity of sympathetic pathways, thereby contending that stress is an important factor in the development of hypertension. Various stressors are known to evoke prominent but temporary elevations of blood pressure. Can these elevations become chronic if the stress persists for longer periods of time? There are indications that this may be the case. Recent studies have shown that a habitual increase in activity of the sympathetic nervous system often accompanies the genesis of essential hypertension. Apparently, long-term hyperactivity of the sympathetic system produces changes in the peripheral vascular bed. In such instances microscopic examinations of skeletal muscle have revealed a twofold decrease in both the number of precapillary arterioles and in their mean diameter. The decreased vascularity increases peripheral resistance, which leads to chronically elevated blood pressure. What mechanism maintains this condition? Normally, arterial baroreceptors are activated by elevations in blood pressure, initiating reflexes that tend to counteract the vasoconstriction. However, habitual increases in arterial pressure can reset the baroreceptor response to a higher level. The baroreceptors are still regulative, but at higher pressures.

Apparently the peripheral catecholamines do not cross the blood-brain barrier; however, the brain has its own central catecholamine pool. Quite recently it has been shown that receptors in the hypothalamus and brain stem are activated by brain epinephrine. This activation leads to a hypertensive response, suggesting a definite involvement of central brain catecholamines in clinical hypertension. Moreover, several studies have shown the concentration of norepinephrine in cerebrospinal fluid to be much higher in patients with essential hypertension than in normal individuals, even when the concentrations of norepinephrine in plasma are similar in the two groups.

Additional mediators have been implicated in the regulation of blood pressure. For example, certain prostaglandins, a family of fatty acid derivatives, are potentially vasoactive. Some are vasoconstrictors, while others such as prostaglandin E_2 (PGE$_2$) strongly oppose vasoconstriction. A decline in the synthesis of PGE$_2$ will induce hypertension. In addition, small peptides known as kinins lower blood pressure by increasing the excretion of water and sodium ions by the kidneys, and by promoting vasodilation. Kinins such as *bradykinin* are produced by the enzyme *kallikrein*. Hypertensive individuals excrete less urinary kallikrein than do healthy individuals, while patients with certain allergies, who suffer from conditions characterized by excess vasodilation, or tissue inflammation, are not

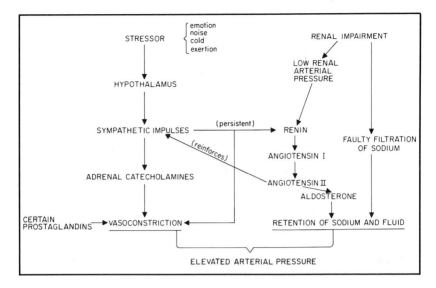

FIGURE 5-11   Physiologic mechanisms that lead to elevations in arterial blood pressure. Various degrees of environmental stress and irregularities in kidney function initiate the process, the former culminating in vasoconstriction, and the latter resulting in an increase in plasma volume. Note, however, that there is interaction between the two mechanisms, in that sympathetic activity maintains renin output, and angiotensin II reinforces sympathetic action.

often hypertensive. The major mechanisms contributing to hypertension are summarized in Figure 5-11.

What part do stresses play in the development of hypertension? Even though genetic factors cannot be overlooked, there is no denying that habitual excitement, chronic emotional tension, noise, high salt intake, inadequate rest, obesity, chronic exposure to cold, and the intake of nervous system stimulants are significant contributors in many cases. It is of interest that blacks in northern cities of the United States show a much greater incidence of hypertension than do southern, rural blacks. As for renal hypertension associated with such conditions as diabetes, infections, immune complexes, and high salt intake, we must acknowledge that some of these associated conditions in themselves may be stress-related in various ways.

Hypertension is a health problem of considerable dimensions. It can exist for some time without symptoms, thereby avoiding detection until arterial damage is well established. The damage occurs in even the smallest arterioles. Arteriole damage in the retina of the eye is readily observed. Such damage is illustrated in Figure 5-12.

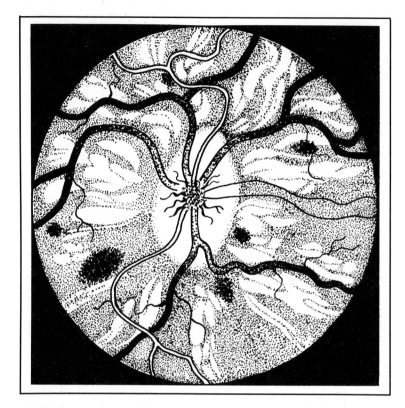

FIGURE 5-12   Appearance of the retina in malignant hypertension.
Exudation of plasma protein is indicated by the light regions, and
hemorrhage is represented by the dark splotches. The light-dark contrast
among various arterioles marks the extreme variation in content and flow
of the blood due to spasm.

The treatment of hypertension traditionally includes the use
of diuretics to inhibit sodium resorption, together with antiadrenergic agents to subdue vasoconstriction. A new drug, captopril,
is being heralded as superior to those in present use. Weight control,
restriction of salt intake, and avoidance of emotional stress also are
strongly advised for those predisposed to hypertension. In fact,
weight loss alone is effective in reducing blood pressure in many
individuals.

Hyperlipidemia and Hyperglycemia

There appears to be little doubt that cholesterol and other blood
lipids are of significance in the development of atherosclerotic le-

sions. There is a substantial correlation between coronary artery disease and chronically elevated serum cholesterol, particularly the fraction associated with low density lipoproteins. In addition, there are statistical data indicating that people consuming a diet high in saturated fat tend to show higher levels of serum cholesterol.

Cholesterol is a ubiquitous substance found in every cell of the body. Its quantity in blood serum is determined by the difference between the amount absorbed and synthesized, and the amount degraded and excreted. Most cells can synthesize cholesterol from acetate, and this synthesis is the primary source of endogenous cholesterol. Liver cells are especially active synthesizers. There is an inverse relation between cholesterol synthesis and dietary intake of cholesterol.

Like most lipids, cholesterol must be combined with protein (forming lipoprotein) to be soluble for transport in the plasma. Lipoproteins vary in size and density. Cholesterol is associated with both low density lipoproteins (LDL) and high density lipoproteins (HDL).[2] However, in vitro studies show that smooth muscle cells from human arteries take up *only* the cholesterol associated with LDL. Moreover, electron micrographs of intimal lesions in the arteries of individuals with elevated LDL and diminished HDL show large deposits of lipid in smooth muscle cells. Lipid deposition in smooth muscle of a human aorta is shown in Figure 5-13.

Recent studies have shown that high density lipoproteins are capable of transporting cholesterol from arterial walls to the liver, where it is degraded to bile acids. Indeed, those individuals having plentiful levels of HDL appear to be less susceptible to coronary artery disease. Regular exercise, weight control, dietary restriction of sugar and saturated fat, freedom from emotional tension, and being female favor a high ratio of HDL to LDL. Today less emphasis is being placed upon the total quantity of serum cholesterol, especially in men over fifty years of age, and more attention is being directed to the amount of HDL in the blood. The relation of HDL levels to estimated risks of developing coronary artery disease is shown in Table 5-1.

Many investigators feel that serum levels of triglycerides also are important in the development of atherosclerosis. There is usually an inverse relationship between serum triglycerides and the level of protective HDL. In many cases of hyperlipidemia, both cholesterol and triglycerides are elevated in the plasma. However, in the two most common classifications of primary hyperlipidemia introduced

2Fat is less dense than protein; therefore, LDL complexes have a higher fat to protein ratio than HDL complexes.

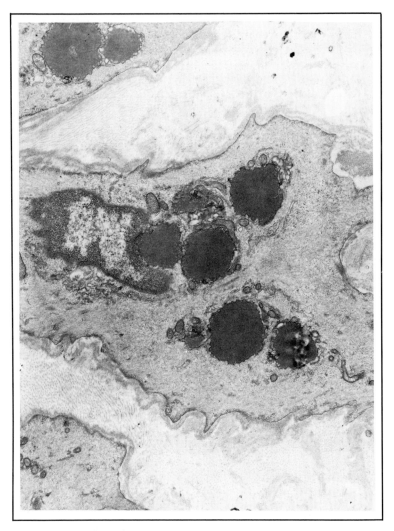

FIGURE 5-13   Electron micrograph of a smooth muscle cell from a human aorta (×6000). The dark inclusions are large droplets of fat believed to be deposited by low density lipoprotein complexes. (Courtesy of Dr. Jack C. Greer, Chairman, Department of Pathology, University of Alabama Medical Center, Birmingham, Ala.)

by Fredrickson (Table 5-2), elevated cholesterol with normal triglycerides characterizes type II, whereas in type IV the triglycerides are always elevated regardless of whether or not the cholesterol is excessive. Type IV is common in persons with a diabetic predisposition. The range of "normal" values for serum lipids is presented in Table 5-3.

TABLE 5-1
Risk Factors for Coronary Heart Disease from HDL Levels

HDL (MG/DL)	RISK FACTOR	
	Men	Women
25	2.00	. . .
30	1.82	. . .
35	1.49	. . .
40	1.22	1.94
45*	1.00	1.55
50	0.82	1.25
55	0.67	1.00
60	0.55	0.80
65	0.45	0.64
70	. . .	0.52
75+	Longevity syndrome	

Source: Clinchem Comments, Clin-Chem Laboratories, Boston, Mass. March–April 1978.
* The average HDL in men is 45 mg/dl, so the standard or average level of risk is set at 1.00. Thus men with an HDL of 25 have twice the average risk, whereas those with 63 mg/dl have only half the average risk. Even an average risk is not necessarily desirable.

Atherosclerotic lesions are usually found in long-standing cases of diabetes mellitus. These lesions, also characterized by deposition of lipid in the arterial walls, may appear earlier than in non-diabetics. In addition, the capillaries are involved, and a thickened capillary basement membrane along with a deposition of hyaline mucopolysaccharide can be demonstrated in this form of angiopathy. Many specialists attribute the development of vascular pathology to chronic elevation of glucose in the circulating plasma. Other physicians claim that abolishing the hyperglycemia will not necessarily prevent angiopathy. However, it must be realized that despite the best efforts, control of glucose intolerance is never perfect; therefore, during each 24-hour period some degree of hyperglycemia is bound to prevail. Very likely, hyperglycemic fluctuations are the rule, even in cases where good blood sugar determinations may be performed on a monthly basis. Futhermore, it should be noted that the organs and tissues most affected by diabetic complications, such as the lens, glomeruli, retina, peripheral nerves, and capillaries, are not insulin-dependent for glucose penetration. Hence they become overloaded with glucose during periods of hyperglycemia.

In animals in which there is no diabetic predisposition, but which are made diabetic by selectively damaging the pancreatic beta cells with alloxan, the resulting hyperglycemia does lead to thickening of the glomerular basement membrane (glomerulonephritis, see Figure 5-10), demyelization of the myelin sheath of nerves (diabetic

TABLE 5-2
Classification of Primary Hyperlipidemia

TYPE	LIPOPROTEIN	TRIGLYCERIDES	CHOLESTEROL
I (rare)	Chylomicra elevated	Elevated	Normal
II	Beta lipoproteins elevated	Normal	Elevated
III	Abnormal beta lipoproteins present	Elevated	Elevated
IV	Pre-beta lipoproteins elevated	Elevated	Normal or elevated
V	Chylomicra and pre-beta lipoproteins elevated	Elevated	Elevated

Source: Modified adaptation from D. S. Fredrickson, 1968. *Hosp Practice* 3:54.

neuropathy), and retinal hemorrhages (diabetic retinopathy). Moreover, in hyperglycemic humans there is a distinct increase in the glucose portion of the disaccharide content that comprises over 10% of the collagen complex of the capillary basement membrane, leading to its thickening and resulting in faulty barrier function of the membrane. In addition, it has been demonstrated that excessive free glucose attaches to various amino acid residues of polypeptides. In this way the glucose can modify the tertiary structure of proteins, thereby altering enzyme function. In fact, excessive glucose readily permeates red blood cells and binds with hemoglobin. Diabetics have significantly higher levels of glycosylated hemoglobin than do normal individuals; indeed, this can be used as an index in evaluating the severity of the diabetic condition. And finally, there is much experimental evidence pointing to the fact that elevations of blood glucose begin to shunt glucose metabolism into accessory pathways, such as the sorbitol pathway, which alters mass action momentum for both carbohydrate and lipid metabolism, resulting in the deposition of mucopolysaccharide complexes and beads of lipid globules in and around the walls of small blood vessels. Accumulation of sorbitol by the lens of the eye plays a role in the development of cataracts and also is involved with diabetic neuropathy.

Diabetics are especially prone to the development of atherosclerosis, and they tend to have elevations of triglycerides and LDL cholesterol in their blood. At the same time their HDL levels are often low. The hyperlipidemic predisposition stems from the loss of control of lipid metabolic regulation, which in turn is due to the impairment of glucose oxidation by way of the hexose monophosphate pathway. Interestingly, in diabetics in which a tight metabolic

TABLE 5-3
Range of Normal* Values for Serum Lipids

AGE (YRS)	TOTAL CHOLES-TEROL (MG/DL)	TRIGLYC-ERIDES (MG/DL)	LDL (MG/DL)	HDL (MG/DL) Male	Female
0–19	120–230	10–140	50–170	30–65	30–70
20–29	120–240	10–140	60–170	35–70	35–75
30–39	140–270	10–150	70–190	30–65	35–80
40–49	150–310	10–160	80–190	30–65	40–95
50–59	160–330	10–190	80–210	30–65	35–85

Source: Section on Lipoproteins, Laboratory for Molecular Disease, National Heart and Lung Institute, NIH, Bethesda, Md., 1974.
* What is considered normal varies among specialists, many of whom consider that at any age total cholesterol >280 and triglycerides >150 constitute undesirable levels.

control has been maintained, the levels of HDL cholesterol may not significantly differ from those of normal individuals.

Is stress an important factor in promoting hyperlipidemia and hyperglycemia? Chapter 4 states that the catecholamines and adrenal glucocorticoids, both of which are secreted in direct response to many stresses, stimulate the mobilization of lipid from fat stores, and enhance the synthesis of cholesterol while suppressing its degradation. The same hormones are responsible for increases in levels of blood glucose, and they impose a resistance to the action of insulin, making greater demands on its output from the pancreatic beta cells. Therefore, stress resulting in an excess of ACTH, growth hormone, cortisol, glucagon, and epinephrine must be seriously considered as a contributor to hyperlipidemia and hyperglycemia.

Hormones such as thyroxin, insulin, and estrogen are known to reduce levels of serum lipid. Thyroid output often diminishes in later years, while at the same time, there is a tendency for levels of serum lipid to increase with age. Thus, chronic hypothyroidism should never be overlooked as a possible contributor to hyperlipidemia.

Tissue Hypoxia

There is mounting evidence that reduced oxygenation of tissues making up the arterial intima plays a significant role in the formation of atherosclerotic plaques by enhancing deposition of lipid in the arterial wall. In vitro studies with arterial tissue demonstrate a proliferation of fibroblasts in response to reduced oxygen tension.

The metabolism of lipid requires more oxygen than does the

metabolism of an equal amount of carbohydrate; therefore, elevated levels of lipid impart a risk of proportionately lowering the oxygen tension in tissue, which in turn would compromise the oxidation of the remaining lipid, leading to a greater deposition of it in the arteries. Among lipids, cholesterol requires the greatest amount of oxygen for oxidation, closely followed by saturated fats, with unsaturated lipid requiring the least. Each unsaturated double bond of lipid requires one less atom of oxygen for oxidation than does a saturated bond. With diets high in saturated fats, the oxygen tension of the arterial wall may be insufficient to effectively oxidize the fat, resulting in an accumulation of some of the lipid in smooth muscle, forming what are known as *foam cells.*

An increased number of fibroblasts, originally arising in response to reduced oxygen, will further deplete available oxygen, and at the same time the deposition of collagen impedes oxygen diffusion. The entire process exemplifies the principle of positive feedback; in this case tissue changes stemming from hypoxia promote additional tissue hypoxia, which in turn leads to greater degrees of atherosclerosis.

Recent in vitro studies clearly show that lowering the oxygen tension of the culture medium decreases the breakdown of the protein portion of LDL, the degradation of which is necessary in preventing undue deposition and accumulation of lipid in the smooth muscle cells of arteries. Also, it is now known that smooth muscle, in other locations besides arterial walls, can show an infiltration of lipid that is characteristic of the specific pathology of atherosclerosis. For example, in toxemia of pregnancy there is formation of foam cells associated with much lipid deposition in uterine smooth muscle. Hypoxia of the cells from the toxemia appears to be the primary cause of these changes.

With tobacco-smoking, there is chronic tissue hypoxia from the inhalation of carbon monoxide. Undoubtedly this is one important reason for the positive statistical relation of smoking to cardiovascular disease.

The combination of hypertension and hyperlipidemia together with chronic tissue hypoxia poses a very high probability of developing progressive atherosclerosis. Hypoxic stress is discussed more fully in Chapter 9.

Platelet Aggregation and Fibrinogenesis

In preceding sections there is allusion to the fact that both platelet adhesiveness and fibrin production are associated with the development of atherosclerotic lesions. Fibrinogenesis leads to thrombus formation. Moreover, the aggregated platelets release serotonin and epinephrine, which maintain vasoconstriction in the small vessels. The entire chain of events appears to be initiated by injury to the endothelium of the artery.

Although platelets tend to adhere to rough surfaces, they do not adhere to the smooth-surfaced endothelial cells of healthy blood vessels. When injury disrupts the endothelium and exposes the underlying collagen, platelets begin to adhere. Another material released from platelets, adenosine diphosphate (ADP), causes their surfaces to become sticky so that new platelets begin to adhere to old ones. This results in a rapid, self-perpetuating aggregation of platelets.

It is well known that many blood clots retract. In fact, when the clotting process is initiated, the fibrin of an incipient clot may be decomposed by *plasmin*, a proteolytic enzyme. It is believed that small amounts of fibrin are constantly being laid down in the normal vascular system, and that plasmin is responsible for keeping the blood stream free of clots. When the balance between fibrinolysis and fibrinogenesis is shifted toward the latter, the additional fibrin favors clot formation in the circulatory system. When fibrin barriers are not removed by natural fibrinolysis, the cells underneath the deposit become hypoxic and are deprived of nutrition, leading to their degeneration.

Recently, a chemical relative of prostaglandins, a *thromboxane* (TXA_2), was discovered and shown to be effective in causing platelets to clump and arteries to constrict. The enzyme that synthesizes TXA_2 also has been identified. More recently a prostaglandin has been discovered that directly opposes the action of TXA_2, thus preventing the formation of blood clots. The substance was first called *prostacyclin*, but it is more commonly known as PGI_2. It is synthesized in human arteries and is formed from endoperoxides in the vessel linings. The endoperoxides in turn are derived from arachidonic acid. It is thought that when platelets come in contact with the linings, they release endoperoxides that are converted to PGI_2, preventing platelet aggregation and subsequent clotting. However, in damaged endothelium the PGI_2-synthesizing enzyme may become saturated, allowing platelet aggregation, which then favors clot formation. Thus, the presence of lipid peroxides in atherosclerotic plaques might be a factor in the clotting problems of patients with atherosclerosis. Recent work has disclosed that therapeutic doses of aspirin destroy the cells' ability to synthesize PGI_2 from arachidonic acid.

It has been demonstrated many times that various stresses lead to an acceleration in the rate of blood coagulation. Platelet aggregation, fibrin deposition, and suppressed fibrinolysis all are enhanced by activity of the sympathetic division of the ANS and the consequent release of epinephrine from the adrenal medulla. In addition, endothelial damage from the stress of hypertension and hyperlipidemia promotes fibrinogenesis. Thus, stresses favor development of cardiovascular pathology by these means as well as through other mechanisms.

MALIGNANT NEOPLASMS

The second leading cause of death in this country is pathology associated with growth of malignant tumors. For this reason the nature of this disease and its stress relationships deserve attention. Controlling malignant growth remains a major challenge to modern medicine. Approximately one in five of us will die of cancer. More frightening is the present trend toward increasing incidence. Of particular interest is the conclusion of the Federal Council on Environmental Quality that between 70% and 90% of all cancer stems directly from environmental causes. Much of the incidence appears to be associated with exposure to an extensive list of manufactured chemical agents (carcinogens). Therefore we must consider cancer to be a preventable disease.

The statistical association of certain forms of malignancy with specific occupational exposures is especially striking. Workers with asbestos, nickel, and chromium have high lung cancer rates relative to the general population, whereas those working with dyes have high rates of bladder cancer. Workers exposed to polyvinyl chloride have shown a high probability of developing cancer of the liver.

Malignant change can occur in any cell. When such a change occurs in epithelial tissue, it is termed a *carcinoma*, whereas cancerous development in connective and supportive tissues is termed a *sarcoma*. Although connective and supportive tissues exceed epithelial tissue in mass by about fivefold, carcinomas arise 11 times more frequently than sarcomas, accounting for about 85% of all malignant growth. One reason for this may be that epithelial tissues line the inner and outer body surfaces and therefore are more directly exposed to carcinogens. In addition, the chances of developing carcinomas increase with age, whereas the occurrence of many sarcomas remains about the same for all age levels.

A malignant growth in itself does not directly harm the body. But when tumor cells monopolize nutrients and oxygen needed by normal tissue, or when the neoplasm obstructs flow, movement, or exchange of necessary materials, the body begins to suffer. Such malignant interferences with normal processes tend to worsen as the tumor grows and spreads. If not permanently checked these interferences culminate in a gradual wasting of the body, ultimately leading to death. Cancerous tumors vary greatly in their rates of growth and their tendency to spread malignant cells to other sites. Surgery, controlled radiation exposures, and chemotherapy with powerful drugs constitute conventional therapy for all forms of malignant growth.

Common Sites of Occurrence

In men the organ where cancer is most likely to develop is the lung (Figure 5-14), whereas in women the breast is the foremost site of occurrence. A recent tabulation of the number of deaths in the United States from cancer of various sites of the body is given in Table 5-4. The proportion of cancers being detected in each organ has undergone changes through the years. The incidence of lung cancer, for example, has shown dramatic increases within the past 50 years. Even though an increase in this form of cancer is continuing, the trend appears to be related to an upswing in the incidence among white women during the past 20 years. The incidence of breast cancer in women also has shown marked increases since World War II. On the other hand, mortality rates for cervical cancer have shown a steady decline since that time, possibly reflecting the value of the Pap test in early detection. Stomach cancer also has been declining at a significant rate.

Before 1930, lung cancer was a relatively rare disease. The widespread adoption of the smoking habit together with the advent of urban air pollution have changed this drastically (Figure 5-15). Occupational exposure to carcinogenic inhalants also has contributed. Some of these stressors are discussed at length in Chapters 13 and 14.

The hormonal secretions of the pituitary-gonadal axis appear to have much to do with the etiology of breast cancer. There has been speculation about the relationship of changing trends in the reproductive histories of modern women to the rising incidence of breast tumors. It is known that childless women, or those who are past 30 years of age when their first full-term pregnancy occurs, stand a higher than average risk of developing breast cancer. More-

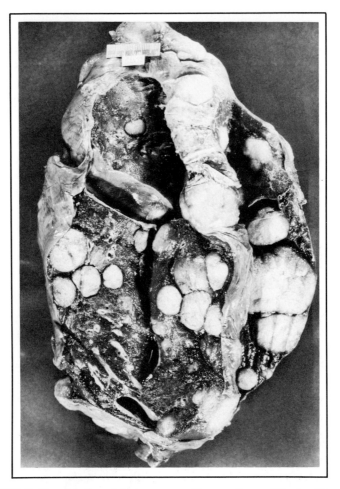

FIGURE 5-14 **Advanced lung cancer.** Observe the multitude of tumors (lighter color) progressively destroying this lung. (Taurus Photos, N.Y.)

over, the incidence of this pathology is six times higher in North America than it is in Asia and Africa. There are additional evidences implicating the female sex hormones in mammary carcinogenesis. Ovariectomized mice and rats show a decreased incidence of breast malignancy, whereas repeated injections of estrogen, progesterone, and prolactin lead to an increased occurrence of tumors in mammary tissue of rats and mice. There are others who consider diet and viral infections to play a significant role in the etiology of breast cancer, and normal breast milk has been incriminated as a source of latent virus particles capable of infecting the next generation and initiating

TABLE 5-4

Approximate Number of Deaths in the United States from Cancer

CANCER SITE	DEATHS IN 1979
Lung	76,000
Colon and rectum	48,000
Breast	33,800
Pancreas	20,000
Prostate	18,000
Urinary bladder	9,200
Oral	7,900
Larynx	3,000

Source: National Cancer Institute.

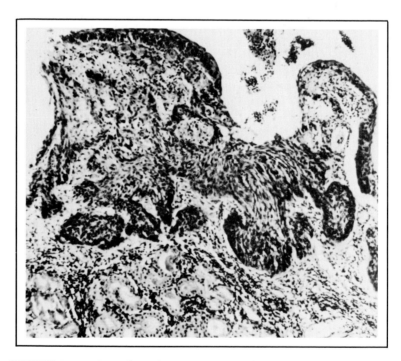

FIGURE 5-15   Bronchopulmonary tissue from a long-term smoker.
The dark ovoid inclusions just below an imaginary horizontal midline of
the photo are masses of rapidly proliferating malignant cells. (Courtesy of
Dr. Oscar Auerbach, Distinguished Physician, Veterans Administration
Medical Center, East Orange, N.J.)

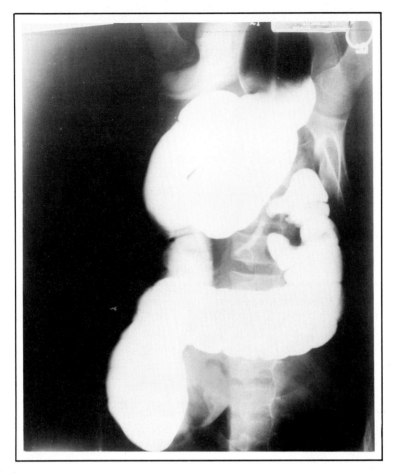

FIGURE 5-16   Cancer of the colon. The proliferation of malignant tissue is seen in the x-ray film as the darkened area invading the ascending arm of the colon. (Courtesy of Eldra P. Solomon, Professor of Life Sciences, Hillsborough Community College, Tampa, Fla.)

malignant changes. Studies with mice have supported this hypothesis, but viruses have yet to be demonstrated in human tumors.

Cancer of the colon and rectum is relatively frequent in both sexes (Figure 5-16). The leading theory regarding etiology is centered around diet. Epidemiologic data implicate a diet high in fat. In addition, some investigators have emphasized that dietary fiber deficiency can be associated with carcinogenesis of the large bowel. Controlled studies comparing a high-meat, high-fat diet with a meatless, low-fat one have shown that the former is associated with an elevated level of fecal bile acids and cholesterol metabolites along with a greater total microflora. Patients with colon cancer often have an increased level of fecal bile acids. Bile acids are believed to be tumor-promoters rather than true carcinogens. Patients with familial polyposis, ulcerative colitis, and adenomatous polyps have an increased risk of colorectal carcinoma, and there are those who believe that chronic constipation may enhance this risk in such patients. Interestingly, it has been shown recently that the element selenium is capable of inhibiting colon cancer by as yet unknown mechanisms.

In view of the results of animal experiments, the most probable types of human cancer caused by a virus are the leukemias, and possibly the lymphomas, although ionizing radiation also must be suspected as a causal factor in these types of malignancy. Leukemias involve an uncontrolled production of leukocytes by the bone marrow. These cancers constitute the most common types of childhood malignancy (Figure 5-17). Lymphomas, of which *Hodgkin disease* is the best known, arise in the lymph nodes and spleen, and involve the production of abnormal numbers of lymphocytes. Leukemias and lymphomas are quite similar in that each involves uncontrolled production of white blood cells. Significant strides are being made in successfully treating both types of conditions. Splenectomy has become routine in many cases of Hodgkin disease. Absence of the spleen significantly reduces lymphocyte production and permits a more normal regulation of lymphoid tissues. Radiation also is standard therapy for Hodgkin disease, whereas chemotherapy is the treatment of choice in leukemias. High dosages of drugs such as adriamycin can be effective in suppressing bone marrow activity. Unfortunately, these drugs are capable of initiating severe cytotoxic reactions.

Tumorigenesis

Any mass of tissue that persists and grows without any adaptive significance to the organism is called a *tumor* or *neoplasm*. Tumors may be *benign* or *malignant*. Benign tumors tend to grow more slowly, and they usually become surrounded by a fibrous membrane that contains them and prevents them from invading surrounding tissue. Malignant tumors often *metastasize*, which means that the growth sheds abnormal cells which can be spread by blood and lymph systems to remote parts of the body. Wherever these cells happen to lodge, they begin to multiply, subsequently riddling the body with dozens of malignant growths at many locations. Cancer cells have distorted nuclei with chromosomes that are often odd and irregular in number and shape. Close contact with normal cells does not ap-

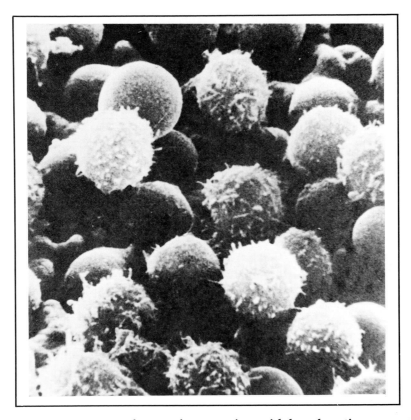

FIGURE 5-17 **Lymphocytes from a patient with lymphocytic leukemia.** Seen with the scanning electron microscope (×4200). In this form of white cell malignancy there is an excessive production of both B and T lymphocytes. Cells with rough surfaces are believed to be B cells, and those with smooth surfaces are T cells. (Courtesy of Dr. A. Polliack, Department of Haematology, Hadassah University Hospital, Jerusalem, Israel.)

preciably retard their rate of multiplication as it usually does in the case with benign tumors. Cancerous cells are depicted in Figure 5-18.

The causes underlying the initiation of tumor growth are complex and not completely understood. In most instances chronic exposures to chemical carcinogens, radiation, or viruses are involved. In addition, a susceptible cell is somehow receptive to the chemical action of the invader. Ability to metabolically activate carcinogens, specific DNA combination, age of the cell, previous damage to the cell, degree of immune competence, and hormonal influences on the nucleus all are significant host variables in deter-

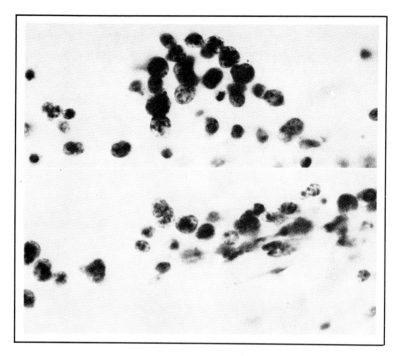

FIGURE 5-18   Cancerous cells from the pleural fluid of a patient with lymphoma. Observe the dense chromatin-clumping, distorted cell shapes, and multinucleate quality. (From J. K. Frost, *The cell in health and disease. An evaluation of cellular morphologic expression of biologic behavior.* Monographs in Clinical Cytology, Vol. 2. Karger: Basel, 1969.)

mining whether or not tumors will arise. Any persistent cellular trauma that disposes the cell to nuclear instability may be of importance. There is a strong parallel between mutagenicity and tumorigenicity.

In addition to exposure to chemical carcinogens, radiation, and viruses, subjecting tissue to elevated temperature and higher than usual oxygen concentrations favors the induction of cellular changes leading to tumorigenesis. Before becoming cancerous, cells tend to pass through stages of change in which the cells are considered *precancerous*.

Suppression of Tumor Development

There are excellent reasons for believing that the initiation of tumor growth is far from an unusual occurrence. Tumors may arise often, but they frequently discontinue further development. Apparently many are nipped in the bud by the body's immune surveillance. In some manner tumorous cells or tissue prompt the so-called natural killer cells of the immune system to kill and destroy malignant cells. This process may be similar to what happens in the rejection of transplanted organs. Perhaps cancerous cells possess antigenic properties that are distinctly different from those of normal cells, although it would appear that the type of cell destruction brought about by natural killer cells does not require priming by exposure to a particular tumor antigen, as does that by cytotoxic T lymphocytes. Moreover, killer cell activity is not specific for any one kind of tumor. Animal studies suggest that both tumor development and metastatic spread are retarded by killer cell activity. Furthermore, it has been shown that natural killer cell activity is far below normal in many cancer patients.

The ability of the immune system to check malignant growth offers a potential means of controlling cancer. Moreover, the role of immune surveillance in preventing cancer development implies that any factor which suppresses immune capability may dispose the individual to the development of malignant tumors. Indeed, those who have had immunosuppressant drugs administered for considerable periods of time to preserve organ transplants have shown a much greater than average incidence of malignant neoplasms. Since it is well established that elevations of ACTH and glucocorticoids suppress immune competence, we must consider that stress in general can be a contributing component in the development of cancer. Data from animal experimentation strongly support this view.

Environmental Carcinogens

It is becoming apparent that our modern environment is rife with carcinogens. They gain access to the body through ingestion, inhalation, and contact with the skin. The carcinogens of most notoriety are organic compounds. Inhaled polynuclear aromatic hydrocarbons such as benzapyrene, the nitrosamines derived from ingested nitrites, and the aniline and azo dyes are some of the major groups of organic compounds associated with carcinogenicity in man. More attention is given to these materials and their sources in Chapter 13.

How do these materials initiate malignant changes in cells? This is presently an area of active investigation. One theory is that certain carcinogens are cytotoxic and capable of suppressing the immune system. Another concept that has considerable support from animal experiments, at least with the polynuclear hydrocarbons, is that the carcinogen must be converted into oncogenic metabolites by the host tissue. In this sense, the environmental agent entering the body is likened to a pro-carcinogen.

Both in vivo and in vitro studies indicate that polynuclear hydrocarbons are metabolized to epoxides by certain actions on the double bonds of the hydrocarbon. The double bonds that are localized to initiate the reaction are termed *K-regions.* Study of human lung preparations have shown that the *K-region epoxides* then bind to DNA. Apparently DNA-binding alters cell regulations normally imposed by the nucleus. In both animal and human cells it has been shown that natural body enzymes, when they occur at higher than normal levels, can allow environmental agents to initiate tumor growth. The enzymes are normally present, but apparently must be induced in higher than normal amounts by exposure to environmental chemicals. It is believed that the enzymes are part of the cell's machinery for detoxifying poisons. One such enzyme, *aryl hydrocarbon hydroxylase,* performs in this manner. Mice bred to produce much of this enzyme readily develop lung cancer when various hydrocarbons are inhaled. Those with less enzyme, but similarly exposed, rarely develop cancer. Apparently the enzyme oxidizes polycyclic aromatic hydrocarbons, and once oxidized, the chemicals can cause cancer. It has been reported that white blood cells from humans vary enormously in the inductability of these enzymes. There is evidence also that cells contain enzymes that can convert carcinogens to noncarcinogens. Ordinarily the two kinds of enzymes may be in some sort of balance. Thus, either a deficiency in the enzymes converting carcinogens to harmless molecules, or a preponderance of enzyme activity producing carcinogenic action, would dispose the individual to tumorigenesis.

Evidence is accumulating to indicate that even though carcinogens alone are capable of initiating tumorigenesis, they are much more likely to do so in the presence of certain other chemicals, which collectively have come to be known as promoters or accelerators. The list of suspected promoters includes the drug phenobarbital, artificial sweeteners, and even bile acids. Thus saccharin and sodium cyclamate may be implicated in tumorigenesis as promoters rather than true carcinogens. Bile acids, being more abundant as a result of diets high in fats, may provide the reason rats on high-fat diets show more colon cancer than do the controls.

Environmental carcinogens are further discussed in Chapters 13 and 14.

Stresses and Susceptibility to Cancer

From the foregoing discussion it is clear that certain environmental ingestants and inhalants serve as chemical stressors at the cell level, initiating a chain of nuclear events that lead to malignancy. Radiation stress also causes these changes. Whereas chemical carcinogens are more likely to promote carcinomas, the penetration of high energy may show a greater association with sarcomas.

The other important relationship of stress to cancer development is the role played by generalized stress reactions capable of suppressing the immune system by way of the pituitary-adrenal axis. Not only may this allow tumors to continue their development, but in addition the immunosuppression permits multiplication of viruses that may be associated with malignant changes.

SUMMARY

Continual exposure to various physiologic stressors plays a paramount role in the development of disease processes. Stress disturbances become pathologic derangements when homeostatic responses to stress are faulty and ineffective.

Atherosclerosis, a degenerative disease, occurs in the walls of arteries and is responsible for most instances of cardiovascular pathology, including coronary heart disease, which is by far the leading cause of death in industrialized regions of the world.

Hypertension is believed to be a foremost factor in initiating and perpetuating the endothelial damage that marks the beginning of atherosclerosis. Perpetual arterial vasoconstriction and faulty glomerular function in the kidney are two of the mechanisms underlying the development of hypertension.

Elevation of low density lipoproteins associated with cholesterol promotes the formation of atherosclerotic plaques. Elevations in plasma triglycerides and glucose also are important in this regard. The metabolic stress from long-term dietary indiscretion, together with the many stresses that stimulate the release of epinephrine and glucocorticoids, is the factor primarily responsible for increases of lipids and glucose in the plasma.

Tissue hypoxia in the arterial walls, as well as platelet aggregation and fibrin production, also contributes to the development of atherosclerosis.

Malignant tumors, the second leading cause of death in the United States, result from alterations in gene action controlling the regulation of cell division. Continual exposure to chemical carcinogens, radiation, and certain strains of infective viruses are responsible for initiating these changes. The appropriate metabolism of the carcinogen on the part of the host cells is necessary in order to bind nuclear DNA.

Many incipient tumors are eradicated by cell-mediated immune reactions. Since the action of ACTH and glucocorticoids suppress immune responsiveness, the many forms of stress that are responsible for the secretion of these hormones warrant consideration as important variables in the development of cancer.

Chapter Glossary

aneurysm   a weakened, bulging wall of an artery or vein

angiopathy   progressive pathology of the capillaries and arterioles

blood-brain barrier   membrane providing some degree of separation of brain circulation from the circulatory system of the rest of the body

desquamation   a scaling off; refers to loss of squamous epithelium

diuretic   any substance stimulating kidney action and the excretion of urine

dyspnea   difficulty in breathing

endothelial cells   flat cells forming the innermost epithelium of the blood vessel walls

fibrinolysis   the dissolving of fibrin networks; the converse of fibrinogenesis

hematoma   a small accumulation of blood within tissue; accompanies rupture of small vessels

in vitro (in glass)   refers to investigations performed with test tube preparations, rather than with intact, living organisms

mutagenicity   the ability of a chemical substance to induce alterations (mutations) of DNA in cell nuclei

oncogenic   tumor-producing

T lymphocytes   a population of white blood cells that are responsible for cellular-mediated immunity as opposed to antibody-mediated immunity

tachycardia   a rapid pulse exceeding 100 beats per minute

triglycerides   neutral fats; the most common form of lipid in the body, found in adipose cells and the blood

For Further Reading

Becker, F. F., ed. 1975. *Cancer: A comprehensive treatise.* New York: Plenum Press.

Benson, H., and Gutmann, M. C. 1974. The relation of environmental factors to systemic arterial hypertension. In *Contemporary problems in cardiology.* Vol. 1. *Stress and the heart.* R. S. Eliot, ed. Mt. Kisco, N.Y.: Futura Publishing Co.

Braun, A. C. 1974. *The biology of cancer.* Reading, Mass: Addison-Wesley.

Brothers, M. J. 1976. *Diabetes: The new approach.* New York: Grosset & Dunlap.

Brown, M. S.; Kovanen, P. T.; and Goldstein, J. L. 1981. Regulation of plasma cholesterol by lipoprotein receptors. *Science* 212:628.

Buehlmann, A. A., and Froesch, E. R. 1979. *Pathophysiology.* New York: Springer-Verlag.

Bunn, H. F.; Gabbay, K. H.; and Gallop, P. M. 1978. The glycosylation of hemoglobin: Relevance to diabetes mellitus. *Science* 200:21.

Fredrickson, D. S. 1968. New drugs in the treatment of hyperlipidemia. *Hosp Practice* 3:54.

Freis, E. D., ed. 1979. *The treatment of hypertension: Current status of modern therapy.* Baltimore: University Park Press.

Frohlich, E. D., ed. 1976. *Pathophysiology: Altered regulatory mechanisms of disease.* 2d ed. Philadelphia: J. B. Lippincott Co. Chapts. 3, 5, 36.

Genest, J.; Koiw, E.; and Kuckel, O., eds. 1977. *Hypertension: Physiopathology and treatment.* New York: McGraw-Hill Book Co.

Gordon, T.; Castelli, W. P.; Hjortland, M. C; et al. 1977. High density lipoprotein as a protective factor against heart disease. The Framington Study. *Am J Med* 62:707.

Groer, M. E., and Shekleton, M. E. 1979. *Basic pathophysiology: A conceptual approach.* St. Louis: C. V. Mosby Co. Chapts. 3, 9.

Gunderson, E. K., and Rahe, R. H., eds. 1974. *Life stress and illness.* Springfield, Ill.: Charles C Thomas Pubs.

Guyton, A. C. 1977. *Basic human physiology: Normal function and mechanisms of disease.* Philadelphia: W. B. Saunders Co. Chapt. 18.

Henry, J. P., and Stephens, P. M. 1977. *Stress, health and the social environment: A sociobiological approach to medicine.* New York: Springer-Verlag.

Iwatsuki, K.; Cardinale, G. J.; Spector, S.; et al. 1977. Hypertension: Increase in collagen biosynthesis in arteries but not in veins. *Science* 198:403.

Kaplan, N. M. 1980. The control of hypertension: A therapeutic breakthrough. *Am Sci* 68(5):537.

Klein, G., and Weinhouse, S., eds. 1979. *Advances in cancer research.* Vol. 30. New York: Academic Press.

Kolata, G. B. 1979. Blood sugar and the complications of diabetes. *Science* 203:1098.

Manning, G. W., and Haust, M. D. 1975. *Atherosclerosis: Metabolic, morphologic, and clinical aspects.* New York: Plenum Press.

Marx, J. L. 1980. Coronary artery spasms and heart disease. *Science* 208:1127.

Oglesby, P., ed. 1979. *Epidemiology and control of hypertension.* Chicago: Year Book Medical Publishers, Times Mirror.

Old, L. J. 1977 (May). Cancer immunology. Sci. Am. Vol. 236: p. 62.

Price, S. A., and Wilson, L. M. 1978. *Pathophysiology—clinical concepts of disease processes.* New York: McGraw-Hill Book Co.

Richards, A. N. 1976. Pathophysiology and therapeutics of myocardial ischemia. In Proceedings of the 18th A. N. Richards Symposium. Jamaica, N.Y.: Special Medical & Scientific Books.

Ross, R., and Harker, L. 1976. Hyperlipidemia and atherosclerosis. *Science* 193:1094.

Samuelsson, B., and Paoletti, R. 1976. *Advances in prostaglandins and thromboxane research.* New York: Raven Press.

Saran, R. K.; Sahugja, R. C.; Gupta, N. N.; et al. 1978. 3-methoxy-4-hydroxyphenylglycol in cerebrospinal fluid and vanillyl mandelic acid in urine of humans with hypertension. *Science* 200:317.

Selye, H. 1976. *Stress in health and disease.* Boston: Butterworths.

Süss, R.; Kinzel, V.; and Scribner, J. D. 1973. *Cancer: Experiments and concepts.* New York: Springer-Verlag.

Vander, A. J. 1976. In Introduction to *Human physiology and the environment in health and disease.* San Francisco: W. H. Freeman and Co. Part 1, article 3.

Wellington, D. G.; MacDonald, E. J.; and Wolf, P. F. 1979. *Cancer mortality: Environmental and ethnic factors.* New York: Academic Press.

PART TWO

STRESS AND DISEASE FROM PHYSICAL STRESSORS

We are constantly being bombarded with energy from our environment, various forms of which are capable of eliciting both localized and systemic effects on the body that can be injurious. With each passing year more and more of this energy is from manufactured sources.

Radiation

Objectives: Upon completing this chapter you should:

1. Be acquainted with the damaging effects on the body from ultraviolet radiation.
2. Be informed of the phenomenon of photosensitization and its pathologic implications.
3. Recognize the dangers of exposure to ionizing radiation.
4. Understand how various dosages of high energy result in malignant changes and accelerated aging.
5. Know about potential body damage from microwaves and laser beams.

About 93 million miles away the sun of our solar system transmutes about 564 million tons of hydrogen into helium each second. The massive thermonuclear reaction showers space with energy, radiating outward in every direction at the speed of light. Various units have been formulated to measure the electromagnetic energy from the sun. Thus we refer to electron-volts, foot-candles, kilocalories/mole, and *photons*, the smallest units of radiation. Wavelength refers to the length of oscillations, a complete oscillation into the magnetic and electric vectors comprising a cycle. Reference to time is incorporated in *frequency*, which is the number of cycles per second. For our purposes here, wavelength is our primary consideration, and it is usually measured in nanometers (nm), which is 10^{-9} meters. A diagrammatic concept of the electromagnetic spectrum is offered in Figure 6-1.

Fortunately, the atmosphere screens out much of the higher energy such as x-rays and some of the ultraviolet rays (UV). Approximately half of the radiant energy reaching the earth is infrared radiation (IRR). The rest is visible light and ultraviolet radiation (UVR). Radiations below 200 nm, which begin just left of 10^1 in the

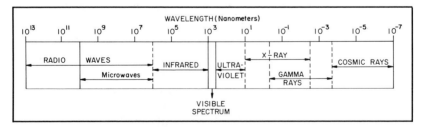

FIGURE 6-1   The electromagnetic spectrum. Wavelengths are progressively shorter with higher energy as one reads the chart from left to right.

electromagnetic spectrum shown in Figure 6-1, are greater than the energy in most chemical bonds, leading to bond disruption and ionization.

Although the physiologic effects of visible light have been widely investigated in animals, the amount of work with humans has been modest in comparison. Apparently light perception does stimulate the hypothalamus and the pituitary-adrenal system. Studies in which hormones have been measured in blind subjects indicate that their levels of ACTH, cortisol, growth hormone, and thyroxin are often significantly below levels of these secretions in sighted persons. For example, a group of blind adults averaged only 1.16 pg/dl[1] of growth hormone compared to 4.08 pg/dl in those with sight.

We are particularly concerned with UVR as an environmental stressor. Only UVR above 290 nm reaches us because molecular oxygen is converted to ozone in the upper atmosphere, and ozone intercepts UVR below 290 nm. There has been much concern over the possibility that the use of fluorocarbons from commercial aerosol sprays and their release into the atmosphere will seriously reduce the protective ozone layer, permitting the stronger UVR to reach the earth. Sunlight breaks down fluorocarbons to chlorine compounds, and it is these that destroy ozone. The destruction of the ozone layer is thought to be occurring twice as fast as was earlier predicted. It is estimated that a 5% drop in ozone concentration will increase the incidence of human skin cancer by 10%, at least in fair-skinned individuals. At present there are about 400,000 new cases of skin cancer each year.

The molecules in our bodies that absorb solar UVR (290 to 400 nm) are those with conjugated double bonds, particularly those with aromatic ring structures such as proteins and nucleoproteins. In fact, the absorption of UVR by proteins in the outer skin offers a measure of protection for underlying tissue.

In considering physiologic stress from radiant energy, we must realize that some exposures are not natural. When Edison perfected the incandescent lamp, we no longer had to rely on natural light. Later cool fluorescent lamps were invented; they are now the most widely used artificial light, and their spectral characteristics differ markedly from sunlight. Ionizing radiation, radio waves, IRR, UVR, and laser beams are some other forms of artificial radiation.

Light perception by the eye and brain may have a number of effects on overall body function. Apparently the hypothalamus can become activated by light, resulting in alterations in endocrine reg-

---

[1]Picograms per deciliter. A picogram is 10^{-12} of a gram, or 10^{-9} of a milligram.

ulation that in turn can affect metabolism, mood, and behavior. Though some of these effects are well documented in animals, they are just beginning to be investigated in humans.

However, in humans there are a number of well-known physiologic effects from radiation; some are harmful and some beneficial. UVR is significant in both instances, and exposures to it are commonplace. Since the skin is the primary organ involved, let us examine the effects of UVR on skin.

ULTRAVIOLET RADIATION AND THE SKIN

Human skin is a complex organ consisting of an outer, thinner epithelial layer, the *epidermis*, and a deep inner connective tissue layer, the *dermis*. Several types of cells are found in the epidermis, which is about 60 to 100μ in depth. Cells at the very suface comprise the *horny layer*, a tough, resistant epithelium containing keratin filaments. These cells progressively die and are shed. They are constantly being replaced by a proliferation of the basal cells that migrate upward. The migrating cells are sometimes called *prickle cells*, and they accumulate granules as they approach the horny layer. The pigment synthesizers (*melanocytes*) are interspersed among the basal cells. A diagrammatic representation of skin is shown in Figure 6-2.

Exposure of the unprotected skin to UVR of 290 to 320 nm produces an inflammatory erythema (sunburn) within a few hours that may persist for several days. The damage is not just a first-degree burn, but has a photochemical aspect in addition to a thermal effect. A given quantity of photochemical reaction produces an equivalent effect whether it is all received in a short time or distributed throughout longer intervals.

In histologic sections of sunburned skin, the cells showing the damage are mostly the prickle cells rather than the basal cells. The damage seems to be more pronounced among differentiating cells rather than mitotic cells. However, some UVR may penetrate to depths of 70μ and reach the capillaries. In skin with lesser pigment, basal layer cells are more easily reached by UVR, and here malignant changes are initiated (see Color Plate 1).

Regardless of how common it is in occurrence, sunburn is a true pathologic inflammation. Blood vessels dilate, reaching a maximum diameter between 8 to 20 hours following exposure. There may be severe blistering, sweat suppression, and much discomfort. Changes in blood vessels can persist for weeks. Furthermore, there may be changes in the blood itself, such as the formation of red

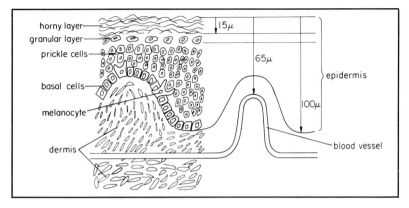

FIGURE 6-2   **A simplified diagram of human skin.**

blood cell rouleaux, causing an elevation in sedimentation rates and leading to obstructed capillaries. Repeated exposures in a short time period produce degenerative injury to both dermis and epidermis, leading to necrosis of the epidermal layers (peeling). Repeated exposures also carry a risk of skin cancer.

The energy dose (intensity multiplied by time exposure) is the significant variable in determining the erythemogenic potential of UVR. Erythema is due to vasodilation. There is also an increase in vascular permeability, and neutrophils begin to appear in the dermis. What is the mechanism of injury? Some have attributed the changes to direct action of photons on small blood vessels. Others have postulated that photons initiate release of mediators such as histamine, serotonin, and bradykinin into the upper dermis.

Recent work indicates that UV photons rupture lysosomal membranes in three critical sites: epidermis, endothelial cells of capillaries, and mast cells. The theory is that release of epidermal lysosomal enzymes leads to vacuolar degeneration of these cells, with eventual necrosis and sloughing of the epidermis. Release of lysosomal enzymes from the endothelium damages the vascular lining, resulting in dilated vessels and increased permeability. Lysis of mast cell lysosomal membranes releases histamine and possibly other mediators which augment and perpetuate the vasodilation and vascular permeability already initiated.

Certain investigators consider that the lysosomal membranes are altered by the chemical action of free radicals rather than by the direct impact of a UV photon. Exposure to UVR does promote the production of free radicals in human skin cells. In fact, the premature aging of skin from sun exposure is thought to be related to lipid peroxidation and the consequent release of lysosomal collagenase.

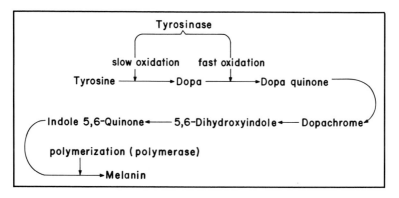

FIGURE 6-3   The synthesis of melanin pigment from tyrosine.

Protective Acclimatization

The amount of melanin pigment synthesized and stored in melanocytes or transferred to keratinocytes is the most important variable in protecting bare skin against UVR. Immediately after exposure to UVR, the amount of pigment in the skin increases, and the skin remains darker for a few hours. The immediate darkening probably results from photo-oxidation of colorless melanin precursors. About 20 to 50 hours following exposure, melanocytes in the epidermis begin to divide and to increase their synthesis of melanin granules. Activation of the enzyme tyrosinase results in the synthesis of melanin from the amino acid tyrosine. The chemical conversion involves several steps (Figure 6-3). Melanin granules are produced in tiny intracellular bodies called *melanosomes*, which are secreted into keratinocytes where the pigment is released. Thus, there is considerable migration of pigment from melanocytes to other regions of the epidermis. This mechanism is illustrated in Figure 6-4.

The exposed skin remains tan for several weeks and offers protection from further damage from UVR. Eventually the pigmented keratinocytes slough off and the tan slowly fades. Skin chronically damaged from UV exposure may show an inadequate pigmentation response. Apparently this is due to a faulty transfer of melanosomes from melanocytes to keratinocytes.

The skin's ability to produce pigment in response to UVR varies considerably and has a strong genetic basis. People of Celtic extraction may have problems with sun exposure. Moreover, extremely fair-skinned people are prime candidates for skin cancer when they are perpetually exposed to UVR. Despite popular no-

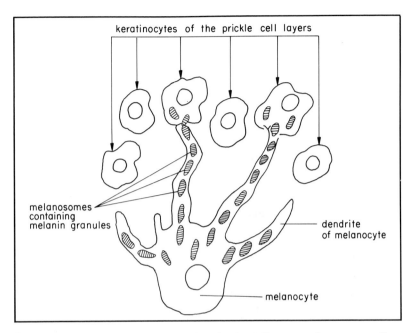

FIGURE 6-4   The mechanism of melanin delivery to the upper cell layers. Sun exposure stimulates the production of melanin-containing melanosomes in the melanocytes. These then form dendrite extensions enabling the melanosomes to be secreted into the keratinocytes. As the keratinocytes move upward and slough off, the tan fades.

tions, a tanned skin is no healthier than an untanned one. In fact, the tanned skin ages much faster than skin that is protected from sun rays.

Beneficial Effects

The synthesis of *cholecalciferol* (vitamin D₃) in the skin is the major beneficial effect of exposure to UVR. The vitamin is formed when its precursor is directly exposed to the same wavelengths of UVR that cause sunburn. In the liver, D vitamins are converted to a compound that is converted in the kidney to yet another compound that binds to the nuclei of intestinal mucosal cells, where it ultimately activates the enzyme effective in transporting calcium ions from the intestine to the blood capillaries.

Before 1920 the defect in calcium absorption, known as *rickets,* was sometimes encountered in young children. Today D vitamins are added to milk and other foods, and rickets has become a rare occurrence. Characteristically, it is the dark-skinned child who is more susceptible to rickets, whereas the light-skinned individual stands a greater risk of hypervitaminosis D. Those who tan their skin through sun exposure are imposing a restriction on their ability to synthesize vitamin D because the UV rays do not penetrate dark skin as effectively.

Other potential benefits of UVR exposure are limited to those with certain skin diseases. In using UVR in diseases associated with microbial invasion, such as certain types of acne, the intent is to produce selective damage to the invading organisms, possibly through inactivation of microbial DNA. In psoriasis there is an excess of proliferating skin cells, and the longer-wave UVR has shown a positive effect in suppressing the proliferation (see Color Plate 2).

PHOTOSENSITIZATION

When photons of around 320 to 400 nm penetrate the skin and their energy is absorbed by various molecules, the excited electrons are transferred to nearby molecules, thereby initiating certain biochemical reactions. This is termed *photosensitization,* and many chemical substances in the skin may serve as photosensitizers. Most of these substances are manufactured; they include numerous drugs, medications, soaps, and cosmetics. Some photosensitizers act through formation of photoproducts with DNA or RNA. Others require the presence of oxygen and are associated with peroxide-formation and lysosomal membrane damage. The overall response in photosensitization is usually phototoxic in nature, although in a few instances it may be allergic, with the presence of cell-mediated hypersensitivity resulting in urticaria and vasodilation.

Among the topical photosensitizers in cosmetics are the essential oils, coal-tar derivatives, and fluorescein derivatives. A number of topical medications such as antibacterial and antifungal preparations also have been incriminated. So have several deodorant soaps. The list of systemic photosensitizers is longer. Sulfonamides, thiazide diuretics, sulfonylurea antidiabetic drugs, tetracyclines, antihistamines, and tranquilizers (phenothiazines and benzodiazepines) are among potential systemic photosensitizers. The toxicity stemming from reactions to these materials often consists of erythema and edema that occur much earlier, are more severe, and last much longer than ordinary sunburn. Either drug or sun exposure must be eliminated. More than one individual being treated for a troublesome sinus infection with tetracycline and anti-

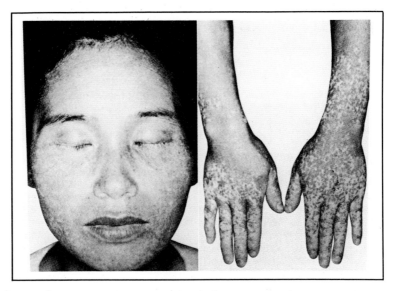

FIGURE 6-5   A clinical example of photosensitization. A skin reaction in a sun-exposed patient taking the antibiotic tetracycline. (Courtesy of Dr. Kihei Tanioku, Emeritus Professor, Department of Dermatology, Okayama University Medical School, Okayama, Japan.)

histamine has yielded to the temptation of sunbathing his or her head and face to obtain the feel of heat on the sinuses. This is a dangerous combination. A skin reaction following sun exposure in a patient on tetracycline therapy is depicted in Figure 6-5, and a list of systemic photosensitizers is provided in Table 6-1.

Endogenous Photosensitizers

In a few instances substances produced by the body may play the role of sensitizers in the skin when the individual is exposed to UVR. Persons with the disease *erythropoietic protoporphyria* produce excessive amounts of porphyrins in bone marrow and liver, and these are released into the blood, where exposure to a radiation of 400 nm produces toxic intermediates. Interestingly, in another condition, *transient neonatal jaundice*, excessive production of bilirubin is counteracted by exposure to light. Thousands of premature infants are successfully treated for this problem by exposing them to phototherapy for 3 or 4 days. Blue light is the most effective. Apparently blue light, through photo-oxidation, converts bilirubin in the skin capillaries to metastable isomers that can be excreted in bile. *Hyperbilirubinemia* afflicts 15% to 20% of premature infants because the liver

TABLE 6-1

Major Groups of Phototoxic Chemicals

Antibacterial creams
  salicylanides

Deodorant soaps
  salicylanides

Sunscreen lotions
  substituted benzoic acid

Antibiotics
  sulfonamides
  tetracycline

Antihistamines
  promethazine (Phenergan)

Diuretics
  chlorothiazides (Dyazide, Hydropres)

Oral hypoglycemic agents
  tolbutamide (Orinase)
  chlorpropamide (Diabinese)

Tranquilizers
  chlorpromazine (Thorazine)
  chlordiazepoxide (Librium)
  diazepam (Valium)

Artificial sweeteners
  cyclamates
  saccharin

has not fully matured.[2] Excess bilirubin tends to become concentrated in the brain, where it produces damage known clinically as *kernicterus*. If the blood level of bilirubin can be kept under 10 mg/dl until the liver matures, there is little risk of brain injury.

Solar Radiation and Autoimmune Disease

Certain autoimmune diseases are exacerbated by exposure to the sun's rays. For example, *lupus erythematosus* (LE), a serious autoimmune malady, is severely worsened by sun exposure, which precipitates new skin lesions and stimulates progressive systemic pathology (Figure 6-6). The disease, found primarily in young women, is characterized by an immune system attack on nuclear DNA. There appear to be two forms, discoid lupus (DLE) and systemic lupus (SLE);

[2]There are two other causes of hyperbilirubinemia in neonates exclusive of the liver maturity factor; they are associated with Rh and ABO blood group incompatibilities.

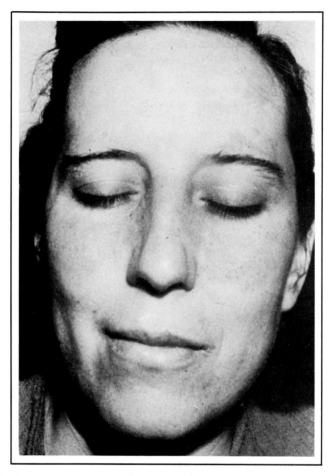

FIGURE 6-6   A patient with systemic lupus erythematosus. Note the subtle discoloration ("butterfly" rash) over the bridge of the nose and along the upper cheeks. (From M. E. Groer and M. E. Shekleton, *Basic pathophysiology.* St. Louis: C. V. Mosby Co., 1979. Courtesy Department of Pathology, University of Tennessee, Memphis.)

the former is characterized by isolated skin lesions (see Color Plate 3), whereas in the latter form, lesions develop throughout many organs, the kidney in particular.

Not only is lupus aggravated by exposure to sunlight, but it is strongly believed by some investigators that radiation exposure is a factor in the original etiology. The mechanism underlying the pathology is not clear, but it has been theorized that in predisposed individuals, either DNA is more susceptible to damage by UVR, or DNA repair capability is not as effective.

UVR and the Eye

The only organ other than the skin that is regularly exposed to solar radiation is the eye. Indeed, our primary sense, vision, is dependent upon the eye being stimulated by that narrow band of wavelength that we call visible light. Visible light of very high intensity may stress the retinal cells and temporarily impair vision. On the other hand, UVR can produce irreversible changes, particularly in the structure of the lens. Experiments with animals have shown that chronic exposure of the eyes to UVR of 290 to 320 nm results in progressive opacity of crystalline lens (cataracts) in about 35% of the specimens. Just how extensive a role UVR exposure plays in producing human cataracts is less conclusive.

Experiments have shown also that the lower wavelengths of UVR are capable of damaging retinal cells. Sunbathers who do not protect their eyes are subjecting both lens and retina to UVR stress. Reading for prolonged periods in bright sunshine is particularly undesirable. With so many light colors and bright, shiny metal structures in our modern urban environment, the reflective glare imposes an unwarranted stress on the visual apparatus.

IONIZING RADIATION

Humans have always been exposed to ionizing radiation from natural sources. However, in this century we have augmented natural sources with our own production and use of high energy to the point that it poses a potential hazard of the greatest magnitude. The severity of the effects of ionizing radiation on our bodies is well acknowledged. Since the turn of the century, employees using radium in the production of luminous paint have suffered from bone cancer and aplastic anemia. Mine workers have shown a high incidence of lung cancer from exposure to radon and uranium. And until recent years there was a notable increase in the incidence of leukemia among radiologists. Improvement in protective techniques and facilities has helped to stabilize this incidence.

It is clearly evident that ionizing radiation is responsible for numerous somatic cellular alterations which may lead to leukemias and other cancers, cataracts, and a reduced life span. This is most unfortunate in view of the fact that artificial sources of high energy have become a part of daily life. A major artificial source is the x-ray

TABLE 6-2
1978 Estimates of Radiation Exposures of United States Population

SOURCE	PERSON-REMS*/YR (IN THOUSANDS)
Natural background	20,000
Healing arts	17,000
Technologically enhanced	1,000
Nuclear weapons (fallout, testing, etc.)	1,600
Nuclear energy	56
Consumer products	6

Source: Summarized by the International Task Force on Ionizing Radiation.
* Person-rems are calculated by multiplying the total number of people exposed by their average individual doses (in rems).

unit employed by the health care professions. Over 200,000 units are in operation in the United States alone, and an average of nearly 2 million patients per year are exposed to their rays. These x-ray units are of indispensable clinical value in diagnostic screening; yet, much caution must be exercised if their abuse is to be prevented. For example, concern has been expressed that periodic, routine mammography for the detection of breast cancer may in itself eventually produce the cancer that the screening is designed to detect. Also, there has been indiscriminate use of x-ray pelvimetry in pregnancy.

In addition to the high energy from x-rays, an average of 30 new nuclear reactors are installed each year. There is concern over these installations in view of the emergency surrounding the reactor accident at Three Mile Island near Harrisburg, Pennsylvania early in 1979. Other sources of exposure to ionizing radiation are summarized in Table 6-2.

Ionizing radiation strips electrons from atoms, thereby disrupting chemical bonds. Much of this radiation results from unstable nuclei of atoms that become radioactive. The structure of the unstable nucleus then stabilizes through a change in nuclear energy, achieved by releasing particles and/or electromagnetic radiation. The particles are either electrons (*beta*) or helium nuclei (*alpha*), whereas radiations originating from atomic nuclei are termed *gamma rays*, and those originating outside the nucleus are termed *x-rays*. This high energy ranges from 10^{-7} to 10^{-11} cm (1 to 10^{-4} nm). Biologic effects result largely from the ionization produced by the energy.

Dosimetry and Measurement

The primary unit in physics for measuring the quantity of ionization produced by x-rays or gamma radiation is the *roentgen*, one such unit being the amount of radiation producing 1 electrostatic unit of ions per cubic centimeter of air. The fact that the roentgen is a measure of interaction with air means that the amount of energy actually absorbed per exposure in roentgens varies in different materials. For this reason a unit of absorbed dose of ionizing radiation, the *rad*, has been introduced. Rads express the quantity of energy absorbed per gram of material from any particular ionizing radiation. For example, an exposure of skeletal muscle to 1 roentgen of gamma rays results in about 0.97 rad.[3] However, the same dose in rads from different types of radiation does not necessarily produce the same degree of biologic effect. Therefore, an additional unit, the *rem*, is employed to express dosage in terms of human effects. To establish a comparison of the dose effect of different types of radiation, a factor called relative biologic efficiency (RBE) is used. It is the ratio of the gamma ray or x-ray dose to the radiation dose in question that produces the same biologic effect. This is termed the *roentgen equivalent for man* (rem) and is derived thus: RBE × rad = rem. The RBE values for various types of radiation are given in Table 6-3.

Effects on Humans

Several variables determine the actual effects of ionizing radiation on the human body. Among these variables are the type and amount of radiation, the structure and density of the target, the tissue type as well as its condition and age at the time of irradiation, and the repair capability of the target tissue. It must be kept in mind that ionizing radiation will disrupt any chemical bond in any molecule of any cell that absorbs the energy from an incident ray. Therefore, observed effects can be quite diverse. Large dosages of ionizing radiation are known to destroy white blood cells, damage skin, produce severe gastrointestinal disturbance, cause internal bleeding, and initiate growth of malignant tumors. Generally, the most rapidly dividing cells are the most sensitive to the energy. Since the blood-cell-forming tissues of the bone marrow and lymphoid structures have high mitotic rates, one of the first recognized effects of radiation is a significant depression in leucocyte count (leucopenia).

In considering biologic effects of high energy, a distinction is often made between localized alterations at the cell level and whole-body disturbances. Recent experiments from tissue cultures in which single human cells were exposed to x-rays indicate that the single

---

3About one rad is the dose a person receives from one chest x-ray or a dental x-ray.

TABLE 6-3
Relative Biologic Effectiveness (RBE) of Several Types of Radiation

FORM OF RADIATION	RBE
Gamma rays and x-rays	1
Beta particles	1–2
Thermal neutrons	2–5
Fast neutrons	5–10
Alpha particles	5–15

cell is much more sensitive to the energy than originally thought. Interest in localized effects on the cell has centered around potential chemical and physical changes in nuclear DNA. A dose of only 40 roentgens will produce at least a single chromosomal break per nucleus, and it is well established that exposure to high energy enhances the probability of both mutagenicity and carcinogenicity.

When considering whole-body effects of ionizing energy, it must be realized that some organs and tissues are much more radioresistant than others. The most radiosensitive structures are mucosa of the gastrointestinal tract, bone marrow, lymphoid tissues, portions of skin epidermis, and lens of the eye. Some degree of damage to the hemapoietic system is always a major consequence of acute radiation exposures. The nondividing small lymphocytes also are extremely sensitive to ionizing radiation. A decrease in the number of these cells in lymph nodes can be detected following total body exposures as low as 10 rads. In fact, lymphocytes are so radiosensitive that they have been used to quantitate radiation exposures. Because of lymphocytic hypersensitivity, ionizing radiation can be expected to interfere with cellular immune response.

The mucosa of the small intestine is quite radiosensitive, and so is the glandular epithelium of the stomach. Gastrointestinal ulcerations, anorexia, reduced nutrient absorption, and diarrhea are common symptoms within a few hours following acute exposures of 100 to 200 rads. Capillaries, germinal layer of skin epidermis, and lens of the eye also are known to be radiosensitive. An increase in capillary permeability as well as hair-follicle damage has been noted, even at low dosages of gamma rays. And individual cells of the lens epithelium become progressively opaque with repeated exposures to low dosages of high energy (Figure 6-7). It must be kept in mind that the effects of ionizing radiation are cumulative. Many small dosages spaced over periods of time may be as damaging as the same amount received in one dose.

There appears to be a strong connection between exposure to radiation and aging. Numerous animal experiments have supported

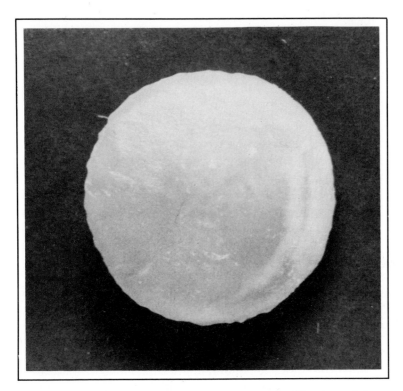

FIGURE 6-7   A human cataract. A cataract is a crystalline lens of the eye that has become opaque and no longer transmits light effectively. Consequently, light does not reach the retina, and vision is seriously impaired. Note the opacity of this lens, which normally would be transparent. (Courtesy Bethesda North Hospital, Cincinnati, Ohio.)

this idea. Survivors of the nuclear explosions in Japan appear to have aged faster than other unexposed Japanese. Two mechanisms are probably operative in promoting changes associated with aging. The increase in mutagenicity from radiation exposure is bound to alter enzyme activity as well as derange patterns of immune reactions. In addition, once again the important matter of production of free radicals and peroxides, which especially accumulate in irradiated cells, figures in the process. These radicals in themselves are damaging to cells and appear to be associated with aging of tissue. The nature of free radicals is explained in Chapter 2.

Cancer

References have already been made to the association of high energy exposure with the development of malignant tumors. Ionizing radi-

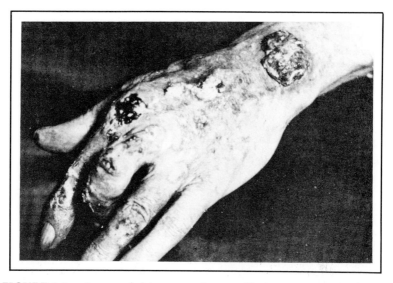

FIGURE 6-8   A case of skin cancer from radiation exposure. Multiple carcinomas appeared in a physician after 15 years of repeated low exposures to x-rays. (From W. A. Meissner and G. T. Diamandopoulos, Neoplasia. In W. A. D. Anderson and J. M. Kissane, eds., *Pathology,* 7th ed. St. Louis: C. V. Mosby Co., 1977.

ation deeply penetrates soft tissue, and it has a reputation for initiating development of sarcomas, leukemias in particular. A higher than average incidence of osteogenic sarcoma (bone cancer) has been found in individuals exposed to cumulative dosages of radiation. Skin cancer also is one of the more prevalent types of malignancy associated with exposure to radiation (Figure 6-8).

Survivors from the Hiroshima and Nagasaki atomic explosions are now showing a much higher than average incidence of leukemias and melanomas (see Color Plate 4). Furthermore, there is a correlation between the incidence of cancers in these individuals and their distance from the site of the blast.

Twenty-eight years after the first announced atomic tests in Utah and Nevada, twice as many children in these two states have died of leukemia than would have been expected statistically. And, of 2,700 soldiers who watched an atomic test in Nevada in 1957, twice the expected number developed leukemia. It is of interest that 91 of the 221 cast and crew members of a movie filmed in 1954 near Yucca Flat, Nevada have since contracted cancer. Eleven atomic blasts had occurred in this region the year before filming. Cancer fatalities among the cast members include such notables as John Wayne, Susan Hayward, Dick Powell, and Agnes Moorehead.

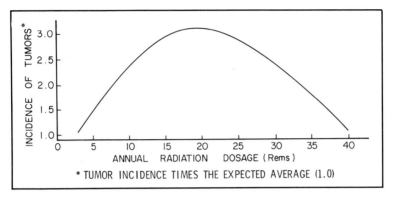

FIGURE 6-9   **The relation of the amount of radiation exposure to tumorigenesis.** Above 2 to 3 rems the incidence begins to exceed the average expectancy, rising to threefold at 20 rems. However, beyond 22 rems the carcinogenic effects progressively diminish due to an increase in lethal effect.

Recent in vitro experiments show, without a doubt, that normal human cells exposed to x-rays are converted to cancerous cells. In the experiments, most of the human skin cells exposed to a dose of 400 rads became malignant. Vitamin A added to the culture prevented some of the radiation-induced malignancy.

Of special concern is the recently discovered fact that the carcinogenic effects of chronic exposure to low doses of radiation (less than 10 rems annually) may be ten times greater than previously estimated. Very high doses are probably not as important as far as cancer is concerned. In fact, when experimental radiation levels become high, carcinogenic effects diminish. This is because higher levels kill cells rather than induce cancerous changes (Figure 6-9).

Small children are more sensitive to ionizing radiation than are adults. For about ten years following World War II, many children throughout the United States were irradiated routinely in the region of the neck and upper chest in order to shrink the thymus gland or the tonsils. To date, about 10% of these individuals have developed thyroid cancer and/or skin cancer. The child's thyroid gland is especially sensitive to radiation.

Radioactive materials readily enter the body through ingestion and inhalation. Radioactive nuclides such as strontium 90, iodine 131, and cesium 137 from reactors and testing may be deposited on the forage of grazing animals and thereby become concentrated in the animal's muscle tissue before being ingested by humans, where they can be carcinogenic. Cancer of the pharnyx, larynx, trachea, and particularly the lung may result from the inhalation of radioactive dusts or gases. Aerosols are more of a problem than the gases because particulates are retained in the lung.

It has been postulated that the threshold intensity for radiation capable of producing leukemia is just below 100 rems. The Federal Radiation Council has established a limit of 0.5 rem per year as the maximum whole-body dosage for an individual. This is exclusive of background radiation and medical sources. Others have proposed that the maximum allowance of exposure from all sources combined should not exceed 250 rems for a lifetime.

Mechanisms of Action

Two different concepts have developed to explain the manner in which ionizing radiation produces its effect on cellular materials. The direct action principle, or *target theory,* has been applied in particular to nuclear alterations such as gene mutation, chromosomal breakage, virus inactivation, and other changes that are known to result from exposures. According to this view, most whole-body effects are based upon the direct, ionizing impact on specific macromolecules, particularly proteins and nucleic acids. Another theory considers that the attack is indirect and is by way of the numerous free radicals such as hydrogen, hydroxyl, O_2H, and H_2O_2 that result from the splitting of water molecules in the cell. Recent evidence suggests that the two concepts are not necessarily contradictory, but are probably complementary. It appears that alterations from direct action are more likely in drier materials, whereas effects from free radicals are favored in very dilute solutions. With nucleic acids (DNA and RNA), the action often centers around pyrimidine modification, and an experimental suppression of free radical production necessitates a larger dose of x-rays to produce the modification. A lowering of oxygen tension likewise renders cells more radioresistant.

LONG–WAVE RADIATION: LASER ENERGY

We are being exposed regularly to wavelengths beyond the visible range. Responses to this energy result from magnetic rather than electronic effects. Absorption of these wavelengths occurs when they produce transient changes in the molecular dipole moment.

Infrared radiation (IRR) can produce headache and fatigue in humans exposed to intensities too low to burn the skin. The same form of radiation can damage the eyes. Posterior cataracts are a well-known effect of long-standing exposure to IRR.

Microwave radiation includes electromagnetic frequencies from 300 to 30,000 megacycles per second. This radiation is similar to IRR in that it heats skin locally, but it penetrates deeper. Animal experiments have shown that microwaves can produce cataracts, actually cook underlying muscle, and eventually result in hyperthermia that may be fatal. Microwaves are propagated into the atmosphere from radiorelay links, television transmitters, and radar antennas. They are employed medically in diathermy devices. However, the greatest likelihood of exposure stems from the popular use of microwave ovens in the home. The main dangers of these ovens are specifically thermal, although another danger is that an electronic device in the body, such as an implanted cardiac pacemaker, could develop malfunctions from exposure to electromagnetic frequencies from a microwave oven.

There has been much concern about microwaves produced by television transmitters like those atop the World Trade Center in New York City. Supposedly the 200-microwatt level there is more than ten times the level that the Soviets allegedly aimed at the United States embassy in Moscow, where one-third of the staff and family members in the embassy were found to suffer blood disorders.

For a number of years there has been a progressive development in laser technology. The basic principle of this energy is *light amplification by stimulated emission of radiation*; hence the name *laser*. One of the chief physiologic hazards of laser radiation is damage to the eye. Retinal injury occurs before the individual is even aware of the danger. Also, several enzymes have been shown to be inactivated by laser emission, and the two porphyrins, hemoglobin and myoglobin, readily absorb laser energy, leading to microthrombosis and disturbances in muscle contractility. In addition, laser radiation is mutagenic and capable of producing striking chromosomal anomalies. On the other hand, laser beams are being put to beneficial use in delicate surgical techniques, particularly in treatment of diabetic retinopathy. The beam is directed at selected microscopic sites.

SUMMARY

Ultraviolet radiation of less than 290 nm does not reach us, but the exposure of unprotected skin to 290 to 320 nm produces an inflammatory erythema within a few hours. The damage stems from the rupture of lysosomal membranes in the epidermis, capillary endothelial cells, and mast cells.

Exposure to ultraviolet radiation also exacerbates certain autoimmune conditions, particularly lupus erythematosus, and it may contribute to the development of cataracts.

Natural protection from UVR is afforded by the synthesis and migration of melanin granules originally produced by melanocytes in the inner epidermis.

A number of drugs, medications, and cosmetics become toxic when they are sensitized in the skin by photons of 320 to 400 nm, either by lysosomal damage from peroxide formation, or by products stemming from reactions with DNA and RNA.

Energy of less than 100 nm, known as ionizing radiation, includes gamma rays and x-rays. Exposures to ionizing radiation are commonly measured in roentgens, although rads account for the difference in absorption among various materials for a given exposure, and rems express variations in human effects from a given quantity absorbed.

The most radiosensitive tissues are small, nondividing lymphocytes, gastrointestinal mucosa, bone marrow, and skin epidermis. Exposures above 150 rads result in a marked leucopenia, acute digestive disturbances, suppressed erythropoiesis, and skin damage. Whole-body exposures exceeding 400 roentgens are fatal.

Ionizing radiation is potentially carcinogenic, particularly with respect to leukemias, other sarcomas, and skin malignancy. In addition, exposure to high energy accelerates aging, probably through mutagenic effects and the production of free radicals in the cells.

Chapter Glossary

anorexia   abnormal loss of appetite for food

autoimmune disease   damage from the body's immune reaction to its own tissues

erythema   reddening of the skin, caused by vasodilation and congested capillaries

hemapoietic (or erythropoietic) tissue   bone marrow in which new red blood cells are produced

hypervitaminosis   unfavorable reactions from the intake of excessive vitamins

keratin   a tough, fibrous protein found in hair, nails, and outer skin epidermis

leucopenia   a substantial reduction in the number of white blood cells

microthrombosis   occlusion of small blood vessels by blood-clot formation

nuclides   species of atoms characterized by their nuclear constitution

rouleaux   plural of rouleau; a roll of cells, as if in a stack, like coins

systemic   spread throughout the body, as opposed to localized

topical   an application to a localized region of the body, usually the body surface

For Further Reading

Coggle, J. E. 1971. *Biological effects of radiation.* The Wykeham Science Series, Vol. 14. New York: Springer-Verlag.

Fitzpatrick, T. B., ed. 1974. *Sunlight and man.* Proceedings of the International Conference on Photosensitization and Photoprotection. Tokyo: University of Tokyo Press.

Folk, G. E., Jr. 1974. *Textbook of environmental physiology.* 2d ed. Philadelphia: Lea & Febiger. Chapt. 2.

Frisancho, A. R. 1979. *Environmental physiology: Human adaptation; a functional interpretation.* St. Louis: C. V. Mosby Co.

Giese, A. C. 1976. *Living with our sun's ultraviolet rays.* New York: Plenum Press.

Grosch, D. S., and Hopwood, L. E. 1979. *The biological effects of radiations.* 2d ed. New York: Academic Press.

Hollwich, F. 1979. *The influence of ocular light perception on metabolism in man and in animals.* New York: Springer-Verlag.

Hutterman, J.; Kohnlein, W.; and Teoule, R., eds. 1978. *Effects of ionizing radiation on DNA: Physical, chemical and biological aspects.* New York: Springer-Verlag.

Lee, D. H. K., ed. 1977. Reactions to environmental agents. In *Handbook of physiology.* Bethesda, Md.: American Physiological Society. Section 9, Chapts. 7, 8.

McDonagh, A. F.; Palma, L. A.; and Lightner, D. A. 1980. Blue light and bilirubin excretion. *Science* 208:145.

MacDonald, G. J. F., chairman. 1973. *Biological impacts of increased intensities of solar ultraviolet radiation.* Environmental Studies Board. Washington, D. C.: National Academy of Sciences and National Academy of Engineering.

Nygaard, O. F.; Adler, H. I.; and Sinclair, W. K., eds. 1975. *Radiation research: Biomedical, chemical, and physical perspectives.* New York: Academic Press.

Slonim, N. B., ed. 1974. *Environmental physiology.* St. Louis: C. V. Mosby Co. Chapt. 7.

Urbach, F. 1969. *The biological effects of ultraviolet radiation.* New York: Pergamon Press.

Vander, A. J. 1976. In Introduction to *Human physiology and the environment in health and disease.* San Francisco: W. H. Freeman and Co. Part 3, articles 11, 12.

7

Temperature Change

Heat Exchange and Thermoregulation
Exposure to Temperature Extremes
Thermal Stress and Disease
Variable Sensitivity to Temperature Change

‖ Objectives: Upon completing this chapter you should:

1. Understand the principles underlying the body's heat exchange with its environment.
2. Be acquainted with the physiologic regulations for balancing heat production with heat loss.
3. Recognize the danger of lowered body temperature (hypothermia).
4. Be informed about the nature of various hyperthermic states such as heat exhaustion, heat stroke, fever, and burns.
5. Recognize the importance of thermal stress and sensitivity to temperature change in promoting and aggravating various disorders.

Ambient temperature change is probably the most frequently encountered stressor. In some respects it may appear that we are relatively exempt from this stress since many buildings and automobiles are heated and air conditioned. However, it is this very convenience that subjects us to unusually abrupt thermal changes when, for example, we walk from 25 C in a heated building to less than 0 C outside, or depart from an air-conditioned building at 21 C and enter the outdoors at 34 C. In addition to the stress from temperature change itself, there can be body disturbances as well from variations in the humidity and movement of the air.

Those of us living in temperate regions are well aware of the pronounced temperature extremes that can occur seasonally within 3 or 4 months. No one in north-central United States will forget the severity of the winters of 1977, 1978, and 1979, nor will those of the central and southern United States forget the summer of 1980. Thermal stress can be a highly significant factor in the health versus disease equation. Its role in promoting and aggravating chronic disturbances within the body is often overlooked. Temperature change is especially stressing to the elderly.

Even a modest change in the temperature of living mammalian tissue profoundly affects the rate of biochemical reactions. Temperature change may alter as well the qualitative character of chemical processes. *Homeotherms,* such as humans, can tolerate a considerable range of ambient temperatures only because they possess remarkable temperature-regulating capabilities. However, compared to the poikilotherm, the homeotherm is extremely restricted in respect to body temperature variation. The temperature of most human tissue and its internal environment is confined to a narrow range of 35 C to 39 C. The upper limit is particularly critical. Higher temperatures entail risks of dehydration, nerve-firing sensitivity to heat (convulsions), and denaturation of protein (enzymes). Above 42 C death becomes imminent.

Despite the restricted variation imposed upon it by thermoregulation, internal body temperature is not constant. It normally varies as much as 2 to 3 degrees in response to activity pattern, environmental temperature, and diurnal rhythm. Body temperature is lowest just prior to arising in the morning, and highest during early evening. This temperature variation is a well-known *circadian,* or 24-hour rhythm. There may be rhythms other than the circadian that are associated with fluctuation in body temperature. For example, in the luteal phase of the menstrual cycle, the rise in progesterone levels is accompanied by a slight increase in body temperature.

HEAT EXCHANGE AND THERMOREGULATION

The human body, as well as any other body, animate or inanimate, is constantly exchanging heat with its surroundings. The capacity of a given quantity of heat to produce alterations in temperature varies with different materials, and forms the basis for the concept of *specific heat.* Water has a much higher specific heat than most substances, a fact of great biologic significance. Body composition is based on solutions and colloidal dispersions that are aqueous. Thus the specific heat of water promotes thermal stability in tissues and the internal environment, which thereby can gain or lose considerable heat without a concomitant change in their temperature.

Heat is exchanged from one body to another by *conduction, convection,* and *radiation.* In conduction, there is a transfer of thermal energy from molecule to molecule, obeying a gradient. In convection, air that gains heat from a warmer body moves away from the body due to its expansion, and is replaced by cooler air which in turn is warmed and moves away. Without convection, only a limited amount of heat would be lost to the air by conduction. All objects radiate heat in the form of electromagnetic infrared rays. Radiant energy, like conduction, follows a gradient, and the rate of heat transfer depends upon the temperature of the radiating surface. Loss of heat from a body also occurs when thermal energy is expended in converting liquid water to water vapor, as in perspiration. The heat required for this is taken from the body surface from which the liquid is evaporating. A general idea of heat exchange of the human body with the environment is illustrated in Figure 7-1.

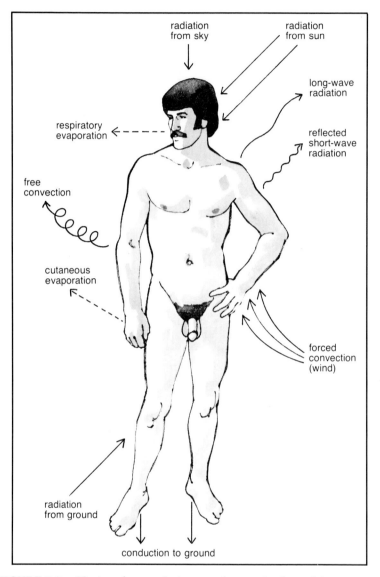

FIGURE 7-1   **Heat exchanges between a human body and its environment.**

Temperature regulation in a homeotherm affords an excellent example of homeostasis. Heat balance is essentially simple in principle, total heat content of the body representing the net difference between heat being produced and that being lost. Accordingly, maintenance of relatively constant body temperature implies that heat production equals heat loss. Physiologic controls govern both variables. Either a net gain or net loss of heat persisting for any time indicates a disturbance in the control of thermal equilibrium and is potentially dangerous. This is immediately true of a net gain of heat.

Accounting for all the actual heat exchanges of the body is not so simple in practice because of the many variables. Thermal physiologists often employ the following equation: $M + E + R + C + K + W + S = O$, in which,

M = metabolic heat production
E = evaporative heat exchange
R = radiative heat exchange
C = convective heat exchange
K = conductive heat exchange
W = work accomplished
S = heat storage

In this equation, the overall transfer of heat is the algebraic sum of the individual components. E, R, C, and K are negative when heat in each of these cases is being lost from the body; in fact, E can never be positive. If a person rests unclad in an ambient temperature of 39 C, then K, C, and R can be expected to be positive (with E negative). In using the above equation, all terms must be expressed in the same units. For energy exchange the units are usually watts per surface area (w/m^2). A watt is 1.163×1 kcal/hr.[1] The average at rest heat production of the body is about 80 to 85 w.

Heat exchange between the environment and the body occurs, of course, at the body surface. However, most of the heat is produced deep within the body, some distance from the skin. The term *shell* is used to denote the portion of the body near the surface, and the term *core* denotes the deeper recesses of the body where most of the heat is produced. Thus, a consideration of body heat exchange must be based upon transfers throughout a continuum of three regions: core, shell, and external environment. Core temperature is normally between 36 and 38.5 C. Shell temperature is more variable and dependent to a greater degree upon environmental temperature. The temperature of bare skin is only 16 to 23 C at an ambient temperature of 0 C, whereas at an ambient temperature of 24 C, skin temperature is between 32 to 35 C.

The balance between production and loss of heat is continually being disturbed, either by the capriciousness of environ-

---

[1] A kilocalorie is the amount of heat required to increase the temperature of 1 liter of water 1 C.

TABLE 7-1
Distribution of Body Heat Production at Rest

ORGAN	PERCENT OF TOTAL
Liver	21
Muscle	20
Brain	18
Heart	12
Kidney	7
Skin	5
Others	17

mental temperature change, which alters rate of heat loss, or by disturbances in metabolism, which influences heat production. A review of each side of the heat balance equation follows.

Heat Production

Metabolism is unavoidably heat-producing. For this reason it is easier to maintain a body temperature that is above ambient temperature than it is to maintain one that is lower than environmental temperature. The human body is more like a stove than a refrigerator. The minimum level of heat production is set by the basal metabolic rate (BMR), which is that metabolism necessary to maintain life at neutral temperatures, exclusive of all activity and feeding. The BMR can be quite variable, depending upon age, sex, body surface area, state of health, and production of certain endocrine secretions, particularly thyroid output. An adult male of average dimensions (65 to 70 kg) requires approximately 15 liters of oxygen per hour just to remain alive. Since 1 liter of oxygen is required for the oxidation of 4.8 kcal of foodstuff, the BMR should approximate 15 × 4.8, or 72 kcal/hr, which is 84 w. This would amount to about 1700 kcal/day, and in respect to body surface area would be approximately 40 kcal/hr/m², or 47 w/m². (An average body surface area is 1.3 to 1.9 m².) The distribution of heat production in the body at rest is given in Table 7-1.

Most of the time we are producing heat beyond the BMR level. Five factors that are thermogenic, singly or in combination, are listed in Table 7-2. Much heat results from the contraction of skeletal muscle, and the first three factors listed in the table involve muscle activity. The first muscle changes in response to cold are imperceptible increases in muscle tone. Increased muscle tone can lead to tenseness in the muscles, as some can attest from the experience

TABLE 7-2
Factors Producing Increase in Body Heat

Exercise
Shivering
Muscle tension
Increase in metabolic rate (hormonal)
Specific dynamic action of food
Fever

of not being able to relax when sleeping in a cold bedroom. Muscle tone is decreased in a warm environment; however, the decrease is a limited means of restricting heat production, since muscle tone normally is quite low.

Heat loss eventually leads to shivering, which is a rhythmic contraction of skeletal muscles, oscillating at about 10 to 20 tremors per second. Vigorous shivering is a substantial producer of heat, capable of increasing the production severalfold in a few minutes. Yet, the efficiency in terms of maintaining body heat is less than 20% since the muscle activity causes an elevation of heat loss from body to environment, because of enhanced blood perfusion of muscle near the body surface. Shivering also promotes heat loss by increasing convection due to body motion. No external work is performed in shivering, so all the metabolic energy appears as heat.

Both shivering and increased muscle tone are reflexive and completely involuntary. Overt body movement is normally voluntary, and this degree of muscle contraction produces much greater quantities of heat than does shivering. Strenuous exercise can elevate heat production as much as 12-fold.

Exposure to cold is known to promote chemical thermogenesis in which chemical mediators elevate the production of heat by increasing the metabolic rate. The major mediators are epinephrine and thyroxin, and there is evidence that the presence of each of these hormones enhances the action of the other. The calorigenic effect of epinephrine is immediate, and a principal target of this action is adipose tissue, where lipid is rapidly mobilized to free fatty acids, which are then oxidized. The resultant energy has been termed the heat of stress, or emotional heat. Thyroxin and triiodothyronine, on the other hand, have a much longer acting, cumulative effect on metabolic rate. Cold stimulates thyrotropic secretion from the pituitary by way of the hypothalamus. Several weeks of exposure to very cold conditions may raise the output of

TABLE 7-3
Factors Promoting Body Heat Loss

Cool ambient air
Decreased insulation (clothing)
Increase in surface radiation
Increased air movement
Increased skin vasodilation
Insensible water loss (lungs and skin)
Sweating

thyroid hormones by 75% to 100%, a level capable of increasing the BMR by 20%. Conversely, it has been shown that prolonged exposure to heat depresses thyroid activity. Exposure to cold also stimulates cortisol response by way of ACTH from the pituitary. Not only does the cortisol promote gluconeogenesis, which provides a key fuel, but the steroid also appears to be permissive for effective action from thyroxin and the catecholamines. A general discussion of various hormone actions is found in Chapter 4.

The ingestion, digestion, and assimilation of food requires an expenditure of energy (heat). The increment in metabolic rate following food ingestion is termed the *specific dynamic action* (SDA) of food. Protein has the highest SDA value because much of the energy in amino acids is not available for adenosine triphosphate (ATP) due to the deamination process in the liver. Also, the protein has a longer lasting thermogenic effect. Therefore, eating a lot of protein warms the body, particularly the liver. For this reason only a low protein meal is permitted the night before a BMR is measured.

Heat Loss

Our ability to regulate body temperature by decreasing the production of heat is quite limited. Hence, heat balance depends primarily upon the regulation of heat loss. In most environments heat is constantly being lost from the skin surface by radiation, convection, conduction, and evaporation. Several factors that singly or in combination promote heat loss from the body are listed in Table 7-3.

In cooler ambient temperatures, heat loss from the skin is primarily by radiation. The practical significance of losing heat by radiation is exemplified when an individual is near a window on a very cold, cloudy day. Even though the air temperature of the heated room may be 24 C, the glass of the window may be only 2 C. Heat

TABLE 7-4
Chill Index Relating Wind Factor to Temperature

AMBIENT TEMPERATURE WITH NO WIND	TEMPERATURE EQUIVALENTS (C) Wind Velocity (mph)			
	5	15	25	35
10 C	8	1	−3	−5
5 C	3	−6	−11	−13
0 C	−2	−11	−16	−18
−5 C	−7	−18	−23	−26
−10 C	−12	−25	−31	−34
−15 C	−17	−32	−39	−42

Source: Modified from charts of the United States Weather Bureau.

radiates at a high rate from the person's body to the glass, which becomes a heat sink. Window drapes help considerably by serving as a radiation shield. Hospital patients near large uncurtained windows in rooms or corridors may unknowingly become stressed by cold despite adequate temperatures throughout most of the room.

Although heat may be conducted from our bodies much of the time, conduction is not highly significant as a heat loss mechanism except in such instances as bathing in cool water or consuming iced drinks. Convection, which actively removes the conducted heat, is more important. Convection becomes a particularly significant heat loss mechanism when there are forced air movements. Wind is a strong facilitator of heat loss. Therefore, relating a given wind speed to a given temperature provides an indication of the particular temperature which alone would produce an equivalent heat loss. This relationship is known as the chill index. It is shown in Table 7-4.

Vascular Regulation

It must be kept in mind that it is the core temperature (37 C) that is being regulated. If skin were a perfect insulator, core heat would never be lost, and the skin surface temperature, exclusive of sun exposure, would equal the environmental temperature. However, the skin only partially insulates; in fact, its effectiveness as an insulator is subject to physiologic control through the regulation of blood flow to the skin.

Exposure to cold increases the core to environment gradient, promoting vasoconstriction which reduces skin temperature, thus restricting heat loss. As much as 99% in reduction of cutaneous

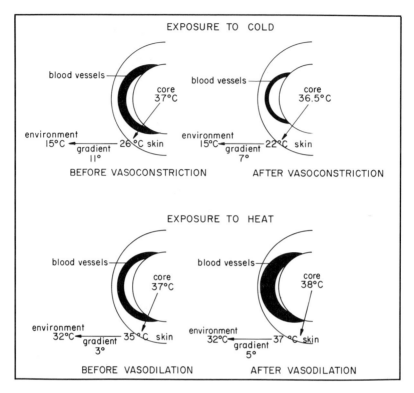

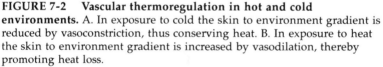

FIGURE 7-2 **Vascular thermoregulation in hot and cold environments.** A. In exposure to cold the skin to environment gradient is reduced by vasoconstriction, thus conserving heat. B. In exposure to heat the skin to environment gradient is increased by vasodilation, thereby promoting heat loss.

blood flow can occur in exposure to extreme cold. Exposure to heat decreases the core to environment gradient, promoting vasodilation which augments the skin to environment gradient, thus facilitating heat loss. These effects are illustrated in Figure 7-2.

Vascular regulation of heat loss is not based only upon arteriole adjustments; changes in vein diameter occur as well. In cold ambient temperatures most of the venous return is through the deeper veins which dilate as superficial veins near the surface remain constricted. Thus, heat loss from the skin is restricted, and the venous blood returning to the heart has suffered little decrease in temperature. In warm ambient temperatures the deeper veins constrict and the superficial veins handle most of the venous return, thereby enhancing heat loss from the skin. This vascular mechanism results in a shrinkage of the functional core area in a cold environ-

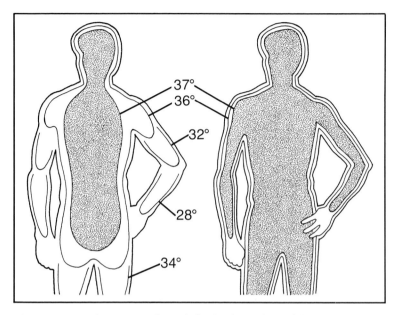

**FIGURE 7-3   The core region of the body under cold and warm
conditions.** *Left,* the core region (shaded) shrinks when the body is
exposed to cold, thereby conserving heat. *At right,* under warm conditions,
the core region expands to a much greater area, promoting heat loss.

ment, and an expansion of this area in warm environments. The effect is depicted in Figure 7-3.

Vasomotor responses to temperature changes are primarily effective throughout a range of environmental temperatures between
about 20 to 30 C. This range is sometimes known as the *zone of thermal neutrality.* With temperatures lower than this, additional reserves, such as increased metabolism, shivering, and voluntary
muscle activity become necessary. On the other hand, with higher
ambient temperatures, an additional mechanism, sweating, is
needed in order to control core temperature.

Insulation and Surface Area

There are two additional variables that are important in determining
the amount of heat loss from the body. The more significant one of
these is insulation, which for us means clothing. The adoption of
clothing as a replacement for fur has been a saving factor in our
ability to withstand substantial reductions in ambient temperature.
How effective an insulation clothing offers depends upon its thickness, type of material, color, and looseness. The thickness of the

trapped air layer is particularly important in cold temperatures. Light color to reflect radiant heat, and looseness to permit air movement for evaporation, are effective in warm environments.

Protection of the head is very important in exposure to cold. Because of the priority of brain function, blood flow to the head remains constant, and there is very little variation in the coefficient of heat transfer. In still air at −4 C, heat loss from the head may exceed 40 w, which represents almost half of the resting heat production. Despite this fact, the habit of going bareheaded during the winter remains strongly ingrained among people of the United States. Head protection can also be important in the heat, especially where there is prominent exposure of the head to the sun. Radiating the bare head in this manner can accumulate a staggering heat load, which entails risks of heat stroke.

A second variable affecting heat loss from the body is the amount of surface area being exposed. In warm environments animals instinctively stretch out, thereby exposing a greater surface area for heat loss. Conversely, curling up diminishes the surface being exposed, and this serves to conserve body heat. A thinly clad individual exposed to cold can reduce body surface area by 50% just by assuming a hunched, sitting position.

Evaporative Heat Loss

The evaporation of water regularly occurs from the lungs and the skin. The vaporization of 1 ml of water requires 0.58 kcal. There is evaporation from the skin even within the zone of thermal neutrality, without the active participation of the sweat glands. This evaporation is termed *insensible perspiration*. Because of the slowness of diffusion and the immediate evaporation, the water is imperceptible, yet, as much as 600 ml/day can be lost in this way.

True sweating results from active secretion of fluid from specific glands in the dermis. Sympathetic stimulation of myoepithelial cells of the glands forces perspiration through a duct and out a pore at the surface. A sweat gland is illustrated in Figure 7-4.

There are two types of sweat glands. Those confined to the axillae and pubic regions are known as *apocrine glands*, and they are not primarily thermoregulatory. It is believed that they originated in conjunction with sexual stimulation. The other sweat glands are the *eccrine glands*, which are much more numerous than the apocrines. The eccrine glands of the palms and soles, like the apocrine glands, are of less importance in the dissipation of heat. The chemical mediator of sweat-gland stimulation, acetylcholine, can activate the ec-

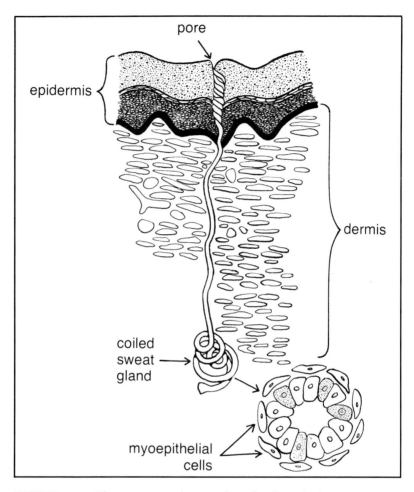

FIGURE 7-4   The structure of an eccrine gland. At the bottom is an enlarged cross-section of the coiled portion showing myoepithelial cells.

crine glands of the palms and soles without an external heat stimulus. The result is the so-called cold sweat associated with emotional states.

Although minimal thermal sweating may occur in a lightly clad individual at comfortable ambient temperatures, perspiration begins to become quite apparent at temperatures exceeding 30 C. At ambient temperatures equaling and exceeding body temperature, sweating is the only highly effective mechanism for heat loss. The relation of variable ambient temperature to the part played by the three major heat loss mechanisms is shown in Table 7-5.

TABLE 7-5

Temperature Variation Effecting Major Means of Losing Body Heat

Ambient Temperature	HEAT LOSS MECHANISMS		
	Evaporation	Radiation	Convection
25 C	23%	67%	10%
30 C	26%	41%	33%
35 C	90%	4%	6%

Neural Mechanisms in Thermoregulation

How does the body know when there are substantial changes in ambient temperature? How is this information transformed into such responses as vasoconstriction, vasodilation, increased muscle tone, shivering, increased rates of metabolism, and sweating? One surmises that there must be a stimulation of temperature-sensitive receptors. This is indeed the case. Receptors fire afferent input to specific hypothalamic nuclei, which then relay efferent output to appropriate effectors (for instance, smooth muscle and glands). Heat loss control is generally mediated by anterior (preoptic) nuclei of the hypothalamus, whereas heat conservation is regulated by nuclei of the posterior areas (Figure 7-5).

There are two distinct groups of temperature-sensitive receptors, the *peripheral thermoreceptors,* located in the lower epidermis and upper dermis of the skin, and the central thermoreceptors, most of which exist in the hypothalamus itself. Certain afferent nerve endings in the skin are stimulated only by lower temperatures (< 30 C), while other groups of endings respond to a higher temperature range (> 37 C). Both groups of receptors have ascending pathways to hypothalamic centers.

Since it is the core temperature that is being regulated, peripheral receptors alone would be insufficient for thermoregulation; hence the importance of central thermoreceptors. These are located in or around the preoptic region of the hypothalamus. The hypothalamic receptors have direct synaptic connections with hypothalamic integrating centers from which descending efferent pathways innervate effectors such as skeletal muscle (shivering) and smooth muscle of blood vessels (vasoconstriction). There are additional sympathetic pathways that separately stimulate release of catecholamines from the adrenal medullae and activate the sweat glands. Any stress promoting an increase in sympathetic activity may result in a contraction of myoepithelial cells of the sweat glands

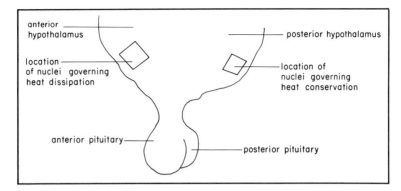

FIGURE 7-5   **Thermoregulatory regions of the hypothalamus.**

located in the palms, soles, and axillae. There is clear evidence that the neurotransmitter responsible for stimulating the myoepithelial cells is acetylcholine, despite the fact that sympathetic pathways innervate the sweat glands. Acetylcholine is the mediator associated with parasympathetic activity.

Animal studies have shown that persistent afferent input to the preoptic nuclei of the hypothalamus induces them to secrete the releasing factors for thyrotropic hormone and ACTH from the pituitary. Output of the former hormone is increased with chronic exposures to cold. ACTH responds to exposures to both temperature extremes, heat as well as cold. The interaction of temperature regulating mechanisms is summarized in Figure 7-6.

The Thermostatic Set Point

From the foregoing discussion it is apparent that certain hypothalamic nuclei serve as the body's thermostat. Is the temperature setting fixed or variable? Apparently it is variable. The best example of variable resetting of the body's thermostat is when fever is induced, as occurs with some infections. Another example is the unstable temperature regulation resulting in so-called hot flashes at the onset of menopause. Fever is a special form of hyperthermia in which temperature-regulating mechanisms are still operative in response to heat and cold, but they do so from a higher temperature setting of the hypothalamic thermostat, the new setting being optimum for handling a condition of infective stress. At onset of fever, the individual feels cold (chills), which induces vasoconstriction and shivering. The resulting heat conservation drives up the body temperature (fever). As the fever breaks, the thermostat is restored to a normal set

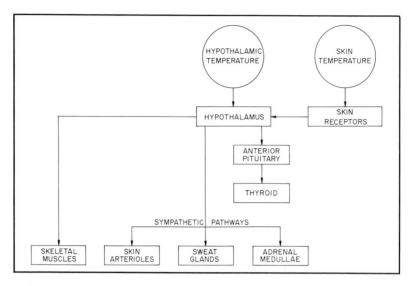

FIGURE 7-6   The neural pathways involved in temperature regulation. Observe the key role of the hypothalamus as an integrator.

point, and the individual feels hot from the heat buildup. Vasodilation and sweating then occur.

Mediators known as *pyrogens* are released in the presence of infection and inflammation, either from host cells or from the microbes themselves. Recent evidence indicates that the pyrogenic effect on hypothalamic thermoregulation is facilitated by local release of prostaglandins. Salicylates, such as aspirin, inhibit synthesis of prostaglandins; hence their antipyretic effect. However, aspirin will not act to lower body temperature to below normal.

Recent data from research with lambs indicated that arginine vasopressin produced by the brain keeps fevers from getting too high. This may be the reason for the fact that most fevers are not extremely high. The brain substance may be of future importance in controlling high fevers.

EXPOSURE TO TEMPERATURE EXTREMES

Cold Exposures

When an individual is exposed to temperatures below the zone of thermal neutrality, the initial response is vasoconstriction. If the exposure to cold continues, skeletal muscle tone is increased, followed by overt shivering. By this time the release of catecholamines from the adrenal medullae has initiated chemical thermogenesis. The sympathoadrenal response to cold is important, not only for elevating the metabolic rate, but for other beneficial effects such as dilating bronchial passageways and increasing cardiac output. The increase in cardiac rate is paradoxical in that blood is moved to the surface faster with a greater risk of heat loss. However, the heat loss from increased rate of blood flow tends to be counteracted by the vasoconstriction. The increased cardiac output plus the vasoconstriction result in an elevation of blood pressure.

It is well known that the amount of body fat is significant in determining tolerance to cold exposure, the metabolic response in both sexes being inversely related to the percentage of body fat. Both deep fat and subcutaneous fat are insulating.

When cold exposure persists for some time, hypothalamic releasers induce the pituitary gland to stimulate the thyroid and adrenal cortex. Secretions from both glands enhance catecholamine action. Hormonal responses play an important role in cold tolerance. For example, it has been shown that asthmatics under cold stress do not mobilize catecholamines as readily as normal individuals. Perhaps this is one factor underlying asthmatics' disposition to bronchoconstriction, or at least their relative inability to counteract it, since catecholamines mediate bronchial dilation. (Exposure to cold air can induce an asthmatic attack.)

Adequate food intake and physical exertion both contribute significantly to cold tolerance. However, voluntary muscular activity cannot be continued for prolonged periods without interruption, or fatigue becomes a problem. Furthermore, strenuous exertion under a high chill index is extremely stressing, particularly to the heart. The occurrence of myocardial infarction is not infrequent in situations where there is strenuous exertion in the cold, as there is with shoveling snow. The pronounced vasoconstriction induced by exposure to cold imposes a strong vascular resistance against an increased cardiac output, subjecting the heart to exaggerated workloads.

When an individual is no longer capable of adequate homeostatic responses to cold conditions, the body temperature begins to fall, a condition known as *hypothermia*. Metabolism, which in itself is temperature-dependent, becomes depressed. This diminishes heat production, which further lowers body temperature. Eventually, the respiratory rate, heart rate, and blood pressure greatly decrease, leading to tissue ischemia. Hypothermia can be a risk in newborns, particularly those delivered prematurely. In neonatal hypothermia there is a demand for increased oxygen consumption as well as risks of acidosis.[2]

Hypothermia can be localized as well as systemic. In cold temperatures with strong convection, there are excessive losses of heat from the extremities (ears, nose, fingers, and toes), especially when they are poorly protected. Such exposures to cold promote extreme vasoconstriction in these regions, almost to the point of cutting off the circulation. The vasoconstriction, of course, conserves core heat as a priority. However, in prolonged exposures, the temperature of the extremities gradually begins to approach environmental temperature until the tissue may freeze. The greatly lowered temperature of the tissue, plus the near-absence of blood perfusion, results in damage known as *frostbite*, characterized by numbness and further impairment of localized circulation. The circulatory occlusion, followed by ischemia, imposes a serious risk of gangrenous necrosis. In thawing tissue, the blood vessels tend to show an exaggerated dilation, and the parts become swollen, red, and extremely painful. Frostbite is never a condition to be taken lightly.

Heat Exposures

When an individual is exposed to temperatures above the zone of thermal neutrality, stimulation of peripheral heat receptors induces vasodilation and enhances blood flow to the skin. A rise in the temperature of blood-perfusing hypothalamic nuclei leads to an increase in cardiac output and initiates sympathetic firing to activate the eccrine glands.

As the exposure to heat continues, the evaporation of sweat assumes the major role in promoting heat loss. Because of this, the ability to withstand high temperatures is greatly dependent upon the humidity content of the air and its motion, dry air currents greatly increasing the rate of evaporation.

Because of the burden of additional heat production, muscular activity is an important contributor to heat stress. Only humans, with their ritualistic habits and compulsions, are likely to be highly active in high heat and humidity. Other mammals rest in the coolest possible spots during the heat of the day. When one exerts on hot days, it must be realized that heat exposure alone stresses the heart by inducing increases in cardiac output. Exercise superimposes an additional workload on the myocardium. The increase in cardiac

---

2Hypothermia can also be a problem in the elderly, about 10% of whom suffer from some degree of hypothermia. In such instances the temperature of vital organs drops below 35 C. Environmental temperatures below 18 C in an at-rest elderly subject risks hypothermia.

output at first is due to an elevation of both heart rate and stroke volume. However, as profuse sweating and hyperventilation proceed, dehydration and loss of sodium lead to hypotension. At this point, the stroke volume decreases, and the cardiac output must depend upon increases in cardiac rate alone.

The venous return to the heart also suffers during exertion in the heat because of the hypotension brought about by both the vasodilation and the hypovolemia. In fact, the major problem in prolonged heat exposure is hypotension. Eventually the reduction in central blood pressure may be characterized by dizziness and fainting.

Sweat output increases about 20 gm/hr for each 1 C rise in air temperature, and continual loss of water cannot be sustained without replacement by drinking fluids. Nevertheless, the rate of sweating is not especially altered by dehydration. The rate at which perspiration is produced is determined primarily by the need for heat dissipation.

Over extended periods of time, continual losses of fluid from prolonged overactivity of the sweating mechanisms produce such degrees of hypovolemia and hypotension that collapse is imminent. This is termed *heat exhaustion*. As a rule, core temperature is not elevated unless the dehydration is severe. Replacement of water and sodium, along with cessation of all physical activity, will alleviate the threat of collapse.

Heat exhaustion is not to be confused with *heat stroke*, which is much more critical. In the latter condition, the heat loss mechanisms have failed, and the core temperature becomes very elevated, a condition termed *hyperthermia*. In some way the heat load in the head induces a functional breakdown of hypothalamic regulatory centers, so that despite the elevated body temperature, the skin is dry. When heat loss mechanisms are inoperative, an excessive build-up of heat occurs rapidly. Heat, in the amount of 0.83 kcal/kg, raises the body temperature 1 C. Thus, a production of only 58 kcal can increase the temperature by 1 C in a person weighing 70 kg. A rise of 6 C in body temperature can be lethal. Such a rise occurs when 348 kcal (6 X 58) of heat has been retained rather than lost. (Normal metabolism requires about 5 hours to produce this much heat.)

Burns

By far the most severe form of thermal stress is when hot material is applied directly to living tissue. Such acute trauma may destroy large areas of skin. Without skin protection body fluids may escape

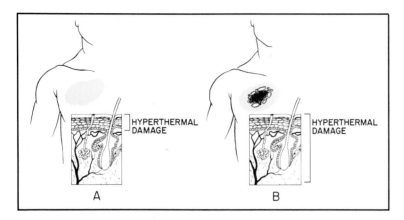

FIGURE 7-7   Partial-thickness and full-thickness burns. A. Partial-thickness burn. Damage is restricted primarily to the epidermis. B. In the full-thickness burn, damage has penetrated deeply into the dermis, sometimes involving subcutaneous tissue, and requiring replacement grafts.

and microorganisms can enter. A direct application of heat to tissue denatures cellular proteins, and if the temperature is extreme enough the heat can physically carbonize tissues. The prognosis depends entirely upon the extent and depth of the burn.

The traditional classification of burns as first degree, second degree, and so on is becoming outmoded. Instead we refer to whether or not epithelializing elements are still present. In what is known as a *partial-thickness* burn, a regrowth of epithelium is possible, and skin grafting is not necessary (Figure 7-7). Even some cells of the dermis can provide the epithelial growth necessary for healing. In *full-thickness* burns even the dermal epithelial cells are irreversibly damaged. In these cases skin grafting is required. The full-thickness burn may involve subcutaneous tissue, often affecting many of the veins. As a rule in burns of this severity there is destruction of the sensory nerve endings resulting in a loss of sensation that may be permanent, although in some instances sensation has been known to gradually return after extended periods of time. (Although nerve fibers themselves can be irreversibly damaged, receptor cells have the power of potential recovery.)

The initial response of tissue exposed to hot (> 60 C) materials is typically inflammatory in nature. Inflammation is immediately followed by cellular infiltration, extreme edema, and surface blistering. When much of the body has been exposed, the imminent dangers are hypovolemic shock, due to a massive shift of plasma from the vascular system to the extracellular spaces, and a rapid spread of infective agents following widespread skin destruction.

When burns are severe, all parts of the body may become involved. Erythrocytes and platelets are heat-lysed, and there is a strong catabolic predominance throughout the body that is associated with negative nitrogen balance, a dramatic increase in BMR, and a depletion of numerous metabolites, especially calcium and phosphorus. The hypermetabolism is associated with an extreme mobilization of catecholamines in response to the stress, whereas much of the catabolism is thought to be due to a surge in release of glucocorticoids. Such an acute alarming stress as burns certainly would strongly activate the adrenal glands.

THERMAL STRESS AND DISEASE

Can chronic exposure to relatively severe changes in ambient temperature result in disease? When thermoregulatory mechanisms are overworked and begin to lose effectiveness, this form of stress certainly becomes a factor in pathogenesis. Moreover, there is no question that thermal stress greatly exacerbates certain forms of pre-existing pathology.

Aside from the obvious acute disturbances (such as burns, frostbite, heat stroke, heat exhaustion), temperature stress possesses less recognizable, more insidious involvements in promoting pathology. These involvements may be difficult to perceive as far as direct cause and effect relationships are concerned; however, statistical correlations are clearly suggestive. Gastrointestinal ulcers and ulcerative colitis characteristically become active with seasonal change (fall and spring), and those with a predisposition to asthma and other bronchial conditions dread late autumn with its change to colder temperatures. Indeed, it has been shown in many asthmatics that a reduction in ambient temperature is more responsible for bronchoconstrictive distress than the presence of such air pollutants as suspended particulates and ozone. These data may be surprising to many of us. Nevertheless they bring out the true significance of temperature change as a stressor of the human body.

Nor should we overlook the role of temperature stress in promoting secretions of ACTH and glucocorticoids. Resistance to infection and tumorigenesis, as well as freedom from the effects of so-called slow and latent viruses, can become diminished when the

TABLE 7-6
Conditions in Which Thermal Stress Is a Contributing and Aggravating Factor

Bronchial asthma

Gastrointestinal ulcers

Ulcerative colitis

Susceptibility to infections (particularly viral)

Autoimmune processes

Hypertension

Arteriosclerosis

Thyroid imbalance

Chronic bronchitis

Myocardial insufficiency

Allergies

Most forms of arthritis

Acne and other skin diseases

Latent viral outbreaks (e.g., herpes)

Sinusitis

Migraine (and possibly other forms of headache)

Mental conditions

Raynaud disease

Neonatal stress (particularly premature deliveries)

pituitary-adrenal axis remains activated—as it tends to be in perpetual exposure to uncomfortable hot or cold temperatures. In addition, these exposures often bring about anxiety and mental anguish. Experiments with animals have shown that persistent exposure to cold or heat can lead to adrenal exhaustion.

One of the most insidious effects of chronic exposure to cold in some individuals could be a progressive development of habitual overdrive of sympathetic responses and the consequent secretion of catecholamines. A consequent elevation in blood pressure from the vasoconstriction, as well as increases in serum lipids and glucose, would pose risks of injury to the cardiovascular system. A list of disorders in which temperature stress is thought to play an important role is provided in Table 7-6.

The relationship of existing disease to further physiologic stress is exemplified by conditions that interfere with normal thermoregulation. Foremost among these conditions are derangements

TABLE 7-7
Disturbances Impairing Thermoregulatory Capability

Thyroid imbalance

Insufficient mobilization of catecholamine response

Arteriosclerosis

Anemias

Peripheral ischemia (diabetes, etc.)

Cardiopulmonary

Malnutrition

Inflammatory erythema of skin (sunburn)

Acute psychologic trauma

in circulation and neurohormonal balance. Metabolic irregularities associated with imbalance in thyroid secretions interfere with normal heat production. Reduced heat production results also from anemias, diminished blood flow, and any other deviation responsible for a restricted oxygen supply to tissue. Of course any condition that interferes directly with sweat gland secretions, or the sympathetic impulses prompting them, is potentially critical in the presence of warm ambient temperatures. Several of the more frequently encountered disturbances that may impair thermoregulation are listed in Table 7-7.

VARIABLE SENSITIVITY TO TEMPERATURE CHANGE

Clinical records, personal experience, and research data all attest to the fact that there is great individual variation in tolerating temperature change. Over 100 individuals died as a consequence of a winter blizzard in midwest United States in January 1979. For the most part these were either patients with hypertensive cardiovascular disease, or were older, weaker individuals who for various reasons were less tolerant of cold stress. Asthmatics, bronchitis sufferers, those with rheumatic complaints, and those with various degrees of arterial ischemia are especially sensitive to a change to cold weather. Indeed, an abrupt change to cold temperatures has been known to incite much vasoconstriction and significantly elevate systolic blood pressures, even in normal individuals. By contrast, persons with elevated blood pressure and kidney problems often find that the vasodilation and fluid loss (sweat) promoted by warm weather can be beneficial to their condition. Yet excessive heat, particularly when humid, can be quite stressing. A heat wave lasting nearly four weeks in the summer of 1980 was responsible for a total of nearly 1200 deaths in Texas, Arkansas, Oklahoma, Missouri, Tennessee, Georgia, Mississippi, and Alabama.

People predisposed to allergy are usually quite sensitive to change in temperature and humidity; indeed, there are some who are actually allergic to cold or heat itself. Such persons may develop urticaria (hives) when subjected to cold water or cold wind.

Some of the better known examples of sensitivity to changes in temperature and humidity are found in persons who suffer from either upper or lower respiratory distress. The nasal and sinus membranes of persons susceptible to rhinitis and sinusitis may swell in heat or cold, and many of the same individuals are especially sensitive to both high and low humidity. As a consequence, the sinuses do not drain and become sites of chronic infection.

Some respiratory distress sufferers are extremely sensitive to rapid cooling of the sinus membranes. When such people's heads are exposed to cold wind or convection currents from an air conditioner, the sinus tissues become stressed and proceed to react. Headache, sinus blockage, and infection may follow. The bronchial passageways of many individuals are also sensitive to fluctuations in temperature and humidity.

Yet there are respiratory distress sufferers who are more free of symptoms in cold weather than during warm seasons. The reason is not directly related to humidity or temperature alone, but is based on allergic sensitivity to pollens and mold spores which are not present in freezing temperatures.

It has long been debated whether or not exposure to heat and especially cold is important in the susceptibility to microbial infections. Recalling that thermal stress stimulates the mobilization of ACTH and glucocorticoids, which in turn can suppress immune response, it is obvious that cold or heat stress can be factors in contracting and aggravating infectious disease, particularly in respect to susceptibility to the viruses causing colds and influenza. Furthermore, thermal stress, like many other stresses, can revive the proliferative activity of dormant viruses such as herpes zoster, the causative agent of shingles.

Stresses of any kind aggravate, and possibly help to initiate, diseases associated with miscarriage of the immune system—autoimmune processes, for example. In many of these conditions, the presence of virus is suspected. It is of interest that several autoimmune maladies, notably rheumatoid arthritis and multiple sclerosis (MS), can be notably worsened by thermal stress. Moreover, incidence of these particular kinds of disorders is lower in the tropics and subtropics, where temperatures remain more uniform.

‖ SUMMARY

We are constantly undergoing heat exchange with our environment, and since body temperature exceeds most ambient temperatures, we generally lose more heat than we gain.

Heat production is regulated by varying the tone and contractility of skeletal muscle, and by modulating the secretions of epinephrine and thyroxin.

Radiation and convection are effective heat loss mechanisms at cooler ambient temperatures. In warm surroundings, evaporative heat loss is the major thermoregulatory mechanism.

Physiologic control of blood flow to and from the skin is an effective thermoregulator with moderate temperature changes. Dilation of blood vessels near the surface dissipates core heat, whereas vasoconstriction conserves core body heat.

Some peripheral thermoreceptors are stimulated by heat, others by cold. Both relay afferent input to hypothalamic nuclei. Thermoreceptors also are located in the hypothalamus itself whence efferent pathways innervate skeletal muscle, sweat glands, adrenal medullae, and smooth muscle of blood vessels.

When thermoregulation is not effective in cold environments, a precipitous reduction in body temperature called hypothermia occurs. Frostbite is a localized hypothermia, usually occurring in poorly protected extremities of the body.

In exposure to high ambient temperatures there is pronounced vasodilation and loss of fluid from sweating; both actions lower blood pressure and can lead to heat exhaustion. Heat stroke is hyperthermia brought on by failure of heat loss mechanisms.

In severe burns there is a high basal metabolic rate associated with marked tissue catabolism. Of particular danger in serious burns is the threat of hypovolemic shock and widespread infection.

There is a significant correlation between ambient temperature change and the activation of gastrointestinal ulcers, ulcerative colitis, asthmatic attacks, upper respiratory distress, hypertension, and rheumatic discomfort. In addition, exposure to temperature change stimulates the ACTH-glucocorticoid mechanism, which may result in heightened susceptibility to viral infections.

Chapter Glossary

adenosine triphosphate (ATP)   compound that supplies ideal quantities of energy necessary for optimum cellular activity

antipyretic   having an effect of reducing elevated body temperature

homeotherm (warm-blooded)   an animal capable of maintaining a constant body temperature, as opposed to poikilotherms

hyperventilation   rate and depth of breathing that are significantly greater than usual

hypotension   lowered blood pressure

hypovolemia   decreased volume of extracellular fluid

negative nitrogen balance   occurs when protein catabolism exceeds protein anabolism

rhinitis   inflammation of the nasal mucosa

thermogenic   heat producing; calorigenic

vasomotor   involving neuromuscular regulation of the caliber of blood vessels

For Further Reading

Edholm, O. G. 1978. *Man—hot and cold.* London: Edward Arnold Publishers.

Folk, G. E., Jr. 1974. *Textbook of environmental physiology.* 2d ed. Philadelphia: Lea & Febiger. Chapts. 4, 5, 6.

Frisancho, A. R. 1979. *Environmental physiology: Human adaptation; a functional interpretation.* St. Louis: C. V. Mosby Co.

Guyton, A. C. 1977. *Basic human physiology: Normal function and mechanisms of disease.* Philadelphia: W. B. Saunders Co. Chapt. 47.

Ingram, D. L., and Mount, L. E. 1975. *Man and animals in hot environments.* New York: Springer-Verlag.

Kerslake, D. M. 1972. *The stress of hot environments.* London and New York: Cambridge University Press. No. 29, monographs of the Physiological Society.

Lee, D. H. K., ed. 1977. Reactions to environmental agents. In *Handbook of physiology.* Bethesda, Md.: American Physiological Society. Section 9, Chapts. 4, 5, 6.

Ramsey, J. M. 1976. The relation of urban atmospheric variables to asthmatic bronchoconstriction. *Bull Environ Contam Toxicol* 16:107.

———. 1977. Time course of bronchoconstrictive response in asthmatic subjects to reduced temperature. *Thorax* 32:26.

Robertshaw, D., ed. 1977. Environmental physiology II. In *International review of physiology.* Vol. 15. Baltimore: University Park Press. Chapt. 2.

Slonim, N. B., ed. 1974. *Environmental physiology.* St. Louis: C. V. Mosby Co. Chapt. 4.

Vander, A. J.; Sherman, J. H.; and Luciano, D. S. 1980. *Human physiology: The mechanisms of body function.* 3d ed. New York: McGraw-Hill Book Co. Chapt. 15.

Wilmore, D. W.; Long, J. M.; Mason, A. D., Jr.; et al. 1974. Catecholamines: Mediator of the hypermetabolic response to thermal injury. *Ann Surg* 180:653.

Yousef, M. K.; Horvath, S. M.; and Bullard, R. W. 1972. *Physiological adaptations: Desert and mountain.* Environmental Sciences series. New York: Academic Press. Chapts. 2, 4, 6, 7.

8

Sound

‖ **Objectives:** Upon completing this chapter you should:

1. Recognize the widespread presence of noise in today's environment.
2. Be acquainted with the role of exposure to noise in producing cochlear damage and consequent hearing loss.
3. Be informed of the stress from neuroendocrine responsiveness to noise.
4. Perceive that chronic exposure to noise in some individuals may contribute to hypertension and altered immune reactivity.

Unlike thermal stress, which has been thoroughly studied for a considerable time, interest in stress from the mechanical energy we call sound is comparatively new, and there is much yet to be discovered about its effects. This may be due to the fact that our environment had always been a relatively quiet one until the last half century. Except for the infrequent occurrence of thunder, hurricanes, tornadoes, and volcanic eruption, the sounds of nature usually do not exceed 80 decibels.

Today, noise is ever present in the urban environment, and within the last three decades the phenomenon has begun to attract the attention of stress physiologists. Noise is defined as unpleasant, unwanted, or intolerable sound, and it has come to be considered a special form of environmental pollution. We are surrounded by the noise from cars, trucks, jet aircraft, television, rock and roll music, huge crowds, vacuum cleaners, automatic dishwashers, power mowers, motorboats, motorcycles, bulldozers, pneumatic riveters, and jackhammers, not to mention an extensive array of specialized machinery employed in industrial operations. It is estimated that over 17 million Americans are exposed to a degree of excessive noise in their work that will prove to be harmful.

It is becoming more evident that chronic exposures to noise not only can produce damage to the ear and impair hearing, but they also may be responsible for widespread disturbances in various physiologic and biochemic activities of the body as well. Moreover, the environment is becoming noisier. The crescendo of perceived loudness of urban sound has more than doubled in the past two decades, and unlike exposure to bright light, where individuals can close their eyes, ears have no protective mechanisms.

The study of responses to acoustic stress is usually divided into two categories: the effects on the auditory structures, and the systemic effects arising largely from activation of the neuroendocrine system. Before these are discussed, let us investigate something of the nature of sound, and discover how it is measured.

CHARACTERISTICS OF SOUND AND ITS MEASUREMENT

The generation of vibratory energy depends upon the displacement of some physical structure. If, for example, one plucks a guitar string, the movement of the plucking finger is the energy input to the source (the string) which is displaced. Before the string is plucked, the air molecules surrounding it are distributed in a uniform manner. Upon being plucked, the string reaches its maximum displacement in a given direction, the magnitude of which depends primarily upon the inertia and elasticity of the string. As it moves to a point of maximum displacement, the string compresses the air molecules in its path of motion, increasing the air pressure at a point near the string. By this time the string's elasticity has prompted its return to its original resting position. However, because of inertia, the string does not stop at this position but continues past it to a maximum displacement in the opposite direction. In this displacement the air molecules are pulled apart by the motion, resulting in a decrease of pressure. Thus, sound waves are characterized by pressure fluctuations above and below the ambient, or prevailing, air pressure. These features are depicted in Figure 8-1. The string will continue to vibrate until the forces of friction absorb all the energy of the original pluck.

Measurement

The major parameters employed in the description of sound waves are *frequency, intensity,* and *duration.* Though all three are significant in our consideration of acoustic stress, foremost attention is given to intensity.

Frequency is the number of wave oscillations, or cycles, per second. One cycle per second is denoted as hertz (Hz). The range of frequencies detectable by humans (audiofrequency) is 20 to 20,000 Hz. Frequencies above this are designated as *ultrasound,* and those below it as *infrasound.* Certain physiologic effects may be frequency-dependent; higher frequencies are usually more irritating and potentially damaging.

Intensity

Sound intensity is the amplitude of sound waves. The ideal measurement would be to determine the motion energy of air particles or their velocity. However, practical techniques are not generally

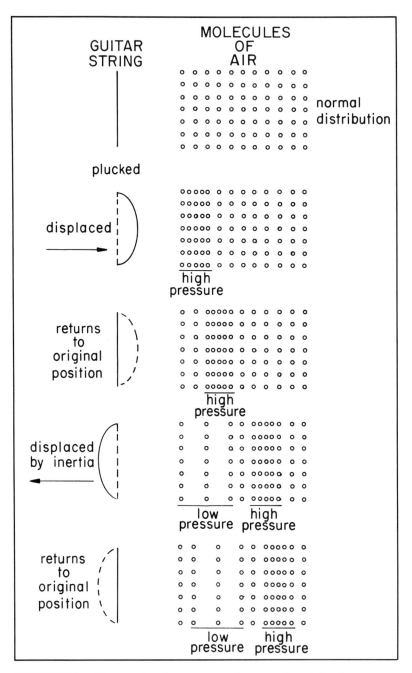

FIGURE 8-1   Changes in air pressure when a guitar string is plucked.

available. The pressure changes can be measured (in watts), yet those associated with most sounds are extremely small quantities; indeed, pressure changes intense enough to damage cells of the inner ear may be less than 0.002 w. Moreover, human hearing can detect a fantastic range of intensities. The maximum sound pressures that can be received without consequent damage are still a million times greater than those of minimum detectability. For this reason, a logarithmic scale is convenient, and sound intensities usually are scaled in *decibels* (db). Since a logarithmic scale has no zero point, intensities must be specified in respect to a standard reference, a decibel in itself being a dimensionless quantity that simply expresses a relation between two sound intensities. Thus, if an intensity is ten times greater than the reference intensity, the logarithm would be 1, and the ratio is designated as 1 bel (10 decibels). A ratio of 100-fold would be 2 bels (20 decibels), and 1000:1 corresponds to 3 bels (30 decibels). A decibel represents an actual increase in intensity of 1.26 times, which is about the minimum amount of change in sound intensity detectable by the human ear.

As a matter of practical convenience in dealing with sound intensity, pressure is the quantity which is actually measured; thus the usual derivation for sound intensity in decibels is given as follows:

$$\text{sound pressure level (SPL)} = 20 \log_{10} P_1/P_0$$

where P_1 is the pressure being determined, and P_0 is the reference pressure.

What value do we employ as a standard reference? Since the least sound pressure level detectable by the human ear is approximately 0.0002 dyne/cm²,[1] which corresponds to 0.0002 millionths of atmospheric pressure (microbar), this value has been adopted as the standard reference ($P_0 = 0.0002$). The relationship of sound pressure in microbars to SPL in decibels is presented in Figure 8-2.

From the view of physiologic effect, the duration of sound exposure can be of the utmost significance. A snap of the fingers can generate a peak level of over 140 db, but since the sound endures only a fraction of a millisecond, it is innocuous. Thus, there is in itself no critical intensity of sound. Only a noise exposure that implies a certain duration can be critical, such as may be experienced near an airport runway, for example. The intensity values in decibels for a variety of sounds are listed in Table 8-1.

---

[1]*Dyne* is the smallest unit for measuring force. One dyne is that amount of force required to move a gram mass half a centimeter during the first second.

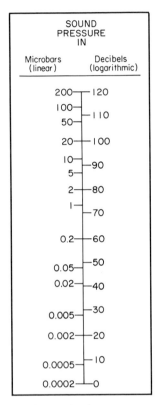

FIGURE 8-2   Linear and logarithmic measurements of sound pressures. One must appreciate that an increase of only 10 decibels (logarithmic) represents a large increment in actual sound intensity.

Sound Reception

Vibratory mechanical energy is not sound until it has been received by specialized mechanoreceptors and transformed to neural impulses. In general, what happens to the mechanical energy when it reaches a human body? How is it received? Is it propagated within the body? Answers to such questions depend on the makeup of particular body structures. When most of the energy is reflected at the body-environment interface, we say there is high *impedance*. On the other hand, structures of the middle ear are adapted for transferring mechanical energy from air to the inner ear fluids; thus the impedance of these structures is low. When there is an input of mechanical energy, certain body structures undergo vibratory displacement much more readily than others, resulting in further propagation of the energy through tissue.

TABLE 8-1

Sound Levels of Common Sources of Noise

SOURCE	DECIBELS	SUBJECTIVE FEELING
Jet plane taking off	140	Painful
Hydraulic press at 3 ft	130	
Rock and roll band (high amp.)	120	
Chainsaw operation at 15 ft	112	Annoying
Thunder	110	
Jet flyover	104	
Power mower at 25 ft	96	
Motorcycle at 50 ft	95	Very loud
Food blender	87	
Diesel truck at 40 mph	86	
Garbage disposal	80	
Passenger car at 65 mph	78	Loud
Dishwasher	75	
Vacuum cleaner	73	
Television	70	Above average level
Air conditioning unit	62	
Average conversation	55	Below average level
Quiet radio	40	
Whisper	22	Quiet
Threshold of audibility	18–20	

EFFECTS ON AUDITORY RECEPTORS

Acoustic stress has been, and is being, studied a great deal with respect to its effects on the ear, and there is no doubting the fact that chronic noise exposure is capable of promoting hearing loss. But before we begin a discussion of this relationship, a very brief review of ear anatomy and auditory function may be helpful. The gross anatomy of the ear is diagrammed in Figure 8-3, in which the outer, middle, and inner ear regions are realistically portrayed. A schematic sketch of the uncoiled cochlear region is presented in Figure 8-4. Although this is not the true appearance of a cochlea, the rendition offers a clearer concept of the associated, functional parts.

The *tympanic membrane* is kept under tension so that sound waves that strike any portion of it are transmitted to the *malleus*. The surface area of the membrane is about 55 mm^2, whereas the surface area of the *stapes* averages 3.2 mm^2. This 17-fold difference times the 1.3:1 ratio of the lever system from malleus to stapes results in 22 times as much pressure on the cochlear fluid as was originally ex-

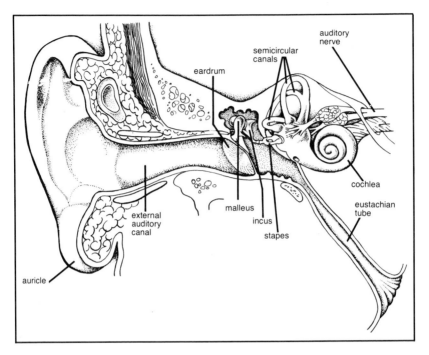

FIGURE 8-3   Gross anatomy of the human ear. Sound waves that are propagated in air through the external auditory canal (outer ear) vibrate the ear drum, 'the waves then being transmitted to the three delicate bones of the middle ear. These mechanical displacements convey the waves into the liquid-filled, coiled cochlea, where specialized hair cells of the organ of Corti transform mechanical energy into the electrochemical energy of nerve impulses along the auditory nerve.

erted against the tympanic membrane. Fluid has greater inertia than air, so this degree of amplitude is needed to adequately transmit vibrations through the fluid.

The inner ear consists of the cochlea and the labyrinth. The labyrinth is not involved in hearing but functions in orienting the organism to gravity (sense of balance). The cochlea is a system of three tubes or canals, coiled tightly side by side. The first two of these are the *scala vestibuli* and the *scala media*, which are often considered together and are separated from the *scala tympani* by the *basilar membrane*. Along the surface of the basilar membrane lies the *organ of Corti*, composed of a series of *hair cells* that are mechanically sensitive (Figure 8-5). The hair cells have sensory hairs at their apexes that project into a gelatinous structure, the *tectorial membrane*. Nerve impulses result from their vibratory movement against the tectorial membrane.

Sound vibrations enter the scala vestibuli from the faceplate,

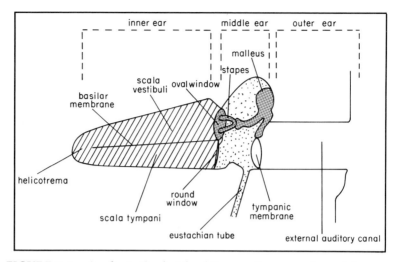

FIGURE 8-4   A schematic sketch of the ear. For convenience this drawing greatly simplifies the cochlea as a straight, uncoiled structure. Sound waves enter the scala vestibuli through the oval window, and the energy is propagated through fluid along the basilar membrane, on which the organ of Corti is situated.

or footplate, of the stapes at the oval window, and the mechanical energy is then propagated along the basilar membrane, through the inner ear fluids surrounding the hair cells (Figure 8-4). The lengths of the 20,000 elastic hairs increase progressively from 0.04 mm at the base of the cochlea to the *helicotrema*, where they are about 0.5 mm. The shorter hairs near the base vibrate at higher frequencies, whereas the long hairs near the helicotrema vibrate at lower frequencies. The transformation from mechanical displacement to the electrochemical energy stimulating neural fibers takes place in the hair cells, which are remarkably sensitive. Deformations as slight as 10^{-11} cm can promote an electrochemical change (nerve impulse).

Noise and Hearing Deficit

There are two distinct impairment mechanisms leading to hearing deficits. In *conduction loss* there is damage to the conducting elements. This loss includes rupture of the tympanic membrane, separation of the ossicular chain of the middle ear, or rupture of the fine membranes (sacs) of the cochlea and labyrinth. As far as sound stress is concerned, it would take an overexposure of intense noise for about a minute to produce such damage. One exposure to an intensity of > 150 db could be sufficient. An exposure of this sort is sometimes designated as a *blast trauma*. Exposure to sonic booms is an

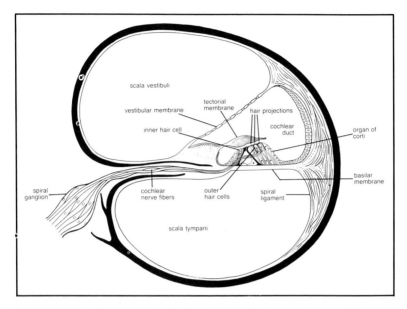

FIGURE 8-5 **The organ of Corti in proportion to the rest of the cochlea.** Observe the highly specialized hair cells and the extremely microscopic hair projections.

example. The intense pressure waves from sonic booms have been known to cause fetal nerve damage. Thunderous sonic booms are generated by supersonic aircraft.

In practically all instances, hearing deficit is a form of *sensorineural* loss, stemming from damage to, and/or destruction of, the sensory cells distributed along the basilar membrane of the cochlea. Typically, this type of deficit is associated with chronic exposures to sound intensities exceeding 80 db—the maximum intensity that ordinarily does not produce sensorineural loss regardless of duration.

At sound levels exceeding 80 db for 8 hours per day, a high percentage of people eventually will begin to show impaired hearing when chronically exposed. For this reason the intensity of noise experienced by industrial workers should not exceed 85 db. However, it is estimated that over 50% of industrial workers are exposed to sound levels exceeding this value. Moreover, many individuals at home, at recreation, and on city streets are exposed at times to noise exceeding 85 db.

Both duration and frequency of the sound also are important. For example, when sound intensity is doubled, the risk of hearing loss will not increase if the duration of exposure is halved. Furthermore, high frequency sounds appear to be more damaging than low frequency sounds. As might be expected, the damage from energy of high frequency is more concentrated in hair cells toward the basal end of the cochlea, where the hairs are shorter.

Evaluation of Hearing Loss

How do we know if hearing loss has resulted from exposure to noise levels? This is usually determined by establishing an *auditory threshold* as a reference point. An auditory threshold is the minimum sound level detectable by the individual. Ideally, the threshold is evaluated before and after an exposure. A difference between the two measurements is termed a *threshold shift* (TS), which can be temporary (TTS) or permanent (PTS). Since there may be reasons for a shift other than sound stress, it may be further specified as a noise-induced TS (NITTS or NIPTS). There is evidence suggesting that men may be more susceptible to NIPTS than women. Other factors capable of inducing TS include variables in the testing instrumentation and procedure, systemic medications and drugs, upper respiratory infections, allergies, and age. Due to hardening of the middle ear ossicular chain, and reduction of vascular supply to the cochlea, almost everyone experiences some degree of PTS with advanced age, a condition termed *presbycusis*. An audiogram illustrating sensorineural hearing loss due to presbycusis is shown in Figure 8-6.

A temporary threshold shift implies that recovery from the hearing loss occurs, and there are several factors underlying the variation in time required for this. With any TTS persisting for more than several minutes after exposure, the noise level and its duration are major determinants of recovery time, high intensity exposure requiring much more time for reversing deficits than lower intensities. In addition there seems to be a wide range of variability among individuals in susceptibility to TTS at a given exposure.

In respect to potential recovery, we may wonder about a relationship between TTS and PTS. Is TTS susceptibility a predictor of PTS? To a certain extent this appears to be true. Repeated TTS over many years, for example in an occupational exposure, can progressively retard recovery time. When TTS caused by one day's noise has not been completely reversed before the next day's exposure, there is an obvious risk of PTS. On the other hand, cases are known in which a particular noise produced considerable TTS at a given frequency, whereas when later PTS did develop, it was in association with an entirely different frequency. Also, where years of noise exposure have transpired, and PTS has developed, it is difficult to assess the role of age as a contributing factor.

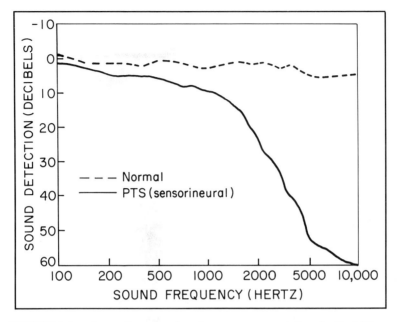

FIGURE 8-6   An audiogram showing a permanent threshold shift (PTS). This is sensorineural impairment commonly found in the elderly. At the higher frequencies, sounds below 50 to 60 decibels become inaudible. (Composed from data contributed by Beltone Hearing Aid Service, Dayton, Ohio.)

The Pathology of NIPTS

It has been established that noise-induced hearing loss is primarily sensorineural, the defect being confined to the cochlea. As a general rule, the frequency spectrum of noise determines the location of damage, whereas the intensity and duration determine the severity of damage. Most of the information relating sound stress to the pathologic insult to the inner ear has been obtained from work with animals. In one experiment, cats were variously exposed from 15 minutes to 8 hours to 115 db at a frequency distribution between 100 and 10,000 Hz. Ninety days later the nuclei of hair cells in the organ of Corti were distorted and enlarged, supporting cells were edematous, and nearly half the hair cells were missing. Essentially the same type of pathology has been demonstrated in numerous other studies where the exposures have varied from a few minutes to 24 hours at about 115 to 130 db.

The specific sites of damage in sensorineural hearing deficit from noise stress are the hair cells. Apparently they are easily in-

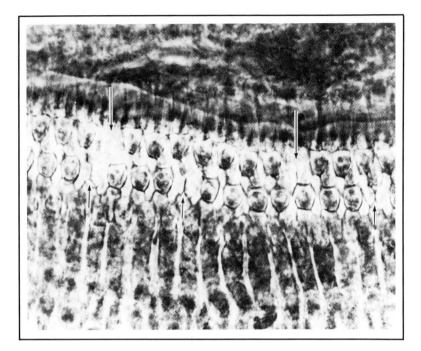

FIGURE 8-7   A badly damaged organ of Corti from exposure to noise. Collapsed cells (small arrows pointing upward) and phalangeal scars (large arrows pointing downward) both are indicative of hair cell necrosis. (From S. A. Falk, Pathophysiological response of the auditory organ to excessive sound. In *Handbook of physiology*, Section 9, *Reactions to environmental agents*, published by the American Physiological Society, 1977.)

jured by prolonged, excessive vibration of the tectorial membrane. Observations with the light microscope invariably show regions of missing hair cells interspersed among the remaining normal ones. This has led to the all-or-none concept, that either a cell will degenerate completely, or survive and maintain a normal appearance. When a hair cell is destroyed, adjacent cells form a scar in its place (Figure 8-7). After noise exposure necrosis of hair cells is not clearly observable with light microscopy until several weeks have passed. With electron microscopy, however, earlier, more subtle changes can be detected. These changes include cytoplasmic vacuolization, mitochondrial swelling, and nuclear distortions. It is thought that excessive mechanical displacement induces extreme vasoconstriction in the organ of Corti, leading to severe hypoxia of the hair cells.

Social Implications of Sound Stress

Exposure to noise has a number of social implications; foremost is its propensity for masking speech signals. All phases of speech communication can be disturbed by noise. Public announcements of importance and telephone conversations frequently are drowned out by other sounds. Huge throngs at sporting events, as well as crowds at large social gatherings of various descriptions, may be completely immersed in sound. Many social events are accompanied by loud music. Speech-masking from noise at social gatherings has become known as the cocktail party effect. People may politely nod affirmatively in response to a spoken comment, while in reality they did not hear what was said.

Attenuation Mechanisms

When considering the effects of sound stress on hearing, it is worthwhile knowing about any protective mechanisms that the ear naturally possesses. There are two mechanisms, but each is restricted in its ability to protect. In the first of these an unexpected sound produces a reflexive contraction of muscles in the middle ear. The contraction can somewhat reduce the conductivity from the ossicular chain to the cochlea. It is estimated that this mechanism can attenuate up to 10 db for lower frequencies, less for higher ones. The reflex is not particularly effective against high intensity levels. The other mechanism is neural and involves efferent pathways from the cerebral cortex to the ear. These fibers synapse with hair cells on the basilar membrane and appear to improve signal-to-noise ratios by imposing some degree of inhibition on the hair cells.

EXTRAAUDITORY EFFECTS OF NOISE

Investigations of the systemic effects of noise have been neither as extensive nor as conclusive as those pertaining to hearing loss. Nevertheless, in recent years such studies have become increasingly frequent. Furthermore, the data suggest that sound can be a significant stressor in respect to the overall body physiology. Most of the effects are indirect, being manifested through activation of the autonomic nervous system and the hypothalamic-pituitary-adrenal axis.

The neural impulses originating from the cochlear hair cells are transmitted by way of the auditory nerve to the temporal lobes of the cerebrum. From there, many neural pathways provide connections with various corticular and subcorticular centers in the brain. Sound reception, continual or intermittent, can strikingly activate subcortical neuronal systems, including hypothalamic nuclei. Thus, we can expect exposure to noise to stimulate autonomic activity and elicit hormonal changes.

Cardiovascular Effects

One of the first detectable physiologic reactions to noise is vasoconstriction. Several investigations with both animals and humans have demonstrated a reduction in blood flow through precapillary arterioles when sound levels of 85 to 95 db were employed. Even placental vessels in pregnant women may constrict, threatening fetal hypoxia. At 110 db as much as a 40% decrease in pulse amplitude of the finger has been demonstrated in human subjects. Moreover, the vasoconstriction response does not adapt with time, but occurs over and over with each exposure at any interval, and the effect often persists after cessation of the sound stimulus. Vasoconstriction as a response to sound has even been observed during sleep.

An expected consequence of pronounced arteriole constriction is an elevation of systolic blood pressure. Rats subjected to an intermittent but chronic audiogenic stimulation of 100 db showed a maximum increase in systolic blood pressure within 8 weeks. Moreover, the hypertension persisted for several weeks after exposures had ceased, possibly due to a resetting of the baroreceptors. Monkeys exposed for 2 to 3 weeks to typical urban noise levels have developed blood pressures 40% higher than values determined while they were in a quiet environment. In still another investigation it was shown that both systolic and diastolic pressures rose significantly in a group of labile hypertensive patients when they were exposed to 30 minutes of noise at 90 db. Furthermore, a substantial number of these individuals demonstrated tachycardia, and the ECG revealed a lengthened QRS segment as well as a diphasic T wave, both of which are indicative of ventricular arrhythmia.

Data from the Federal Health Agency of West Berlin recently produced findings that are now being carefully studied by the World Health Organization. The West Berlin investigators monitored blood pressure of workers in a bottling plant where the noise level is maintained at 95 db. Workers transferred to this environment developed hypertensive levels of blood pressure within 2 weeks. There has also been suspicion of heart damage among some of the exposed workers who had been working in the plant for more than a year.

Perhaps the most convincing evidence of the role of noise exposure in hypertension comes from a recent and extremely well controlled study with rhesus monkeys. In this investigation, moderate levels of realistic noise experienced for several days produced sustained elevations in blood pressure without producing any significant changes in auditory sensitivity. Furthermore, the blood pressure did not return to baseline values after the noise ended. Apparently blood cholesterol levels and atherosclerotic changes also may be related to noise stress. A much higher serum cholesterol level was found in rabbits exposed to 102 db of sound for 10 weeks than was shown in the controls despite identical diets. In addition, the exposed animals began to show atherosclerotic changes in the aorta after 10 weeks.

Persistent exposure to noise is not to be taken lightly as a contributing factor to the arterial vasoconstriction believed to play a role in the development of hypertension. Evidently the hypothalamic induction of sympathetic impulses and the resultant release of catecholamines from the adrenal medullae are the responsible mechanisms.

Other Autonomic Effects

Two other physiologic responses mediated by autonomic pathways can be induced by noise exposure, especially in certain types of individuals. It has been shown that gastrointestinal motility can be increased when an audiogenic stimulus is raised from a low to moderate level. Conversely, motility decreases after the sound level has been lowered. Typically, the motility progressively increases until it reaches a maximum after a few hours of exposure. Sound stress also can affect the gastrointestinal mucosa by way of hormonal mediation. It is recalled that one of the three effects that Selye observed in the generalized stress syndrome of his rats was the development of duodenal ulcers, and one of the stressors he employed was noise (110 db for 48 hours). Selye attributed the ulceration to excessive secretion of glucocorticoids (see Chapter 3).

In many individuals sound exposure of high intensity lowers electrical skin resistance, an effect usually taken as an indicator of sympathetic activation. However, it is not known whether this effect of sound can occur without involving the centers of the cerebral cortex associated with the subjective reactions of alarm, irritation, or excitability.

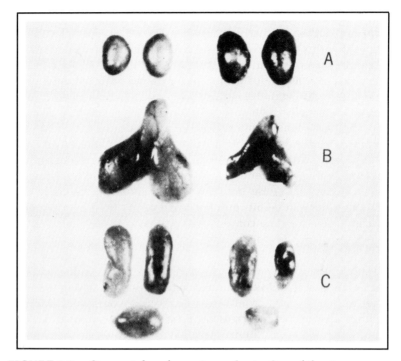

FIGURE 8-8   Organs taken from stressed rats. One of the stressors employed was 110 db of sound for 48 hours. The structures shown on the left are from unexposed controls. Those on the right are from exposed animals. A. Adrenal glands. Note the hypertrophy of those on the right. B. Thymus gland. C. Lymph nodes. Observe the shrinkage and atrophy of both these structures in exposed animals. (From Hans Selye, *Story of the adaptation syndrome.* Courtesy Acta, Inc., Montreal, 1952.)

Effects on the Immune System

Another of the three effects that Selye obtained in his rats when he subjected them to a sound level of 110 db for 48 hours was a pronounced shrinkage of the thymus gland (Figure 8-8). Since Selye's experiment it has become well documented that ACTH and glucocorticoids possess potent immunosuppressive capability. We would expect exposure to noise to be effective in promoting generalized stress responses because of hypothalamic stimulation.

In mice it has been demonstrated that only 3 hours' exposure to a sound level of 120 db produces a distinct leucopenia shortly after the onset of the stress. This effect is not observable in exposed mice that have been adrenalectomized. Moreover, the noise exposure appears to dispose the mice to a greater susceptibility to such viral infections as herpes simplex, poliomyelitis, and Coxsackie B. This degree of audiogenic stress also retards the production of interferon, and results in a notable absence of characteristic inflammatory responses. Other studies in which mice were inoculated intravenously with vesicular stomatitis virus have shown that those exposed to noise are more susceptible to the virus than those unexposed to noise. In addition, mice infected with polyoma virus, then subjected to sound stress, develop more tumors than do nonstressed animals.

Just how reliably the results with mice can be extrapolated to humans is difficult to assess. In the first place, there is probably much greater variation in susceptibility to these effects among people than among mice. Yet, in combination with other stressors, chronic exposure to noise must be looked upon as potentially contributive to alterations in immune reactions, at least in some individuals.

Neuromuscular Responses

Several kinds of electrical measurements have indicated that changes in neural and skeletal muscle functions are among the most sensitive responses to sound exposure. Electromyographic (EMG) recordings demonstrate increased muscle action potential at any sound level exceeding 70 db. A steady noise of 90 db notably increases tension in practically all skeletal muscle, and sounds above 90 db tend to promote hyperactive, exaggerated reflexes. As one would expect, change in electroencephalograph patterns (EEG) constitutes the most sensitive indicator of physiologic response to sound. Even when sound levels are not intense enough to disrupt the relative unconsciousness of sleep, they are still capable of disturbing the sleep patterns associated with adequate rest and relaxation. Without these patterns, irritability and fatigue are experienced after waking.

There is evidence that senses other than hearing may be affected by sound. Exposure to 85 to 115 db sounds lowers the fusion-frequency threshold for blinking lights (flicker fusion) when compared with the fusion-frequency thresholds without sound stimulation. Also, the vestibular sense is often affected by intense, chronic noise. The result is dizziness and loss of balance. This effect is not surprising in view of the anatomic proximity of the vestibular structures to the cochlea.

Metabolic Effects

Brief exposures of laboratory animals to sound levels exceeding 100 db can result in serum elevations of free fatty acids, triglycerides, cholesterol, and glucose. The mobilization of lipid from adipose tissue, as well as the increase in blood glucose, is caused in part by the action of epinephrine. Apparently this hormone is responsive to loud sounds, even when they are of short duration. Studies with limited numbers of human subjects suggest that noise elevates the metabolic rate. Whether this effect is entirely due to the calorigenic effect of epinephrine is not known with certainty. Prolonged increase of muscle tension may be a factor, and of course alterations in thyroid output should not be overlooked.

Hormonal Responses

From the preceding accounts of the effects of noise exposure on blood pressure, immune competence, and metabolism, one might expect to find an elevation of catecholamines and glucocorticoids in the blood and urine of those exposed to excessive intensities of sound. Substantial experimental data from both humans and animals bear out this expectation. Sound-induced (90 db for 30 minutes) increases of plasma 17-hydroxycorticosteroids and urinary epinephrine have been found in normal subjects as well as in patients suffering from various cardiovascular and psychologic disorders. When rats are exposed to 130 db, the secretion of corticosterone from the adrenal cortex is doubled in 30 minutes, and trebled in 60 minutes, a truly remarkable increase. It is no wonder that the adrenal glands of Selye's rats showed a marked hypertrophy when exposed to noise at 110 db for 48 hours (Figure 8-8). Catecholamine response to noise exposure appears to be even more sensitive. Exposure of rats to noise at 120 db (20,000 Hz) for durations as brief as 5 seconds has resulted in a tenfold increase in urinary epinephrine!

NOISE, PSYCHOLOGIC STRESS, AND SOUND–SENSITIVE GROUPS

Are the systemic physiologic effects of noise mediated through the cerebral cortex, as is the case with so-called psychosocial stimuli? Noise can be annoying, irritating, and capable of producing decrement in performance; hence it can lead to an altered subjective state which in turn can effect neural relays to the hypothalamus. In this sense the original sound stress is compounded by psychologic stress. However, what actually happens when auditory neural input reaches the brain depends upon many variables. There is experimental evidence that in some instances the ANS can respond to sound with a minimum of corticular involvement, as when vasoconstriction occurs in a sleeping subject. In fact, there is reason to believe that the activation of hypothalamic nuclei by some sound stimuli can be independent of corticular intervention.

However, even when the physiologic effects involve corticular activation, these effects represent the end of a chain reaction beginning with a unique environmental stimulus, mechanical energy. Therefore, there is justification for separating discussion of acoustical stress from discussion of the stress induced purely by psychosocial stimuli. Despite this separation, it is acknowledged that there are important psychologic components involved in producing the physiologic changes associated with noise exposure. Since human beings are subject to conditioning, many of us become tolerant of noise with repeated exposures. Accordingly, this conditioning should be accompanied by less physiologic disturbance. In fact, some individuals perform more effectively under continual, moderate forms of noise exposure, and premature infants eat better and gain weight faster in response to artificial heartbeat sounds played in incubators. On the other hand, there may be cases in which conditioning to noise can result in increased physiologic reactions. Whenever there is a dreaded expectation of noise, psychologic reactions to stimuli become intensified.

Variables such as age and state of health, as well as individual differences in physical and psychologic makeup, largely determine how well we tolerate noise. Anyone who is particularly sensitive to other physical changes, such as people with allergies and those with finely tuned senses and nervous systems, usually tolerate noise poorly. For example, a sensitive orchestra conductor would be at risk if forced to operate a pneumatic riveter for any length of time. Probably the greatest concern should be for those with preexisting disorders. Individuals already suffering from hearing loss, epilepsy, migraine headaches, hypertension, heart disease, gastrointestinal ulcers, and psychosis certainly can do without excessive acoustic stimulation. Hospitalized patients and those in pain are particularly vulnerable.

‖ SUMMARY

Noise is becoming increasingly significant as a stressor in today's world. Although frequency and duration of sound are important parameters, the most significant quality is intensity, which is determined by comparing the pressure of sound waves with a standard pressure. The units of the derived logarithmic scale are termed decibels. Hertz is the unit of frequency.

The principal form of pathology attributed to noise exposure involves auditory receptors of the inner ear. The damage is characterized by a sensorineural type of hearing deficit which will eventually develop when there are repeated exposures to sound levels exceeding 80 db. This level of exposure is commonly exceeded in today's industrial, urbanized environment.

In animals exposed to sound levels of 115 to 130 db from 1 to several hours, a number of the hair cells of the organ of Corti in the cochlea are injured and destroyed.

Exposure to noise also can elicit generalized stress disturbances in the body by way of neuroendocrine mediation. Auditory nerve impulses to the brain are relayed to the hypothalamus, which activates the pituitary-adrenal axis and the sympathetic division of the autonomic nervous system.

Increased vasoconstriction and muscle tension begin to occur with sound exposures of only 85 db. Relatively brief sounds of around 90 db prompt the release of epinephrine, resulting in further vasoconstriction and elevations of serum lipids and glucose. Such effects, when persistent, increase the risks of hypertension and atherosclerosis.

When noise exceeds 100 db, for a period of time, serum cortisol levels become quite elevated. The resulting immunosuppression may raise susceptibility to infections and tumorigenesis.

Psychologic variables are important in determining the degree of physiologic response to noise. Foremost among individuals intolerant of noise are the high-strung and those with preexisting disease.

Chapter Glossary

amplitude   the extent to which a vibratory wave departs from a mean position

electrical skin resistance   impedance to electrical conduction along skin surface (an assessment of sympathetic nerve activity)

electromyograph (EMG)   measures electrical change during various degrees of muscle contraction

flicker fusion   a test in which light flickers on and off at adjustable rates. The determination sought is the flicker speed at which the human subject can detect flicker rather than sense what appears to be steady light.

17-hydroxycorticosteroids   hormones from the adrenal cortex
interferon   a protein produced by the body that conveys non-specific antiviral activity
labile   easily changeable, unstable
ossicular chain   the series of three tiny bones in the middle ear (malleus, incus, stapes)
precapillary arteriole   microscopic artery that introduces blood to a capillary bed
sensorineural   refers to the primary receptor cells in the cochlea that initiate auditory nerve impulses

For Further Reading

Broner, N. 1978. The effects of low frequency noise on people: A review. *J Sound Vib* 58(4): 483.

Burns, W. 1973. *Noise and man.* Philadelphia: J. B. Lippincott Co.

Chaffee, E. E., and Greisheimer, E. M. 1974. *Basic physiology and anatomy.* 3d ed. Philadelphia: J. B. Lippincott Co. Chapt. 10.

Glass, D. C., and Singer, J. E. 1972. *Urban stress: Experiments on noise and social stressors.* New York: Academic Press.

Howell, R. W. 1978. A seven-year review of measured hearing levels in male manual steelworkers with high initial thresholds. *Brit J Ind Med* 35: 27.

Knipschild, P. 1977. Medical effects of aircraft noise: Review and literature. *Arch Occup Environ Health* 40(3): 201.

Lambert, D. R., and Hafner, F. S. 1979. *Behavioral and physiological effects of noise on people: A review of the literature.* National Technical Information Service. Rep. No. Nosc/Td-267. Rev. 1, 48 pp.

Lee, D. H. K., ed. 1977. Reactions to environmental agents. In *Handbook of physiology.* Bethesda, Md.: American Physiological Society. Section 9, Chapts. 1, 2, 3.

Lipscomb, D. M. 1974. *Noise: The unwanted sounds.* Chicago: Nelson-Hall Co.

Peterson, E. A., Augenstein, J. S., Tanis, D. C. and Augenstein, D. G. 1981. Noise raises blood pressure without impairing auditory sensitivity. *Science* 211: 1450.

Selye, H. 1976. *Stress in health and disease.* Boston: Butterworths.

Singh, R. P. 1980. *Anatomy of hearing and speech.* London: Oxford University Press.

Slonim, N. B., ed. 1974. *Environmental physiology.* St. Louis: C. V. Mosby Co. Chapt. 5.

Welch, B. L., and Welch, A. S., eds. 1970. *Physiological effects of noise.* New York: Plenum Press.

PART THREE

STRESS AND DISEASE FROM NATURAL CHEMICAL STRESSORS

Part Three is devoted to a discussion of chemical substances in the environment that are required by the body, foremost of which are oxygen and a variety of nutrients. Stress is incurred and disease becomes imminent when body cells are provided with either too little or too much of these materials.

9

Oxygen

|| Objectives: Upon completing this chapter you should:

1. Recognize the significance, causes, and classifications of tissue hypoxia (oxygen insufficiency).
2. Have a thorough understanding of altitude sickness.
3. Be informed of the widespread presence of carbon monoxide and know about the pathologic consequences of its inhalation.
4. Be acquainted with the nature of various pulmonary diseases as common causes of hypoxia.
5. Understand the basis of the various forms of anemia.
6. Be aware of the dangers of hyperoxia (too much oxygen).

Everyone is aware that molecular oxygen (O_2) is absolutely essential in maintaining human life. When it becomes unavailable to tissues, for whatever reasons, life ceases within minutes. Even when it is available, there are numerous instances in which the supply is suboptimal for peak metabolic efficiency. On the other hand, there are infrequent cases in which cells can be overloaded with O_2.

The phosphate bond of adenosine triphosphate (ATP) represents energy storage in the cell, and impaired production of ATP constitutes a fundamental stress that has widespread effects throughout all systems of the body. Production of ATP is particularly significant in tissue such as muscle that requires a high expenditure of energy. Adequate ATP is also crucial for the rapid integrative functions performed by the nervous system.

The primary role of cell mitochondria is to couple with ATP synthesis nearly 40% of the energy released during the oxidation of organic molecules. In the electron transport system within the inner membranes of the mitochondria, hydrogen electrons are passed through an oxidation-reduction series of cytochromes. However, if O_2 is not available at the end of this series, ATP is not formed in the mitochondria, where normally 95% of ATP is produced. Thus, O_2 is by far the most fluctuating and limiting variable among cellular components that are essential for ATP production.

A deficiency of O_2 at the tissue level is termed *hypoxia,* and there is reason to believe that chronic forms of this stress are rather widespread. As indicated in Chapter 2, hypoxia is considered to be the primary cause of tissue damage, especially those forms characterized by cellular edema. The swelling results from diminished active transport of sodium and potassium, which in turn is based upon inadequate ATP production. Moreover, there is risk of cellular acidosis from accumulation of lactic acid. Both these effects lead to injury of lysosomal membranes, resulting in a release of their enzymes, the action of which further promotes cellular disorganization and destruction.

How effectively oxygen is supplied to cells also plays an important role in regulating the overall metabolism of the body. For example, in Chapter 12 it is pointed out that the amount of O_2 made available to cells is a significant variable in determining whether one's food becomes energy or fat.

After birth, the source of O_2 is the atmosphere, where there is a rich oxygen content of 20.95 volume percent. The biochemical end-point for the gas is reached when it becomes the final hydrogen electron acceptor in the mitochondrial respiratory chain of each cell. Although there is a plentiful supply of O_2 in the atmosphere, forces are required to get it to the mitochondria. Molecular diffusion, as well as pressure gradients underlying the bulk flow of air and blood, constitute these forces. Diffusion suffices for microscopic distances, whereas bulk flow is required for distribution over greater distances.

When the demand for O_2 by tissue exceeds its supply, a state of tissue hypoxia exists. The critical oxygen tension (PO_2) within most cells is about 1.5 to 5.0 torr. In the interior of mitochondria, it is probably less than 1 torr. If the intracellular utilization of O_2 is impaired despite adequate delivery of appropriate quantities of O_2 to the cells, the condition is termed *histotoxic hypoxia*. A good example of this is the inhibition of the enzyme mitochondrial cytochrome oxidase by cyanide.

The tissue demand for O_2 varies considerably with different conditions. In strenuous exercise, O_2 consumption may increase 30-fold. Likewise, demands are altered in respect to temperature changes and other stressful conditions, often in response to hormonal influences, particularly the secretions of thyroxin and catecholamines.

How are hypoxic stresses incurred? Moreover, how does the body respond to hypoxia, and how is this form of stress related to disease? In preparing to address these questions, let us briefly review how O_2 reaches the mitochondria from the atmosphere.

COMPONENT VARIABLES IN TISSUE OXYGENATION

A prime variable is atmospheric pressure. The higher one goes above sea level, the less the amount of total pressure of the gases impinging upon the earth. An adequate pressure gradient is essential for O_2 delivery by diffusion. Therefore, a reduction in *atmo-*

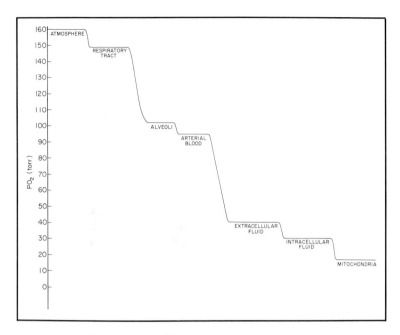

FIGURE 9-1   Oxygen pressure gradient from the atmosphere to cell mitochondria. If oxygen is to reach the mitochondria, a significant gradient is essential.

spheric oxygen pressure (PO_2) contributes to shallow gradients, which in turn promote tissue hypoxia. The cascading gradient of PO_2 from the atmosphere to the mitochondria of the cells is illustrated in Figure 9-1.

The ventilation of the lungs constitutes the next set of variables. Ventilation depends upon a bulk flow of air produced by pressure changes which result from alterations in the thoracic volume. Muscle contractions responding to nerve impulses produce these alterations. If for any reason an adequate volume of air does not flow at an appropriate rate through air passages, the necessary matching of alveolar gas with perfusing blood in the pulmonary capillaries does not occur. In such instances the PO_2 of the alveoli is reduced, and the usual oxygen diffusion gradient to the blood is diminished, resulting in a reduction of the PO_2 in the arterial blood. Pulmonary physiologists refer to the hypoxia resulting from a reduced arterial PO_2 as *hypoxic hypoxia,* regardless of whether it stems from exposure to higher altitudes, or from ventilatory impairment.

Molecular oxygen is not very soluble in water. Therefore, as it diffuses at normal pressures into the blood of the lung capillaries from the alveoli, it dissolves to a limited extent only. With a normal alveolar PO_2 at body temperature, only 3 ml of O_2 dissolves in each liter of arterial blood. However, the free energy of the dissolved molecules creates a pressure or tension (PO_2). Whenever there is reference to blood PO_2, or PO_2 gradients, we are speaking only of the O_2 in solution.

It is apparent that there is a great deal more O_2 in the blood than the amount dissolved in the plasma. This is because once oxygen is in the lung capillaries much of it enters red blood cells in solution. Within each red cell there are immense numbers of hemoglobin molecules. A specific site of the hemoglobin structure has an affinity for O_2. The degree of this affinity is subject to many variables in subtle and complex ways. The association of O_2 with hemoglobin enables the blood to carry 70 times the O_2 that could be transported otherwise. In actuality hemoglobin (Hb) serves as a sink for O_2, because once O_2 is associated with Hb, that particular O_2 is no longer free in solution and therefore does not contribute to the PO_2. This concept is illustrated in Figure 9-2.

Obviously Hb capacity is an important variable in respect to potential tissue hypoxia. A reduced amount of circulating Hb, or diminished numbers of red cells, is termed *anemic hypoxia*. In such cases the arterial PO_2 is usually normal. The relation of O_2 to hemoglobin in particular and to red blood cell chemistry in general is quite intricate; hence, this complex matter is discussed more fully in the next section of this chapter.

Once O_2 has entered the blood in the pulmonary capillaries and returned to the heart, it is conveyed to various organs and tissues by means of the bulk flow of arterial blood. Therefore a major variable in tissue oxygenation resides in how effectively the blood is circulated. For this reason cardiac output is of the utmost importance in supplying sufficient O_2 to the various tissues. Tissue hypoxia stemming from an inadequate perfusion of blood is called *stagnant hypoxia*, or *ischemic hypoxia*. Cardiovascular impairment, whether organic or functional, results in some degree of tissue hypoxia. Tissues that are particularly susceptible include cerebral cortical neurons, myocardium, and cells of renal tubules. Indeed, a greatly diminished level of O_2 delivered to cerebral centers and the heart muscle is very dangerous.

Of course tissue hypoxia is very much a matter of degree, and its seriousness depends upon this variation, as well as upon the duration of time and the particular tissue involved. Generally the first tissues to reflect a state of hypoxia are nerve and muscle tissues constituting the dynamic response system of the organism.

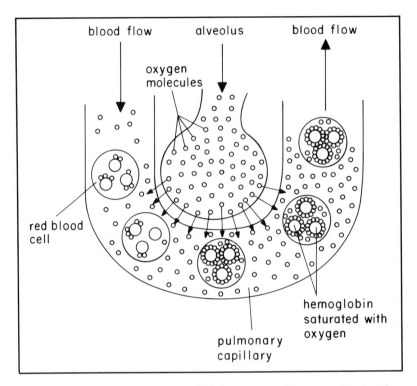

FIGURE 9-2   Hemoglobin as a sink for oxygen. Once associated with hemoglobin within red blood cells, the oxygen no longer contributes to the PO_2. This perpetuates a reduced oxygen pressure in the capillary blood, thereby maintaining a strong alveolar-capillary O_2 gradient.

THE SPECIAL ROLES OF HEMOGLOBIN AND RED CELL CHEMISTRY

In the preceding section it was pointed out that the association of O_2 with Hb is responsible for most of the content of O_2 in the blood. The strength of this association depends upon a number of variables, the most significant of which is the PO_2. Respiratory physiologists describe the relation of the PO_2 to the affinity of Hb for O_2 by graphing the two variables. Such a graph is known as the *oxygen dissociation curve* (ODC), and it is illustrated in Figure 9-3. An accepted point of reference in detecting shifts in the ODC is the particular PO_2 which will saturate half the available hemoglobin (P_{50}). In Figure 9-3 the P_{50} is 26 to 27 torr (mmHg).

A number of additional variables can affect the affinity of Hb for O_2. One such variable is the relative amount of hydrogen ion

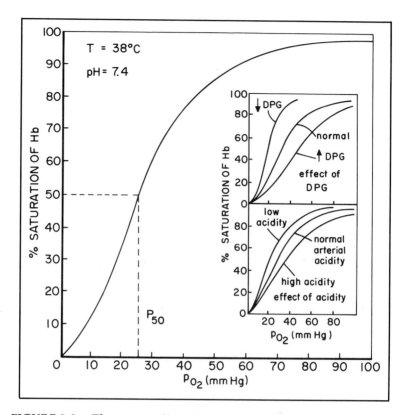

FIGURE 9-3   The oxygen dissociation curve (ODC). Increases in hydrogen ion, temperature, and 2,3-DPG shift the curve downward and to the right, indicating that under these conditions oxygen is more readily released from hemoglobin to tissue. This curve is for human hemoglobin A.

present. Note the lower inset in Figure 9-3. The more hydrogen ion in the red cell, the less the affinity of Hb for O_2. Also, since elevations in temperature are known to disrupt chemical associations, we would expect temperature to affect O_2 to Hb affinity. Indeed, a higher temperature, such as can be found in contracting muscle, increases the P_{50}.

In recent years a common chemical component of red blood cells has been shown to modulate the affinity of Hb for O_2. Mammalian red cells have much greater levels of 2,3-diphosphoglycerate (2,3-DPG) than do most other mammalian cells, and it has been shown that this organic phosphate is an important allosteric effector of hemoglobin's affinity for O_2, meaning that the greater the level of 2,3-DPG, the less the affinity of Hb for O_2. 2,3-DPG is a substrate of red blood cell glycolysis, and it can bind reversibly to deoxy-hemoglobin (Hb not associated with O_2). When binding occurs, this reduces the amount of free 2,3-DPG in the cell, and since 2,3-DPG exerts feedback inhibition on glycolytic enzymes, this lesser quantity of free 2,3-DPG reduces that inhibition, thereby stimulating glycolysis to increase production of 2,3-DPG. Such an occurrence would increase the level of 2,3-DPG in the red blood cell. An elevation of red cell pH also stimulates production of 2,3-DPG, whereas a sustained acidosis depresses it. This happens because many of the glycolytic enzymes are activated at higher pH values.

As indicated above, an increased amount of 2,3-DPG in red cells weakens the affinity of Hb for O_2, whereas diminished levels decrease the P_{50}. Observe the higher inset in Figure 9-3. Indeed, without average levels of 2,3-DPG, the P_{50} would only be about 10 torr instead of 27 torr, which means that without 2,3-DPG there would be a problem in unloading O_2 to tissues. Fetal hemoglobin must have an appreciably higher affinity for O_2 than maternal Hb so that fetal blood can take O_2 from the maternal blood. This difference in affinity is primarily due to the fact that 2,3-DPG has much less effect on fetal Hb than adult Hb.

Hypoxia from altitude exposure, anemias, and ventilatory impairment all are associated with increases of red cell 2,3-DPG which elevate the P_{50}, thereby providing some compensation for the hypoxia.

In stored blood such as is used in blood banking, glycolysis in red cells progressively diminishes, resulting in decreased levels of 2,3-DPG. This can create a problem when blood stored for longer than a few days is used in transfusions. In a recipient who is already hypoxic, the inability of the Hb of the stored blood to dissociate O_2 aggravates the hypoxia.

The effect of 2,3-DPG on the expression of the oxygen dissociation curve sometimes overrides opposing effects from other variables. For example, the immediate effect of reduced blood pH is an elevated P_{50}, yet persistent acidosis eventually reverses the elevated P_{50} by way of a decrease in 2,3-DPG. It is apparent that there are a number of checks and balances within the red cell that operate in maintaining an optimum P_{50} for delivery of O_2 to tissue.

Regulation of Red Blood Cell Production

Since the volume of hemoglobin in the blood is a significant variable in tissue oxygenation, hemoglobin capacity must be regulated in some manner. Certain cells of the kidney cortex (and possibly cells elsewhere) synthesize a glycoprotein hormone termed *erythro-poietin*, which influences the rate of production and maturation of red blood cells in the bone marrow. The hormone also stimulates Hb synthesis in the maturing erythrocytes. Normally the number of circulating erythrocytes fluctuates very little despite a high turnover of cells in which their production tends to balance their destruction. Apparently there is a basal level of erythropoietin always circulating to maintain the proper production rate of red blood cells and Hb for adequate O_2 transport. However, hypoxia induces an elevation of erythropoietin in the blood, and the increase in the hormone accelerates the production rate of red blood cells and Hb. Of course erythropoiesis requires the necessary construction materials. Hence there are dietary variables that are significant in maintaining normal rates of erythropoiesis. Iron, cobalamin (vitamin B_{12}), folic acid, ascorbic acid, and protein are essential nutrients involved in the synthesis of red blood cells.

Studies have shown that it takes about 48 hours of hypoxia before there is a significant erythropoietic response as judged by an increase in the percentage of *reticulocytes* in the circulation. Although an increase in the red blood cell mass is compensatory in hypoxia, such a change is not always an entirely advantageous adaptate. Elevations in red blood cell counts bring about an increase in blood viscosity, which heightens resistance to blood flow, thus elevating blood pressure and imposing an additional workload on the heart muscle.

How does hypoxia come about? The most frequently encountered causes include exposures to high altitude, inhalation of carbon monoxide, and the presence of certain diseases. The basis of stress from exercise is also hypoxic in nature. However, exercise stress is important enough in itself to warrant a special treatment in Chapter 10.

ALTITUDE SICKNESS

If you have ever visited locations that are more than a 1.6 kilometers (1 mile) above sea level, chances are you didn't feel quite the same, at least for a while. You may have noticed some drowsiness and fatigue, even at altitudes of less than 2 kilometers. An individual may also be confronted with altitude hypoxia during air travel. Ascending rapidly to altitudes above 3 kilometers invariably produces some degree of so-called mountain sickness in most individuals. Yet more

TABLE 9-1
Altitudes Decreasing Partial Pressure of Ambient Oxygen

ELEVATION ABOVE SEA LEVEL		PO_2 (TORR)
Km	Ft	
0	0	159
0.6	2,000	146
1.2	4,000	135
1.8	6,000	124
2.4	8,000	115
3.0	10,000	106
3.6	12,000	98
4.2	14,000	90
4.8	16,000	83
5.4	18,000	76
6.0	20,000	70
6.6	22,000	64
7.2	24,000	58
7.8	26,000	53
8.4	28,000	50

than 10 million of the world's people live at altitudes above 3.6 kilometers. Apparently there are acclimating mechanisms that tend to compensate for the hypoxic effects.

It already has been pointed out that atmospheric PO_2 diminishes with increasing elevation above sea level. However, the relation between altitude and barometric pressure is not linear, since atmospheric density diminishes by half with each 5.4 kilometers of elevation. On Mt. Everest, whose peak is about 8.7 kilometers above sea level, the barometric pressure is 245 torr and the atmospheric PO_2 is about 49 torr, as compared to about 156 torr at sea level. The atmospheric PO_2 to be expected at progressively higher points of elevation above sea level is given in Table 9-1.

What happens when one is exposed to a hypobaric atmosphere? This category of oxygen deficit is hypoxic hypoxia, in which the arterial PO_2 is diminished and the PO_2 gradient from the arterial end of the tissue capillary to the cells is depressed. At sea level this gradient for someone at rest is about 95 to 30 torr, a difference of more than 60 torr. If the atmospheric PO_2 is only 100 torr (at about 3.3 kilometers), the alveolar PO_2 would be approximately 60 torr,[1]

---

[1]There are two reasons for the alveolar PO_2 being considerably lower than the atmospheric PO_2. For one, the respiratory tract is saturated with water vapor, and its partial pressure contributes to the overall gas pressure reaching the alveoli. Secondly, the diffusion of O_2 out of the alveoli and into the blood maintains a lower alveolar oxygen pressure.

and the arterial PO_2 only about 55 torr. This does not allow for a significant pressure gradient to the tissues, and hypoxic stress is incurred. A sudden tissue hypoxia of this degree is likely to produce what is known as *acute mountain sickness,* characterized by symptoms of breathlessness, palpitations, headache, nausea, fatigue, disturbances in vision, mental confusion, and impairment of both short-term memory and motor function. Many of these symptoms are the result of an inadequate supply of O_2 to nerve tissue.

The rapidity of onset of mountain sickness varies with the rate of ascent as well as with individual differences. Symptoms usually develop gradually over a period of hours, with a maximum severity reached after 24 to 48 hours. For those remaining at high altitudes, symptoms tend to subside even more slowly, usually disappearing by a week's time. Symptoms of the sickness are prominently exacerbated by exertion. Also, consumption of alcohol may increase rapidity of onset as well as severity. For reasons not understood, women and children experience less severe symptoms than men. Nearly all individuals experience symptoms at 4.2 kilometers or higher, whereas a few that are more sensitive to hypoxia may notice effects at half this altitude.

What are the homeostatic responses to altitude hypoxia? Almost immediately there are increases in the minute volume of ventilation due to the stimulation of the carotid and aortic chemoreceptors by the decreased arterial PO_2. A reduction in arterial PO_2 below 60 torr (about 3.3 kilometers) initiates increases in ventilation. The hyperventilation improves blood oxygenation in two ways. First, the alveolar O_2 concentration is increased in proportion to the decrease in alveolar carbon dioxide (CO_2). Doubling the rate of alveolar ventilation decreases alveolar PCO_2 from 40 to 20 torr, yet raises the alveolar PO_2 by an equal amount. Secondly, in hyperventilation some alveoli that ordinarily are rather poorly ventilated in normal breathing show much improved ventilation, establishing a better ventilation-perfusion ratio. However, the magnitude of the hyperventilatory response is tempered by the hypocapnia (reduced CO_2) induced by hyperventilation. The respiratory center in the medulla oblongata is extremely sensitive to changes in arterial PCO_2. In hyperventilation the pumping of excessive CO_2 from the alveoli diminishes arterial PCO_2 (hypocapnia), thus imposing a limitation on hyperventilation.

A consequence of hyperventilation is a respiratory alkalosis due to a decrease in PCO_2, which in turn reduces the amount of hydrogen ion in the blood. As the individual begins to acclimate, the alkalosis is controlled to some degree by a gradual increase in renal elimination of alkaloid bicarbonate ions.

Another immediate response to altitude hypoxia is an increase in cardiac output. An acceleration of cardiac rate rather than a greater stroke volume accounts for this response. At 3 kilometers and above, tachycardia is to be expected. Hypoxia in the central nervous system appears to increase activity of the sympathetic cardioaccelerator nerves that stimulate beta-adrenergic receptors in the heart. For any given workload the heart rate is faster during exercise at altitude than at sea level. The fact that the initial elevation of cardiac output in hypobaric exposures tends to subside despite the persistence of increased cardiac rates suggests that there has been a decrease in stroke volume. Some investigators attribute this decrease to altitude-induced hypoxic impairment of myocardial contractility. Apparently increased cardiac output is not as permanent a feature of altitude adaptation as hyperventilation.

Blood pressure in the pulmonary artery is usually elevated at high altitudes, both in newcomers and natives. At substantial elevations above sea level there is always some degree of functional right ventricular hypertrophy. It may be that the increase in pressure is beneficial in promoting blood flow in lung regions, such as the upper lobes, that ordinarily are not as well perfused.

In the preceding section of the chapter the oxygen dissociation curve and the concept of the P_{50} were explained (Figure 9-3). With the decreased arterial PO_2 characterizing altitude hypoxia, we find that the P_{50} is increased. For many years the mechanism underlying this phenomenon was unexplained. In fact researchers wondered why the respiratory alkalosis from altitude exposure did not result in a shift of the ODC to the left (decrease the P_{50}). It is now concluded that 2,3-diphosphoglycerate (2,3-DPG), referred to in the preceding section, is the responsible variable. An increase in the quantity of deoxyhemoglobin and an elevated arterial pH both begin to stimulate the production of 2,3-DPG, which in turn promotes dissociation of O_2 from Hb, resulting in the increase in the P_{50}. There are considerable data indicating that exposure to hypobaric atmospheres is associated with increases in red blood cell levels of 2,3-DPG.

During the first few days at high altitude, concentrations of red blood cells and Hb increase. However, this initial hemoconcentration results from a decrease in volume of the blood plasma rather than from increases in red cells themselves. Thus the red blood cell mass increases only by proportion. This early reduction in blood volume may be brought about by changes in capillary permeability to plasma proteins and by a diminished volume of water resulting from hyperventilation. The reduction in blood volume can

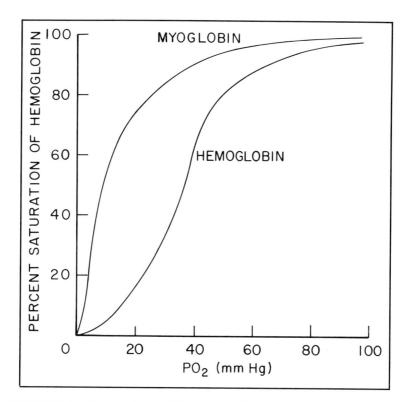

FIGURE 9-4   **Comparison of the oxygen dissociation curves for hemoglobin and myoglobin.**

be associated with decreased cardiac output, and this may be a factor in returning the cardiac output toward normal after its initial increase.

After 48 to 72 hours of hypoxia, newly synthesized erythropoietin has had time to accelerate the rate of erythropoiesis. At this point there is usually no further reduction in plasma volume, and the additional red matter returns the blood volume to normal; or it may even result in some increase in total blood volume.

A potential response to altitude hypoxia that presently is being researched involves the role of myoglobin, another hemoprotein that is associated with skeletal and cardiac muscle. A molecule of myoglobin (Mb) is somewhat like one-fourth a molecule of hemoglobin, in that it has just one heme moiety and one polypeptide chain, whereas hemoglobin has four of each. The oxygen dissociation curve for myoglobin is a rectangular hyperbola, much above and to the left of that for Hb (Figure 9-4). Myoglobin's strong af-

TABLE 9-2
Homeostatic Responses to Physiologic Effects of Altitude

INDUCED EFFECT	COUNTERACTING RESPONSE
Decreased alveolar PO_2	Hyperventilation
Decreased arterial PO_2	Increased cardiac output
Diminished arterial-tissue PO_2 gradient	Elevated red cell 2,3-DPG
	Increase in red cell mass
	Increase in capillary density
	Elevated pulmonary blood pressure
Respiratory alkalosis	Increased elimination of
(due to hyperventilation)	bicarbonate (kidney)

finity for O_2 is adaptive in that Mb can take O_2 from Hb and thereby serve as an O_2 reservoir in muscle, where demands for O_2 can suddenly become quite high. Of course, a very low PO_2 is required to dissociate O_2 from Mb. However, in muscle, where the PO_2 at times can approach zero, the dissociation of O_2 from Mb is not problematical. In addition, there is evidence that myoglobin in some way facilitates the diffusion of O_2, a very appropriate homeostatic mechanism in tissue hypoxia. It has been shown that concentrations of Mb tend to increase in both cardiac and skeletal muscle as a result of prolonged and pronounced hypobaric exposures.

In addition to acute mountain sickness, there is a condition known as *chronic mountain sickness*, which represents some degree of failure in acclimating to altitude hypoxia. Therefore, the only recourse in alleviating the condition is to remove the sufferer from the low pressure environment. It has been proposed that for some reason these individuals do not experience the usual degree of hyperventilation. Symptoms vary but are primarily neural in origin. A summary of the physiologic consequences of altitude hypoxia and the characteristic responses to them are given in Table 9-2.

PATHOLOGY FROM INHALATION OF CARBON MONOXIDE

Most people are unaware of the prevalence of hypoxia from inhalation of carbon monoxide (CO).[2] It is true that most exposed individuals do not become unconscious or die. However, all of us

---

[2] Strictly speaking, carbon monoxide is a man-made chemical stressor. However, since its action promotes oxygen deprivation, a discussion of CO is appropriate in this chapter.

inhale CO at one time or another; indeed, most of us inhale it every day. Low to moderate levels of CO are ever present in the urban atmosphere. The gas is particularly concentrated around city traffic routes and intersections, parking lots, garages, and service stations. A more important source of still greater amounts of CO is tobacco smoke.

Everyone has carbon monoxide in his or her blood exclusive of exogenous sources. When the heme of Hb is catabolized in the liver, one of the substances produced in minute amounts is carbon monoxide. Therefore, endogenous gas is being produced continuously, and exhaled in trace quantities. Ordinarily this is of no health significance; the percent saturation of Hb from this source amounts to about 0.3 to 0.8, except in certain anomalies such as hemolytic anemia when heme catabolism is accelerated and endogenous CO may saturate as much as 1.5% to 2.8% of Hb. However, in sustained rebreathing of the same air, CO can accumulate in the recycled air supply. This problem must be taken into account in administering closed-circuit anesthesia, or in sealed, small-volume cabins or capsules such as those employed for submarine and space travel.

Like O_2, carbon monoxide associates with the ferrous ion of the heme moiety of Hb, and therefore competes with O_2 for this position. However, the competition is extremely one-sided, the affinity of Hb for CO in humans being about 210 times greater than its affinity for O_2. For this reason it is apparent that very little CO can replace considerable amounts of O_2 in blood gas transport. The dissociation curve for CO with Hb is illustrated in Figure 9-5. Note that the shape of this curve is similar to that of the ODC (Figure 9-3). The essential difference between the two graphs is that the partial pressures of CO (PCO) required to progressively saturate Hb are approximately $1/210$ of the corresponding PO_2 values found in the ODC.

Carbon monoxide hypoxia is an anemic hypoxia. Hemoglobin is present but it is not functional in O_2 transport. Moreover, in addition to functional anemia there is another way in which CO inhalation promotes tissue hypoxia. When some of the Hb is associated with CO, the O_2 that is associated with the remaining Hb dissociates less readily than would be expected. The ODC is shifted to the left. This reduction in the P_{50} means that the unloading of O_2 in tissue capillaries is restricted at a given PO_2, and that the cardiac output must be increased to maintain tissue oxygenation. The reduction of P_{50} at several levels of carboxyhemoglobin (COHb) is illustrated in Figure 9-6.

Although CO combines reversibly with Hb, the strong affinity between them means that a considerable time is required to

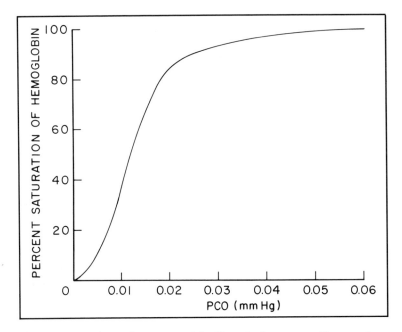

FIGURE 9-5   The carbon monoxide dissociation curve. Observe the
extremely small PCO values in proportion to the percents of Hb saturated.

clear CO from the blood. Hyperventilation accelerates clearing but
not nearly so quickly as the inhalation of 90% to 100% O_2. In individuals who have been overcome by CO inhalation, a therapeutic
mixture of 95% O_2 and 5% CO_2 is recommended. The CO_2 stimulates
the neural breathing center.

In contrast to hypoxic hypoxia, the arterial PO_2 is usually not
diminished in anemic hypoxias. However, since a lower PO_2 is required to dissociate O_2 from Hb when CO is in the blood, the PO_2 of
venous blood draining the tissue capillaries is always diminished in
CO hypoxia. Because of the close correspondence in values of the
two pressures, venous PO_2 is an indirect index of the tissue PO_2.
Hence a diminished PO_2 of venous blood is indicative of tissue hypoxia.

How serious a matter is the tissue hypoxia induced by inhalation of CO? It depends on the CO concentration being inhaled and
the duration of exposure. When the individual first begins to inhale
substantial concentrations of CO, the Hb takes it up at a rapid rate.
Since the CO to Hb association is reversible, some of the CO will
begin to dissociate. When the amount of CO dissociating from Hb
and leaving the body with exhaled air equals the amount being in-

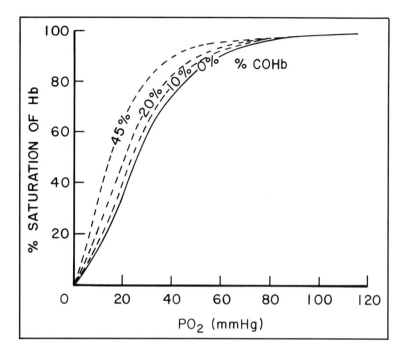

FIGURE 9-6   Modification of the ODC in the presence of carbon monoxide. Note that the more CO present, the greater the curve shifts upward and to the left.

haled and associating with Hb, a point of *equilibrium* has been reached. The time required to reach equilibrium depends primarily upon the concentration of CO being inhaled; thus the higher the concentration, the sooner the equilibrium point is attained. A person continuously breathing 70 parts per million (ppm) CO would require about 5 hours to reach equilibrium. Most exposures to CO, such as smoking or being in congested auto traffic, are intermittent rather than continuous; therefore, as a rule the level of carboxyhemoglobin (COHb) is still rising (preequilibrium) by the end of the exposure period. Habitual smokers may have between 5% to 12% COHb levels by the end of a day, meaning that 5% to 12% of their Hb is carrying CO when it could be carrying O_2.

Many individuals do not experience symptoms below COHb levels of 15%. At or beyond this level there may be frontal headache, dizziness, nausea, and palpitations. When the COHb reaches 30%, visual disturbances, ataxia, and mental confusion are experienced. The ears, lips, and tip of the nose may show the cherry color of capillary carboxyhemoglobin concentration. Beyond 45% COHb the individual rapidly approaches unconsciousness, and a COHb of 65% to 70% is fatal within a few minutes.

The majority of us who inhale CO each day in an intermittent fashion do not accumulate COHb percentages above 3% to 10%. Are these levels harmful? It depends chiefly upon the individual. If one is a young, healthy adult living near sea level, the hypoxia may be considered tolerable. This is not meant to imply that one is otherwise just as physiologically efficient. However, if someone is a small child, or pregnant, or over 50 years of age, or anemic, or has any form of pulmonary and/or cardiovascular ailment, then COHb levels above 4% could very well pose a threat to health and performance; indeed, in some cases of advanced cardiac disease this amount of hypoxic stress can be fatal.

Several studies have been conducted to determine the relation between lower levels of COHb and functional impairment of the nervous system. Some investigations indicate that there can be reversible decrements in visual acuity, psychomotor function, and mental performance at COHb levels between 4% and 15%. Other investigations have not supported these contentions.

Perhaps more concern is warranted in respect to the relation of chronic, low level CO exposures to progressive cardiovascular impairment. In hypoxic confrontations most tissues extract more O_2 than usual from the arteriole capillaries, expanding the arteriovenous (AV) difference in O_2 content. After all, there should be ample O_2 reserve to draw upon because the resting venous PO_2 of around 40 torr maintains an Hb saturation of 70% to 75%. However, cardiac muscle is not as capable as other tissues in drawing off additional O_2 beyond a given AV difference. Therefore, in hypoxia the myocardium must depend upon an acceleration of coronary flow rates. Such an acceleration may pose a problem when compromise in vascular function already exists.

Another factor in the CO-cardiovascular disease relationship is the evidence from animal studies that chronic exposures to modest levels of CO promote atherosclerosis, probably by maintaining hypoxia in the endothelium and smooth muscle of the arterial walls. A third consideration in the relation of CO to cardiovascular impairment is derived from data indicating that chronic inhalation of CO stimulates erythropoiesis. As mentioned previously, an increased red blood cell mass means an elevation of blood viscosity, which promotes peripheral vascular resistance and creates an additional workload for a myocardium that may already have impaired performance.

Of special concern is carbon monoxide inhalation by pregnant women. Repeated exposures throughout pregnancy maintain a state of tissue hypoxia in the developing fetus, resulting in reduced birth weights and possible derangements in the development of the nervous system. Such neural disturbance may well lead to postnatal impairment of mental function. Indeed, litters of rats from mothers exposed intermittently to CO throughout the gestation period are significantly slower than controls in establishing effective operant behavior.

What are the counteracting responses to CO hypoxia? Human beings are not as equipped with acclimating devices to CO as they are for dealing with altitude hypoxia. This is not surprising in view of the fact that people have been visiting and inhabiting mountainous regions for a much longer time than the twoscore years they have been exposed to cigarettes and automobiles. Two of the most significant compensating responses to altitude hypoxia, hyperventilation and the important increase in P_{50}, do not occur in hypoxia from CO inhalation. Since arterial PO_2 is not significantly decreased in low level exposures to CO, it is not surprising that the inhaler of CO does not hyperventilate. In addition, there is very little desaturated Hb in arterial blood because hemes not associated with O_2 are occupied by CO. Then, too; arterial pH tends to remain stable in CO hypoxia because hyperventilation does not occur, and this means that the production of 2,3-DPG is not stimulated. Therefore, the mechanism that increases the P_{50} in altitude hypoxia is not operative in CO inhalation.

There are only two acclimating responses to be considered in CO hypoxia: elevated cardiac output and increases in the red blood cell mass. Both responses may play a role in acclimation to CO, although the degree of response from each mechanism is proportional to the level of COHb. Single exposures to low levels of CO do not produce elevations in either response. However, chronic exposure to CO does stimulate erythropoiesis. Smokers tend to have higher Hb levels than nonsmokers.

Since we do not have a very broad spectrum of compensating responses to CO inhalation, and since this form of hypoxia is characterized by a P_{50} that further aggravates tissue hypoxia, chronic exposure to CO warrants more concern in regard to potential pathology than do some of the other hypoxia-producing conditions.

HYPOXIA DUE TO DISEASE

The fact that physiologic stress can lead to disease is the underlying theme of this book. Disease in turn is stress-producing, and specific diseases result in specific types of stress. For many individuals, particularly those of middle age and older, certain forms of pathology continually impose hypoxic stress on the body tissues; hence the incidence of hypoxia induced by disease is much greater than realized.

The diseases most responsible for hypoxia are those resulting in ventilatory impairment, cardiovascular insufficiency, and the anemias. A substantial proportion of such diseases are chronic and incurable. The central feature of potential incapacitation from these disorders resides in the ensuing tissue hypoxia; hence the patient should avoid other hypoxia-inducing conditions such as inhalation of carbon monoxide, hypobaric atmospheres, and strenuous exertion.

Pulmonary Diseases

There are a number of pathologies leading to impairment of ventilation. Obstructive bronchial disease alone accounts for several major ailments that significantly impair alveolar ventilation. Chronic bronchial inflammation is a common clinical problem that can be both persistent and severe. In this type of condition there is hypersecretion of mucous, edema of the bronchial epithelium, and heightened tion of mucous, edema of the bronchial epithelium, and heightened susceptibility to respiratory infection. Atmospheric pollution, climatic changes, and tobacco-smoking are among the major factors that promote and aggravate bronchitis. Severe degrees of chronic bronchitis are associated with a disturbance in the ventilation-perfusion ratio and a diminished arterial PO_2. In long-standing cases there may be pronounced dilatation and distortion of the bronchi and bronchioles extending through the submucosa into the muscular coat. This complication, called *bronchiectasis*, results in poorly ventilated lungs, a reduced arterial PO_2, and hypercapnia (CO_2 retention).

Bronchial asthma is characterized by a functional, paroxysmal reduction in the diameter of the airways. The bronchial constriction is provoked by vagus nerve impulses, which in turn respond to allergic, thermal, and emotional stressors. In asthmatic episodes the inspired air is not uniformly distributed, and the arterial PO_2 is often reduced. Various references to bronchial asthma are found in Chapters 7, 15, 17, and 18.

By far the most devastating of the obstructive pulmonary diseases is *chronic obstructive emphysema*, in which there is progressive, irreversible bronchial obstruction, a permanent overdistention of the alveoli, and a degeneration of alveolar septa. The consequences of these deviations are pronounced air-flow resistance, a profoundly disturbed ventilation-perfusion ratio, diminished lung compliance, and reduced diffusing capacity of the alveoli. In emphysema gaseous exchange through the walls of the alveoli is impaired, and not only is there a reduced arterial PO_2, but usually hypercapnia as well. Tissue hypoxia is unavoidable. The emphysema patient experiences persistent dyspnea (labored breathing) and an increase in rate of breathing. The increase in breathing rate results from the drive imposed by the elevated arterial PCO_2. In response to the hypoxia the emphysema patient is often polycythemic and may show increases in cardiac output. Such patients must avoid exertion and conserve energy, most of which is spent in breathing effort. Progress of the disease often results in hypoxia severe enough to require periodic oxygen therapy. The prognosis for emphysema is usually unfavorable. Cardiopulmonary complications eventually tend to develop, leading to death.

Current concepts of the pathogenesis of emphysema indicate that it results from an imbalance of elastase and antielastase activity within alveolar structures. Damage is a consequence of attack on the alveolar connective tissue by elastolytic proteases from lung leucocytes and macrophages. Normally the tissue is protected against elastase-mediated attack by the antiprotease, *alpha-antitrypsin,* present in alveolar epithelial fluid. An inherited deficiency of this antiprotease results in emphysema that requires less environmental provocation and can occur before middle age in some cases. However, practically all emphysema patients have normal concentrations of alpha-antitrypsin, at least at the beginning of the disease.

It has now been shown that cigarette-smoking inactivates alpha-antitrypsin through oxidation. Thus the principal risk factor for developing emphysema in practically all persons is environmental rather than genetic. Both tobacco-smoking and exposure to air pollutants have been implicated. Brief inhalation exposure of rats to 3 to 6 puffs of cigarette smoke significantly decreases elastase inhibitory capacity per milligram of alpha-antitrypsin in lung lavage fluid. Samples of human serum obtained immediately after smoking also show decreased elastase inhibitory capacity per milligram of alpha-antitrypsin. Moreover, determination of antielastase activity of alpha-antitrypsin obtained from the lungs of smoking and nonsmoking individuals revealed a twofold reduction in the activity of this antiprotease in the lungs of the smokers. A comparison of the emphysematous lung with normal tissue is shown in Figure 9-7.

Even when air is conveyed normally through the bronchi and bronchioles, there are diseases in alveolar tissue itself that can result in a diminished arterial PO_2. Sometimes these pathologies are considered together under the heading of *pulmonary parenchymal dis-*

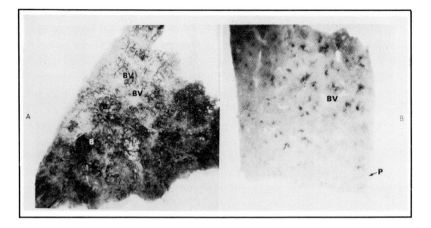

FIGURE 9-7 **Comparison of emphysematous and normal lungs.** A. Observe the gross features of the lung at left, from a patient with long-standing emphysema. B. The lung is normal. BV = blood vessel. B = emphysematous bleb. P = pleural membrane. (From G. L. Waldbott, *Health effects of environmental pollutants*, 2d ed. St. Louis: C. V. Mosby Co., 1978.)

ease. In *atelectasis* the alveoli tend to remain collapsed. This may arise from unusual external pressure from air or fluid in the pleural cavity, or when there is a chest deformity such as *kyphoscoliosis*. On the other hand, atelectasis could be due to an occlusion at a terminal bronchiole. *Pulmonary consolidation* results in alveolar tissue that loses its airy consistency and becomes fluid-filled or solid-like. Causes of pulmonary consolidation include tumors or cysts, the pulmonary congestion secondary to heart and kidney disease, and the alveolar inflammation from pneumonia. One of the more common alveolar diseases is *pulmonary fibrosis,* in which the major problem is a resistance to the diffusion of O_2.

Pulmonary vascular disease can affect the ventilation-perfusion ratio and thereby promote tissue hypoxia. When the systolic pulmonary pressure exceeds 30 torr, and the diastolic pressure exceeds 15 torr, pulmonary hypertension exists. This can stem from several causes such as an elevated left atrial pressure from mitral valve disease, or from left ventricular failure, or from increased pulmonary blood flow due to a ventricular septal defect. However, pulmonary hypertension more typically is a response to hypoxia rather than a cause of it.

Pulmonary embolism, pulmonary edema, pulmonary arteriovenous aneurysm, and pulmonary tuberculosis are other disease entities that can result in hypoxia. Though not as frequently encoun-

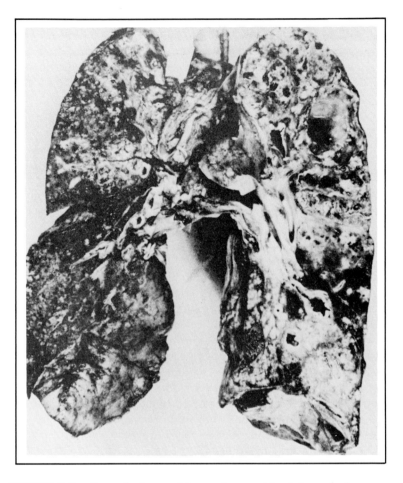

FIGURE 9-8   Gross features of lungs damaged by tuberculosis.
Observe the large areas of destruction. (From W. Boyd and H. Sheldon, *An introduction to the study of disease*, 7th ed. Philadelphia: Lea & Febiger, 1977.)

tered as in the past, tuberculosis remains as one of the more dreaded, incapacitating forms of lung pathology (Figure 9-8).

Some infrequently encountered respiratory ailments, such as pleural disease or diaphragmatic disease, can impair ventilation. Certain diseases of the nervous system also can suppress both the rate and depth of ventilation. It can be seen that the type of hypoxia found as a consequence of pulmonary diseases is typically hypoxic hypoxia characterized by a diminished arterial PO_2. A list of the major hypoxia-producing respiratory diseases appears in Table 9-3.

In hypoxia resulting from respiratory disease, there is usually

TABLE 9-3
Major Hypoxia-Producing Respiratory Diseases

Chronic bronchitis
Bronchiectasis
Bronchial asthma
Chronic obstructive emphysema
Atelectasis
Pulmonary fibrosis
Pulmonary hypertension
Pulmonary embolism
Pulmonary arteriovenous aneurysm
Pneumoconiosis

some degree of hyperventilation stemming from diminished arterial PO_2. In addition, there can be an appreciable amount of desaturated Hb which tends to stimulate production of 2,3-DPG in red blood cells. Many patients with chronic ventilatory impairment indeed show an elevation of 2,3-DPG in their red blood cells. However, the elevation is not as striking as it is in cases of altitude hypoxia—perhaps because the hypercapnia sometimes associated with lung disease tends to suppress the respiratory alkalosis resulting from hyperventilation. Preventing a rise in blood pH could restrict the production of 2,3-DPG. Other compensatory responses to the hypoxia from respiratory disease include the stimulation of erythropoiesis and increases in cardiac output.

Cardiovascular Disease

Stagnant hypoxia was mentioned in an earlier section of the chapter. Any anomaly or disease process impairing the delivery of an adequate volume of blood contributes to stagnant hypoxia. There are numerous cardiovascular deviations that lead to hypoxia of the tissues. It is reasonable to assume that a majority of individuals beyond 50 to 55 years of age experience some degree of impaired blood perfusion regardless of whether a specific disease process is recognized.

Since an ailment that in any way results in circulatory insufficiency is thereby a hypoxia-producing disease, those conditions resulting in various degrees of *shock* deserve attention. Shock is characterized by a very low-perfusion circulatory insufficiency leading to a pronounced imbalance between metabolic needs of vital organs and available blood flow. Hemophilia can produce hypovolemic shock. Thrombosis of the minute vessels can introduce a progressive shock, and diseases of the nervous system, particularly those damaging brain centers, can result in neurogenic shock. Reduced cardiac output and hypotension stemming from depression of the vasomotor center of the medulla oblongata sometimes accompany allergic stress; and of course various degrees of circulatory failure stem from heart diseases. Foremost among cardiac disorders are disease of the coronary arteries and valvular heart anomalies such as aortic and mitral stenosis.

Diseases of the blood vessels constitute the major cause of stagnant hypoxia in those over 50 years of age. Venous dilation and pooling of venous blood affects cardiac output by restricting venous return. However, arterial disease is both more widespread and more conducive to chronic hypoxia than are vein problems. It is pointed out in Chapter 5 that progressive atherosclerosis in modern society is so frequent that it is expected in the majority of individuals past middle age. The entire progression of this disease is typified by a vicious cycle, in that the resulting resistance to arterial blood flow creates hypertension, which in turn is a factor in further damage to the arterial walls, thus promoting further the resistance to blood flow. The ensuing ischemic hypoxia continues to make matters worse by furthering the development of atherosclerosis and by compromising the contractility of a myocardium already strained by the entire process.

It has been mentioned that atherosclerosis may become a problem in diabetes mellitus. Arteries may become diseased, and capillaries as well. Atherosclerosis is likewise a complication in long-standing, untreated hypothyroidism. It is no coincidence that an impairment of short-term memory is a common characteristic of both senile persons and sufferers of mountain sickness. In each case the individual is experiencing cerebral hypoxia.

In stagnant hypoxia there is usually no appreciable reduction in arterial PO_2; therefore, compensatory hyperventilation is not to be expected. Also, the amount of desaturated Hb may be limited and the blood pH is relatively stable. Therefore, little compensation is expected from 2,3-DPG, although actual data pertaining to this point are equivocal. Increases in cardiac output may offer compensation for ischemic hypoxia, but such increases would only augment the stress on a heart with impaired mechanisms. One of the few consistent homeostatic responses is stimulation of erythropoiesis; yet the potential compensation here may be nullified by the tendency of an increased blood viscosity to aggravate the reduced flow rates already existing in stagnant hypoxia.

Hypoxia resulting from cardiovascular disease affords an excellent example of positive feedback: the hypoxia aggravates the cardiovascular condition, which then is responsible for additional hypoxia.

Anemias

Anemia is defined as a subnormal number of circulating erythrocytes, a subnormal quantity of circulating hemoglobin, and a reduced volume of packed red blood cells (hematocrit value). Most hematologists consider a red blood cell count below 4 million per cubic millimeter of blood, or a hemoglobin content of less than 13.5 grams per 100 milliliters of blood, or a hematocrit value of less than 39% to be diagnostic of anemia in an adult male. Adult females normally have less red matter in the blood, in part because the male hormone, testosterone, promotes erythropoiesis. Red blood cell counts of less than 3.5 million per cubic millimeter of blood, Hb levels of less than 12.0 grams per 100 milliliters of blood, and hematocrits below 34% are suggestive of anemia in the adult female. However, the precise cutoff point for normalcy is somewhat arbitrary. Other hormones, notably those from the thyroid, stimulate erythropoiesis, and mild anemia is often a characteristic feature of hypothyroidism.

Anemia itself is not a disease but is a manifestation of some underlying abnormality. Hence there is a lengthy list of types of anemia, and most of these can be classified in six or seven categories. Such a classification is presented in Table 9-4. As noted there, the major causes are hemorrhage, dietary deficiencies, mutant hemoglobins, infections, toxins, drugs, autoimmunity, and complications from other diseases such as malignancies, myxedema, and uremia. In anemias from any cause there is risk of tissue hypoxia, and the cardinal symptom of anemia is fatigue. In addition, there may be complaints of nervousness, not being warm enough, and loss of strength.

In dietary anemia the most critical deficiencies are those of iron and cobalamin (vitamin B_{12}). Pernicious anemia is a chronic, severe condition related to deficiencies in vitamin B_{12} and folic acid. In this type of anemia an adequate diet alone is not enough. Sufferers from this macrocytic form of anemia become deficient in a substance from gastric secretion (intrinsic factor) necessary for the

TABLE 9-4

Causes of Anemia

I. Hemorrhage
   a. injuries
   b. excessive menstruation
   c. gastrointestinal ulcers
   d. ulcerative colitis
II. Dietary Deficiencies
   1. Simple deficiencies
      a. iron
      b. vitamin B_{12} and folic acid
      c. other B vitamins
      d. protein
      e. ascorbic acid
      f. vitamin E
   2. Pernicious anemia (due to insufficient gastric secretion promoting B_{12} absorption)
III. Erythrocytic Membrane Instability
   Premature hemolysis due to:
      a. infective agents
      b. damage from lipid peroxidation
      c. hereditary defects (deviant surface antigens)
      d. drug toxicity
      e. autoimmunity
IV. Endocrine Deficiencies
      a. gonadal steroids
      b. thyroid hormones
      c. adrenal hormones
V. Hemoglobinopathies
   Inherited mutant hemoglobins
      a. sickle-cell anemia
      b. thalassemia
VI. Specific Diseases
      a. leukemias
      b. other malignancies
      c. uremia (kidney damage supresses erythropoietin synthesis)
VII. Bone Marrow Damage
      a. from ionizing radiation
      b. from drugs
      c. lead toxicity

absorption of vitamin B_{12} into the blood. This form of anemia is effectively treated by injections of vitamin B_{12} and folic acid directly into the bloodstream.

In *hemolytic anemia* the red blood cell is not able to maintain its cellular organization and membrane structure for the usual period of time (around 120 days), and the membrane ruptures. Thus

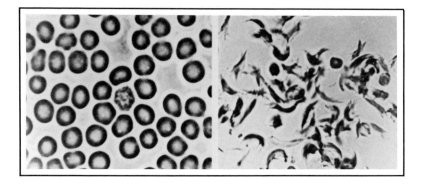

FIGURE 9-9   Red blood cells from a victim of sickle-cell anemia.
Left, normal cells. *Right,* the sickle cells are deoxygenated cells which are much more distorted than oxygenated ones. Very few corpuscles have retained a normal shape. Their severe distortion causes them to aggregate and break easily. (Courtesy of Dr. Anthony C. Allison.)

erythrocytic destruction is premature, and when the rate of destruction exceeds the rate of production, the consequence is anemia. There are various causes of membrane fragility ranging from infections to drug use to autoimmunity. Hemolytic anemia is often characterized by elevated levels of bilirubin in the blood and urine, due to the excessive hemoglobin breakdown. An abnormal accumulation of bilirubin in blood and tissues results in *jaundice.*

Sickle-cell anemia is representative of the hemoglobinopathies, conditions in which mutant genes transcribe for alternate sequences of amino acids in the polypeptide chains of Hb. Not only does the difference affect the relationship of O_2 with hemoglobin, but the abnormal Hb, when deoxygenated, greatly distorts the shape of the red blood cells and affects their normal dispersion in the plasma (Figure 9-9). For example, hemoglobin S of sickle-cell anemia may cause an aggregation of the sickle-shaped red cells. Clumps of aggregated cells create obstruction of smaller blood vessels, thus hindering blood perfusion. The resulting ischemia is known as *sickle-cell crisis.*

In another group of inherited hemoglobin disorders, the globins have a normal amino acid sequence, but the globin chains are reduced in length. These are the *thalassemias.* This form of anemia is frequently found in persons with Mediterranean ancestors. One of the problems for victims of thalassemia is that their bodies metabolize iron poorly. Rather than salvaging and reutilizing iron in the normal way, thalassemia patients receiving transfusions experience a buildup of iron in vital organs (namely, heart and liver).

Because of this, only the youngest red blood cells should be used in transfusions, because reticulocytes last much longer before hemolyzing and depositing their iron.

Anemia is an eventual outcome in the leukemias and Hodgkin disease, as well as in many other malignancies. Severe hypoxia stemming from anemia is quite often the fatal blow for patients with these malignancies.

A number of prescription drugs, including some of the broad-spectrum antibiotics, are capable of retarding erythropoiesis, ultimately resulting in mild degrees of transient anemia. Moreover, the ingestion or inhalation of lead compounds can interfere with heme synthesis, and this leads to diminished levels of Hb.

The arterial PO_2 is not usually diminished in anemia, so ventilation is not significantly increased. However, the P_{50} is increased, which appears to be due to an elevation of 2,3-DPG. Indeed, the level of Hb in red blood cells is inversely proportional to the amount of 2,3-DPG. Normally the two substances are of equimolar concentrations in red blood cells. When there is less Hb, the dilute red cell cytoplasm enhances action of glycolytic enzymes, thereby promoting 2,3-DPG production. Another compensation in anemia is an increase in cardiac output with an acceleration of flow rates in the vascular system. The thin blood of an anemic creates much less than the usual vascular resistance to flow.

Of the three major groups of diseases contributing to tissue hypoxia, the respiratory diseases show the most compensatory responses, and the cardiovascular diseases show the least. Of course there are other, less frequent diseases that may cause hypoxic stress. For example, in thyrotoxicosis, hypoxic stress may be imposed by the unusual tissue demand for O_2.

HYPEROXIA

Until this point in the chapter concern has been with insufficient oxygenation of tissue. Excessive oxygenation (hyperoxia) is not often encountered, but it can be quite toxic, thereby imposing a stress of its own. Oxygen is very reactive, and mitochondrial systems are designed for handling only so much of the gas per unit of time. If one recalls that the hemoglobin of a normal individual near sea level is about 97% saturated, then it is obvious that inhaling higher percentages of O_2, or inhaling it at higher pressures, is essentially of no benefit.

Under what circumstances can hyperoxia occur? One risk occurs in exploration of unusual environments, as in deep sea diving or space travel where O_2 is artificially packaged, and gas pressures are atypical. Also, in certain clinical procedures, heart surgery, for example, the pressure of inhaled O_2 is substantially increased, sometimes to 3 atmospheres for restricted periods of time. Hyperbaric O_2 may be employed in the radiotherapy of certain types of tumors, since it is known that higher O_2 tensions increase the radiosensitivity of neoplastic cells.

Acute Toxicity

Oxygen clearly becomes toxic to living cells after prolonged exposure to twice the normal PO_2. Exposures to pressures of more than 3 atmospheres can produce pronounced cellular toxicity within a few hours. The first symptoms are mucous membrane irritation, pulmonary congestion and edema, nausea, dizziness, muscular twitching, and visual disturbance. Eventually there can be ocular damage, convulsive seizures, and coma. Physical activity increases the susceptibility to the toxicity.

There appear to be three mechanisms underlying the toxic effects of hyperoxia on pulmonary and neural tissue. Excessive O_2 can inactivate oxidative enzymes, interfering with their ability to form high-energy phosphate bonds. Also, hyperoxia promotes vasoconstriction and a decrease in blood flow, thus restricting the availability of nutrients required by neural tissue and jeopardizing the removal of CO_2 and nitrogenous end-products. In addition, excessive O_2 leads to high cellular concentrations of free radicals that oxidize many essential cellular elements, thereby creating the possibility of structural damage to mitochondrial systems and nuclear materials. It has been revealed recently that even normal pressures and volumes of O_2 in cells can produce the reactive superoxide radical as a product of the usual biologic reduction of O_2. A group of enzymes normally protect against the hazard of these radicals. However, in hyperoxia these enzymes become saturated and their capacity for handling substrate is exceeded.

Chronic Toxicity

In acute O_2 poisoning the inhaled PO_2 is elevated, thus allowing the PO_2 of all tissues to rise. When an individual is exposed to a higher than normal volume of O_2 ($>21\%$), but at normal atmospheric pressure, acute O_2 toxicity does not develop. However, if the volume of

O_2 is high (near 100%), pulmonary distress is progressively experienced within a few days. Pulmonary edema represents localized damage, resulting from oxidation of essential compounds in the respiratory epithelium. Other tissues of the body are protected, however, because O_2 is being delivered to them at a normal PO_2, the hemoglobin of the blood serving as a buffer system for the elevated volume of O_2 in the inspired air. The localized pulmonary effect of hyperoxia is termed *chronic O_2 toxicity*.

|| SUMMARY

Hypoxic stress is incurred whenever the tissue demand for oxygen exceeds its supply. The source of oxygen is the atmosphere, and forces such as bulk flow and diffusion gradients are required to move the gas to the mitochondria of the cells.

Because of the low solubility of oxygen in blood, hemoglobin is necessary in maintaining a substantial content of O_2 in blood transport. The principal variable in the association and dissociation of Hb with O_2 is the blood oxygen pressure (PO_2). Elevations in three other variables (temperature, hydrogen ion, and red blood cell 2,3-DPG) enhance the dissociation of O_2 from Hb, and thus can be compensating in hypoxia.

A common response to hypoxia is an increase in red blood cells and hemoglobin brought about by the influence of the hormone erythropoietin on the production and maturation of cells in the bone marrow.

Exposure to high altitudes results in hypoxic hypoxia, leading to both acute and chronic forms of mountain sickness. The diminished arterial PO_2 stimulates hyperventilation and leaves the Hb partially desaturated. Both the alkalosis from the hyperventilation and the desaturated Hb promote an elevation of 2,3-DPG, which permits delivery of O_2 at a higher PO_2. Additional compensation is afforded by an increase in erythropoiesis.

Inhalation of carbon monoxide, which competes with oxygen for association with Hb, results in an anemic hypoxia. Particular attention should be given to the role of CO in producing and aggravating pathology because: (a) many individuals inhale it regularly; (b) there is no compensation from either hyperventilation or elevated 2,3-DPG; and (c) the presence of CO in the blood additionally promotes tissue hypoxia by restricting the dissociation of O_2 from Hb.

Chronic tissue hypoxia is a consequence of many diseases, chiefly those of the respiratory and cardiovascular systems, as well as those producing anemia. Among these categories the stagnant hypoxia from cardiovascular disease has the most limited compensation.

The enzyme systems of mitochondria are adjusted to handle only so much oxygen at a time. Consequently, inhaling air with an elevated PO_2 leads to oxygen toxicity.

Chapter Glossary

alveoli the terminal microscopic air sacs of the lungs in which respiratory gases enter and leave the blood of the pulmonary capillaries

atmosphere a term used to denote the amount of atmospheric pressure at sea level, which is 760 torr. Two atmospheres describes a pressure twice this amount

ataxia staggering, uncoordinated locomotion

deoxyhemoglobin hemoglobin not associated with oxygen (reduced hemoglobin)

erythropoiesis production of new red blood cells and hemoglobin in the bone marrow

hematocrit the percentage of whole blood that is cellular as opposed to plasma

heme an iron containing porphyrin that is associated with polypeptide in forming hemoglobin and myoglobin

hypercapnia excessive carbon dioxide in the blood (opposite of hypocapnia)

hypobaric significantly less gas pressure than usual, for example, as occurs at high elevations (opposite of hyperbaric)

kilometer 1000 meters; equivalent to about 3300 ft, or 0.6 mile

lung compliance the elasticity or stretchability of the lungs and chest wall

macrocytic cells that are larger than usual

polycythemic having significantly greater numbers of red blood cells than normal

red blood cell mass the total amount of circulating erythrocytes

reticulocytes newly produced red blood cells entering the circulation

ventilation-perfusion ratio ratio of volume of alveolar gas to the volume of capillary blood perfusing the lungs

For Further Reading

Bank, A.; Mears, J. G.; and Ramirez, F. 1980. Disorders of human hemoglobin. *Science* 207:486.

Buehlmann, A. A., and Froesch, E. R. 1979. *Pathophysiology.* New York: Springer-Verlag.

Coburn, R. F., chairman. 1977. *Carbon monoxide.* Subcommittee on Carbon Monoxide. Committee on Medical and Biological Effects of Environmental Pollutants. National Research Council. Washington, D.C.: National Academy of Sciences.

Fridovich, I. 1978. The biology of oxygen radicals. *Science* 201:875.

Frisancho, A. R. 1979. *Environmental physiology: Human adaptation; a functional interpretation.* St. Louis: C. V. Mosby Co.

Gadek, J. E.; Fells, G. A.; and Crystal, R. G. 1979. Cigarette smoking induces functional antiprotease deficiency in the lower respiratory tract of humans. *Science* 206:1315.

Green, J. H. 1978. *Basic clinical physiology.* New York: Oxford University Press. Chaps. 6, 8, 9, 10.

Grote, J.; Reneau, D.; and Thews, G. 1976. Oxygen transport to tissue II. In *Advances in experimental medicine and biology.* Vol. 75. New York: Plenum Press.

Hillman, R. S., and Finch, C. A. 1974. *Red cell manual.* 4th ed. Philadelphia: F. A. Davis Co.

MacLean, N. 1978. *Haemoglobin.* Baltimore: University Park Press.

Ramsey, J. M. 1973. Effects of single exposures of carbon monoxide on sensory and psychomotor response. *Am Ind Hyg Assoc J* 34:212.

———. 1975. The hematological effects of chronic, low level exposures to carbon monoxide in rats. *Bull Environ Contam Toxico* 13:537.

Ramsey, J. M., and Casper, P. W., Jr. 1976. Effect of carbon monoxide exposures on erythrocytic 2,3-DPG in rabbits. *J Appl Physiol* 41:689.

Rifkind, R. A. 1979. *Fundamentals of hematology.* Chicago: Year Book Medical Publishers, Times Mirror.

Robertshaw, D., ed. 1977. Environmental physiology. In *International review of physiology.* Vol. 15. Baltimore: University Park Press. Chapt. 7.

Robbins, S. L., and Cotran, R. S. 1979. *Pathologic basis of disease.* 2d ed. Philadelphia: W. B. Saunders Co.

Ruch, T. C., and Patton, H. D., eds. 1974. Circulation, respiration, and fluid balance. In *Physiology and biophysics.* Vol. 2. Philadelphia: W. B. Saunders Co.

Slonim, N. B., ed. 1974. *Environmental physiology.* St. Louis: C. V. Mosby Co. Chapt. 9.

Vander, A. J. 1976. In Introduction to *Human physiology and the environment in health and disease.* San Francisco: W. H. Freeman and Co. Part 3, Article 10.

Vander, A. J.; Sherman, J. H.; and Luciano, D. S. 1980. *Human physiology: The mechanisms of body function.* 3d ed. New York: McGraw-Hill Book Co. Chaps. 11, 12.

Wintrobe, M. M. 1976. *Clinical hematology.* 7th ed. Philadelphia: Lea & Febiger.

Stress from Physical Exertion

Physiology and Biochemistry of Exercise
    Muscle Metabolism
    Lactic Acid Production and Oxygen Debt
    Oxygen Consumption
    Cardiovascular Response to Exercise
    Pulmonary Response to Exercise
    Endocrine Response and Metabolic Alterations
Exercise and Disease Prevention
Injuries from Physical Activity
    Skin
    Muscles
    Joints
    Bone Displacements and Fractures
Other Pathologic Consequences of Strenuous Exertion

|| Objectives: Upon completing this chapter you should:

1. Understand the metabolic operations of contracting muscle.
2. Be informed about the physiologic demands of exercise, especially the role of the cardiopulmonary system.
3. Be acquainted with the various forms of muscle, ligament, bone, and tendon injuries that can result from physical activity.
4. Recognize the role of regular exercise in promoting health and preventing disease.

It would appear that modern, industrial men and women have rediscovered the therapeutic benefits of exercise. The habit of exercising has become surprisingly popular during the past decade. There certainly is not a more natural stress. The healthy body is marvelously adapted for physical activity.

The stress of exertion is basically hypoxic in nature in that the essential problem is providing muscle mitochondria with sufficient oxygen for generating the adenosine triphosphate (ATP) utilized in muscle contraction. Of our classifications of hypoxia we would consider the form associated with exertion as mostly ischemic in nature, since the primary factor limiting required muscle oxygenation is cardiac output. Along with the hypoxia, an associated requirement in exercise is providing the muscle with adequate fuel, most of which is in the form of glucose and fatty acids.

The widespread adoption of the exercise habit warrants consideration of its role as a stressor. As a stress, physical activity is unique because it is capable of bestowing benefits as well as risking harm.

PHYSIOLOGY AND BIOCHEMISTRY OF EXERCISE

Work physiology has been extensively studied for some time, and practically all systems of the body are known to be involved in the response to physical demands. However, it is the metabolic adjustments in the operation of skeletal muscle that are fundamental to overall regulation, so a review of muscle metabolism follows.

Muscle Metabolism

The operations of both the contractile and recovery phases of skeletal muscle require immense quantities of ATP, especially when the exertion is strenuous and prolonged. ATP is not stored in large amounts, though in muscle there may be small reserves incorporated as *creatine phosphate* that can accumulate during rest. However, only several seconds of contractility can be supported by this reserve. Sustained physical activity is impossible without a high, continuous level of ATP production. Working maximally, muscle uses 10^{-3} moles of ATP per gram of muscle per minute.

When muscle is stimulated repeatedly at rates of once per second, or more, the contractile power eventually diminishes and each recovery is slower and less complete. The diminished irritability is called *fatigue*. Chemical analysis of fatigue states reveals that muscle glycogen is nearly depleted, and ATP concentration is very low. Also, the interior of the muscle shows an acidic reaction (accumulated lactic acid). If a period of rest is allowed before stimulation is continued, ATP level and pH both rise, and the muscle renews its ability to contract. This is because ATP production has had time to catch up with its expenditure during the rest interval. To avoid a substantial degree of fatigue, muscle must produce ATP at least as rapidly as it is being utilized.

The energy of ATP is provided by oxidative phosphorylation of acetate in the mitochondria, at least at moderate degrees of muscle activity. However, with intense exertion, ATP breakdown is so rapid that the time required to deliver oxygen to muscles becomes limiting for the oxidative production of ATP. The threshold is approached when exercise reaches about 50% of maximum capability. At this time anaerobic glycolysis in the muscle cell cytoplasm begins to contribute to the production of ATP. Although the glycolytic pathway produces very minute quantities of ATP, compared to that generated from the same amount of glucose by the oxidative pathway, glycolytic production of ATP takes much less time. Glycolysis of 32 molecules of glucose can produce 64 molecules of ATP in the same amount of time that oxidative phosphorylation produces 36 ATPs from 1 molecule of glucose. Thus glycolysis is a comparatively fast operation, though it is effective only if large quantities of glucose remain available. Indeed, the high fuel to energy ratio is a major factor in severely limiting glycolysis as an ATP producer. The pathways that generate ATP in muscle are displayed in Figure 10-1.

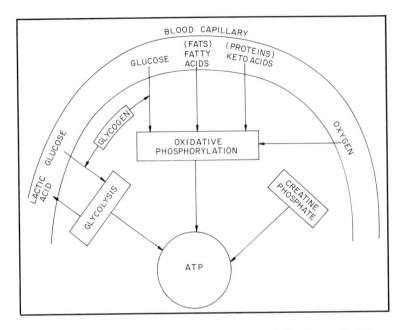

FIGURE 10-1   Pathways that generate ATP in skeletal muscle. The essential provider is oxidative phosphorylation.

Lactic Acid Production and Oxygen Debt

When anaerobic glycolysis becomes necessary for muscle contractions, *lactic acid* begins to accumulate in the muscle. The formulation of lactic acid from pyruvic acid represents a metabolic dead end. The lactate molecule still contains over 70% of the free energy of the original glucose. To be of any use, the lactate must be further oxidized in body tissues to CO_2 and H_2O, or be reconverted to glucose in the liver and kidneys. Oxygen is required for the first option, and additional ATP energy is required for glucose synthesis. As lactate accumulates it tends to diffuse from the muscle into the venous circulation, where values of 0.5 to 1.0 millimoles per liter at rest may increase to as much as 10.0 millimoles per liter when there is acute, strenuous exertion.

When one exercises at a level of activity where the O_2 required for ATP production and lactic acid oxidation is more than the O_2 being consumed, an *oxygen debt* is incurred. This means that after exercise ceases, one's O_2 intake will remain above that required at rest until the debt is repaid. This is why one breathes as heavily for awhile after exerting as one did during the activity. For example, if a certain level of exercise requires 4 liters of O_2 per minute, but the

TABLE 10-1

Two Types of Skeletal Muscle Fibers

	LOW OXIDATIVE	HIGH OXIDATIVE
Color of fibers	White	Red
Diameter of fibers	Large	Small to intermediate
Major source of ATP	Anaerobic glycolysis	Oxidative phosphorylation
Glycogen content	High	Low to moderate
Rate of ATP utilization	Fast	Slow to moderate
Myoglobin content	Low	High
Fatigue rate	Fast	Slow to moderate
Capillaries per gram	Few	Many
Mitochondria	Few	Many

maximum O_2 consumption (VO_2 max) can supply only 3 liters per minute, each additional minute of exercise is incurring 1 liter of oxygen debt. There is a limit to the amount of oxygen debt that can accumulate, and when this limit is reached, the body is incapable of further effort. In the example above, if 10 liters is the maximum O_2 debt allowable, then 10 minutes would be the extent to which that particular workload could be maintained.

Since the O_2 debt is associated with elevated levels of blood lactate, which tend to diminish as the debt is repaid, it had been presumed that the O_2 payment serves to oxidize the lactate. Although some lactate oxidation does occur upon cessation of exercise, it may amount to only a portion. It is now known that it is possible for O_2 debt to occur without much lactate accumulation, and that the quantity of one is not necessarily a reliable measure of the other. The ratio of pyruvate to lactate is a more accurate index of the degree of anaerobiosis.

Skeletal muscle fibers roughly fall into two groups according to both their capacity for producing ATP and their rate of using it. In one type of fiber, ATP utilization is slow to moderate, but the oxidative production of ATP is high, whereas another type of fiber shows a fast ATP utilization, but the oxidative ATP production is low. Some interesting differences between the two types are listed in Table 10-1. Endurance performance, such as distance-running, is associated with the high oxidative fibers, whereas high intensity performance of short duration, such as weight lifting, depends upon the low oxidative fibers with fast ATP utilization. Generally speaking, *isometric* contractions involve the low oxidative fibers. In isometrics no work is done, but much heat is produced. This form of muscle activity is advocated for developing bulging muscles. Pushing against a wall is an example of isometric performance; straining at stool is another example of isometric contractions.

In *isotonic* contractions work is accomplished (force multiplied by distance), and usually there is a greater employment of the high oxidative fibers. Isometric contractions in many respects are more stressing to the body than isotonic work. Comparative studies have shown that blood pressure increases more in isometrics and the heart appears to work much harder. Moreover, lactate levels are usually higher, and the pH of the blood is lower than is the case with isotonics. Apparently the great force and resistance involved in isometrics compresses blood vessels until blood perfusion is severely diminished, thereby creating a substantial degree of tissue hypoxia. Perhaps this is why many coronary attacks occur in predisposed individuals while straining at stool in the bathroom.

One must realize that the best training for a specific physical task is to perform and practice that particular task. Weight lifting will not necessarily produce a better swimmer, but swimming will. Weight lifting tends to increase the muscle mass, but some forms of athletic performance do not benefit from such development.

Oxygen Consumption

In exercise the oxygen-consuming capability is obviously a key variable in delaying and reducing the need for anaerobic glycolysis, thereby restricting the amount of O_2 debt and lactate accumulation. Thus one of the foremost parameters measured in the work physiology laboratory is O_2 consumption (VO_2). This is the most convenient way of studying energy expenditure. The VO_2 may be measured by either the open-circuit technique, or the closed-circuit method (Figures 10-2 and 10-3).

When workloads are progressively increased, the amount of O_2 consumed by muscle increases linearly until a limitation causes it to stabilize despite a continuing increase in the workload. The point of leveling off represents the maximal O_2 consumption, or VO_2 *max*, and it is identified in Figure 10-4. Beyond this point anaerobic glycolysis must furnish the additional ATP. However, glycolysis leads to a rapid depletion of fuel (glycogen and glucose) and therefore is a brief process.

What sets the limit on O_2 consumption? There are two ways in which exercising muscle obtains more O_2. One is through an increase of blood flow to muscle, and the other is by means of increasing the extraction of O_2 from the arterial blood. It is estimated that each of these adjustments accounts for approximately one-half of the

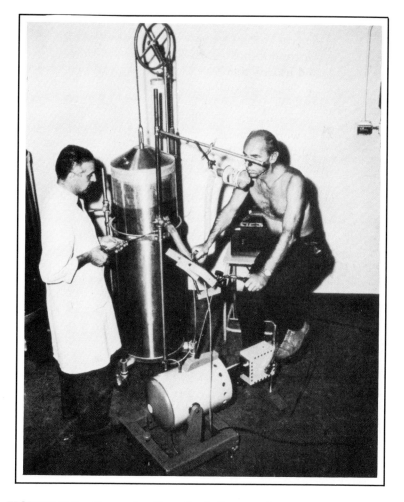

FIGURE 10-2   Open-circuit method of measuring oxygen consumption. The technician at left draws a sample of exhaled air from a Tissot gasometer. The percentage of O_2 in this air is compared with the percentage of that in room air; thus the oxygen utilized can be calculated. (From L. E. Morehouse and A. T. Miller, Jr., *Physiology of exercise*, 6th ed. St. Louis: C. V. Mosby Co., 1971.)

VO_2 max. However, it is the inability to get blood to the muscles fast enough that ultimately limits the VO_2.

The measurement of VO_2 max provides a valuable index of the cardiovascular fitness of an individual. The point at which some degree of anaerobiosis is required not only varies from individual to individual, but from time to time in the same individual. The aver-

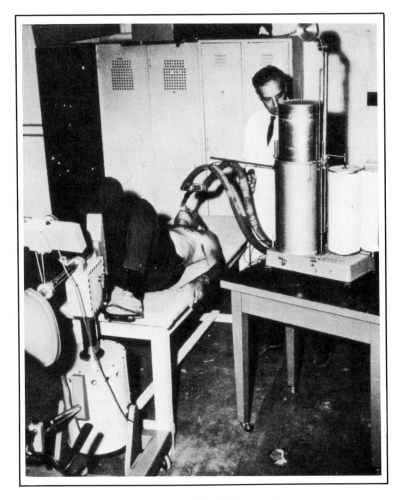

FIGURE 10-3   Closed-circuit method of measuring oxygen consumption. The subject pedals a bicycle ergometer and breathes in and out of a 13.5-liter respirometer, the bell of which has been loaded with pure O_2. The volume of O_2 removed is recorded on chart at far right. (From Morehouse and Miller, *Physiology of exercise.*)

age VO_2 max for untrained, young adults is about 3 liters per minute. Marathon runners can consume twice this amount. To improve the VO_2 max, training must be of the endurance type in which the respiration is largely aerobic. In Table 10-2 exhausting exertion from treadmill-running is compared to strenuous exercise on a bicycle ergometer. The measurement of the VO_2 max, plasma lactate, and pulse rate in 25 young, adult males affords the basis for the comparison in the table.

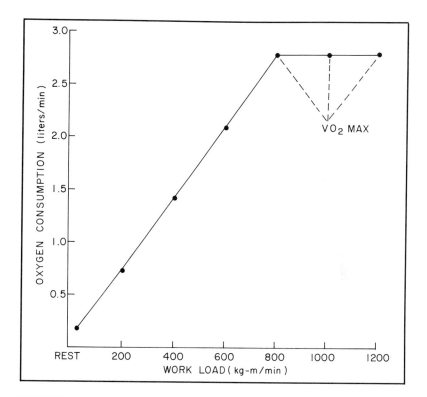

FIGURE 10-4   Quantitative relation of oxygen consumption to workload. The VO_2 increases linearly with increasing workloads until the cardiovascular system reaches its limit in supplying additional O_2. This point represents the maximal O_2 consumption of the individual.

Cardiovascular Response to Exercise

It was stated in the foregoing subsection that muscle obtains more O_2 during exercise by expanding the arteriovenous (AV) O_2 difference, and by increasing the arterial blood flow. The former accommodation involves the dissociation of O_2 from hemoglobin, and the latter change rests upon adjustments in cardiac output and vasomotor regulation of arterioles.

At the high rate of O_2 utilization in exercise, the PO_2 of muscle is drastically reduced, approaching 0 torr in many instances. This, of course, greatly increases the rate of O_2 dissociation from both hemoglobin (Hb) and myoglobin (Mb). From the discussion of Hb to O_2 dissociation in Chapter 9, it may be recalled that below a PO_2 of 60 torr the dissociation curve is very steep, enabling a large quantity of O_2 to be released as the O_2 tension decreases. In addition, active muscle releases large amounts of CO_2 to the blood, and

TABLE 10-2

Effects of Exhausting Exercise on Oxygen Consumption, Venous Lactate, and Pulse Rate in 25 Young Men*

Form of Exercise	VO$_2$ (Liters/min)	LACTATE (mM/l)	PULSE RATE (Beats/min)
Bicycle ergometer	2.66 ± 0.82	11.2 ± 1.8	182 ± 10
Treadmill	2.98 ± 0.73	12.4 ± 2.2	191 ± 7

Source: Unpublished data from the laboratory of the author.
*Untrained.

this elevates the hydrogen ion concentration. The lowered pH raises the P$_{50}$, thus enhancing the oxygenation of muscle by releasing oxygen at a higher PO$_2$. The P$_{50}$ is also increased by the elevated temperature of active muscle.

Whether or not the 2,3-diphosphoglycerate (2,3-DPG) mechanism is effective in improving muscle oxygenation during exercise has not been resolved. Some studies have shown an increase in 2,3-DPG during exercise, whereas others have shown either a decrease or no significant change at all. There are indications that when high lactate levels persist during prolonged exercise, the sustained decrease in blood pH suppresses 2,3-DPG synthesis. Thus the 2,3-DPG mechanism would appear to be more beneficial to trained athletes who possess a greater VO$_2$ max and therefore generate less lactate. It has been shown that trained athletes do have higher resting levels of 2,3-DPG.

Not only does exercise promote an expansion of arteriovenous O$_2$ difference but the blood transport capacity itself is increased. The values for hematocrit and hemoglobin content become higher within a few minutes of strenuous exertion. Since the action of erythropoietin is not effective in such a short time, the increase in red blood cell mass is a proportional one, because of plasma loss from hyperventilation and sweating.

Physical exertion induces localized chemical changes in arteriole smooth muscle, resulting in the vasodilation of vessels perfusing skeletal muscle. At the same time arterioles perfusing the kidneys, liver, and gastrointestinal tract are constricted. The result is a pronounced regional redistribution of blood.

In exercise the organs of priority are skeletal muscle, heart, and as always, brain. Blood flow to most other regions can be drastically reduced. The comparison of blood perfusion to various organs at rest with the redistribution found in exercise is presented in Table 10-3.

TABLE 10-3

Blood Perfusion of Organs at Rest and with Strenuous Exercise

| Organ | % OF CARDIAC OUTPUT | | Change |
	Rest	Work	
Skeletal muscle	21	63	Substantial increase
Lungs	6	7	Not appreciable
Skin	8	10	Not appreciable
Heart	4	4	None
Brain	12	12	None
Stomach and intestines	10	3	Substantial decrease
Liver	18	6	Substantial decrease
Kidney	18	4	Substantial decrease
Others	3	1	Not appreciable

Without question the variable most responsible for increasing blood flow to exercising muscle is the cardiac output. Both heart rate and stroke volume increase. However, the increase in rate is much greater than the increase in force; indeed, both cardiac output and heart rate are linearly related to metabolic demands at all but the very highest workloads, whereas the stroke volume reaches a maximal value at about one-third of the aerobic capacity. Thus the cardiac output of exercise is dependent primarily on an increased heart rate. The measurement of heart rate serves as a valuable indicator of the physiologic strain associated with exertion.

From a resting value of 5 liters per minute, cardiac output in exercise can increase to as much as 30 liters per minute in trained individuals. As a rule, cardiac output increases more than peripheral resistance decreases, resulting in a mild elevation of mean arterial blood pressure. This elevation is based upon a steep rise in systolic pressure (pulse pressure). A summary of values for a number of cardiovascular functions at three levels of exercise is shown in Table 10-4.

What initiates cardiovascular adjustments to exercise? A facilitation of sympathetic impulses together with an inhibition of parasympathetic impulses constitutes the basis for most of the cardiovascular response to exercise. Apparently there is activation of sympathetic pathways descending from specific hypothalamic centers. However, sources of the afferent input to these centers have not been identified with certainty. One probable source is the motor area of the cerebral cortex.

High levels of cardiac output cannot be maintained without an adequate return of venous blood to the heart. Otherwise the end-

TABLE 10-4

Average Values for Cardiovascular Functions at Rest and with Exertion

FUNCTION	AT REST	MILD EXERTION	MODERATE EXERTION	MAXIMAL EXERTION
Cardiac output (liters/min)	5.5	10.5	15.5	22.5
Heart rate (beats/min)	70	105	140	190
Heart stroke volume (ml)	80	100	111	115
Systolic blood pressure (mmHg)	125	155	175	200
Diastolic blood pressure (mmHg)	75	77	80	85
Vascular resistance (mmHg/liter/min)	16	10	7	6
Oxygen consumption (liters/min)	0.3	1.0	2.0	3.2
(AV) oxygen difference (vol %)	5	10	13	15

Source: Unpublished data from the laboratory of the author.

diastolic volume progressively falls, which results in a depressed stroke volume. It is this effect that limits cardiac output during exercise. As previously stated, stroke volume does not increase to the same degree in exercise as does heart rate. At extremely rapid heart rates, the time for diastolic filling of heart chambers is severely restricted, and the peripheral factors promoting venous return cannot elevate the venous pressure enough to maintain ventricular filling during such short diastoles. Now it becomes clear why trained athletes tend to have a combination of slower heart rates with higher stroke volumes. With training, the heart muscle is strengthened, allowing the stroke volume to assume a greater role in cardiac output, permitting a slower heart rate. The result is a more effective ventricular filling time, which also serves to enhance the stroke volume.

In recent years cardiovascular response to exercise is being employed in diagnostic screening of patients in whom coronary atherosclerosis is suspected but whose resting ECGs are normal. The *stress ECG* is recorded while the subject performs on a treadmill. It is true that when cardiac reserve is called upon an impairment of cardiac function is more likely to be detected through ECG examination. However, even a normal stress ECG finding does not rule out coronary atherosclerosis.

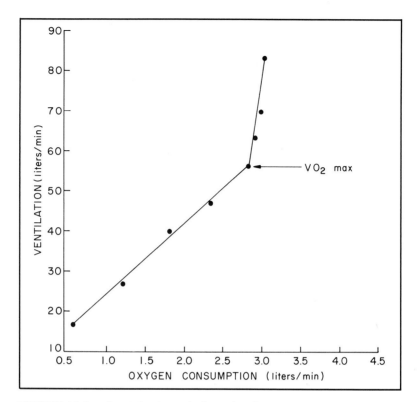

FIGURE 10-5   Quantitative relation of pulmonary ventilation to oxygen consumption. An increase in the two variables shows a linear relationship until the VO_2 max is reached. It is obvious that it is not ventilation capacity that limits the VO_2.

Pulmonary Response to Exercise

There are increases in ventilation during and after exercise. The increase is proportional to the level of O_2 consumption until the VO_2 max is reached. Beyond this point the ventilation becomes excessive and no longer bears a constant relation to VO_2 (Figure 10-5). The excess ventilation serves no useful purpose since by this time the delivery of O_2 has become limited by the cardiac output. In moderate exercise most of the increase in ventilation comes from an elevation in volume, whereas severe exertion may demand an increase in respiratory rate as well.

During physical activity the alveolar PO_2 rises progressively with increasing workloads. In fact, when exertion becomes exhausting, alveolar ventilation has been known to increase 20-fold. The arterial PO_2 may decrease slightly in moderate exercise. However, it can actually increase in heavy exertion, when the alveolar ventilation begins to show a disproportionate increase to VO_2. In moderate physical activity the alveolar PCO_2 shows little change, but with the increased ventilation from heavy exercise it may be reduced.

Endocrine Response and Metabolic Alterations

As pointed out, physical exertion is a stress requiring a multitude of adjustments. Hormonal secretions mediate much of the body's response to exercise. Hypoxia from any cause stimulates the sympathoadrenal system, and exercise is no exception. Numerous investigations with both laboratory animals and humans have verified that the foremost hormonal response in exercise is the release of catecholamines from the adrenal medullae. How is the response mediated? Experimental evidence indicates that a center in the hypothalamus acts through descending sympathetic pathways. It is thought that motor areas of the cerebral cortex provide the necessary afferent input to the hypothalamus.

Even though plasma catecholamines increase markedly in response to exercise, it has been shown that training results in much less output of catecholamines and glucagon during exercise than is characteristic of untrained individuals.

Of course, other stress hormones would be expected to increase during exercise. This is true of ACTH, glucocorticoids, growth hormone, and glucagon. The adrenal cortex is particularly reponsive to prolonged periods of physical activity, especially when other stressors such as cold, heat, and anxiety coexist. Studies have shown that in exercise the numbers of circulating eosinophils and lymphocytes become temporarily reduced. A reduction in numbers of these leucocytes suggests immunosuppression, and it is believed to be due to an increase in glucocorticoid secretion.

Several investigations have shown that levels of aldosterone and antidiuretic hormone become elevated during and immediately following strenuous exercise. Thyroid changes are less predictable. In some cases serum T_4 (thyroxin) has decreased during exercise. This has been interpreted as a result of a shift of T_4 into the cellular compartment because elevated cellular metabolism during exercise would involve increased T_4 utilization. This idea brings up the point that blood measurements of a substance as an indication of what is going on in the body tissues can be misleading. Whether the substance be glucose, a hormone, a vitamin, or any important biochemical component, the measurement of it in the blood does not necessarily tell us what it is doing in the cells. For example, the measurement of blood levels of histamine is often useless, since this mediator can be extremely concentrated locally, despite low serum levels. Likewise, a normal glucose level in the blood does not always guarantee normal utilization of the sugar in cells. Before the advent of insulin therapy some diabetics remained semistarved in order to achieve normal glucose levels in the blood. Despite normoglycemia there was an inevitable deficit in energy production resulting from an insufficient cellular utilization of glucose.

It has been shown that blood insulin levels decrease during strenuous exercise. This is probably due to the increase in catecholamine secretions, which are known to inhibit insulin release. On the other hand, it is well known that much less insulin is required by an individual undergoing muscular activity. The two tissues most dependent upon insulin for cellular uptake of glucose are skeletal muscle and adipose cells. This dependency becomes significantly reduced for skeletal muscle when it is contracting. Just how glucose uptake is facilitated when muscles are active is not well understood. There is evidence that exercise in some way increases binding of insulin to skeletal muscle receptors. Accordingly a given amount of glucose uptake would require less than the usual quantity of insulin.

Although glucose uptake by muscle is significantly enhanced in exercise, blood glucose levels may not be appreciably reduced. This is because of hepatic conversion of glycogen to glucose promoted by the elevation of catecholamines in response to exercise. Also, gluconeogenesis from glucocorticoid activity may result from prolonged exertion. Indeed, many individuals under certain forms and durations of exercise show an elevation in blood glucose, despite an increased rate of removal of the sugar into the muscles.

Although glucose is utilized preferentially by exercising muscle, considerable quantities of fatty acids are oxidized as well. In exercise lipids are mobilized, and there is an increase of free fatty acids in the blood, whence they undergo increased rates of oxidation in the cells. Their increased utilization means a metabolic shift from lipogenesis to lipolysis, which eventually results in a reduced concentration of blood lipids such as triglycerides and the low density lipoproteins associated with cholesterol. Some of the hormonal actions related to physiologic regulations in exercise are depicted in Figure 10-6.

Carbohydrate is usually considered the most economical fuel in exercise in view of its rapid availability to muscle as well as its indispensability in anaerobic glycolysis. Because of preparatory processes, protein is slow in reaching muscle in fuel form. Protein also has a high specific dynamic action (SDA) as far as heat production is concerned. This is pointed out in Chapter 7. For this reason

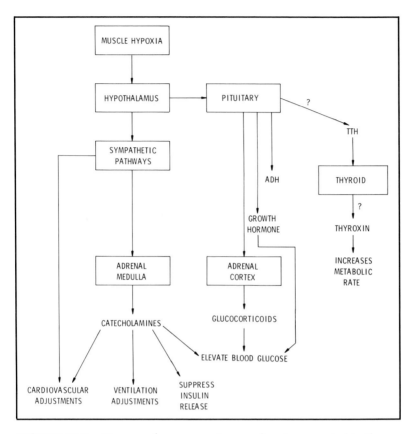

FIGURE 10-6 Hormonal responses to exercise. As suggested in the figure, the role of the thyroid is not totally clear.

protein intake can be troublesome in warm environments. During heavy exercise body heat production may rise as high as 960 kcal/hr, which is a 12-fold increase above resting levels. The slow digestion and absorption of dietary lipid delay its reaching the muscles as acetate. Moreover, fatty acids cannot support anaerobic glycolysis.

EXERCISE AND DISEASE PREVENTION

In view of the increasing number of individuals that are becoming devoted to such activities as jogging, tennis, bicycling, racquetball, and swimming, a discussion of both the benefits and dangers of strenuous exercise is in order.

The purported benefits of strenuous exercise range from the prevention of hypertensive cardiovascular disease, to just feeling better. In between are convictions that the habit will promote weight loss, reduce emotional tension, bestow a better physical appearance, improve sexual performance, and reduce susceptibility to many common infections such as colds and influenza. Such benefits are more likely to be realized by participants who are relatively free of preexisting disease, and are knowledgeable about the necessary precautions in undertaking strenuous exertion.

It is true that certain forms of strenuous exercise, such as running, are capable of increasing the VO_2 max by 20% to 25%. The practice also promotes an increase in cardiac stroke volume and a decrease in cardiac rate. In addition, regular physical activity significantly enhances tissue oxygenation, reduces serum lipid levels, lowers mean arterial blood pressure, and promotes relaxation, all of which are important in preventing atherosclerosis and consequent heart disease. Furthermore, habitual exercise appears to increase levels of protective high density lipoproteins, at least in men (see Chapter 5). However, to be effective, exercise must be taken regularly and should be of the endurance type associated with the high oxidative muscle fibers. This kind of exercise has been termed aerobics, because it encourages predominance of oxidative activity over anaerobic glycolysis (Figure 10-7). Exercise is believed to delay many of the deteriorating aspects of aging. It can retard the loss of muscle tissue and prevent the conversion of lean body mass to fat. In addition, recent work has shown that exercise can retard the loss of bone that characterizes old age demineralization processes, and even increase the size of bones, thereby strengthening them. Skeletal demineralization associated with aging is discussed further in Chapter 18.

Probably the greatest everyday value of exercise in today's world is the release of nervous tension. In emotion the entire muscular and hormonal systems are prepared for the action of fight or flight. Without action, tension progressively builds up and it may be sustained for prolonged periods of time. Eventually this tension can dispose certain individuals to gastrointestinal ulcers, high blood pressure, recurrent headaches, insomnia, and depression. In adult-onset diabetes, glucose tolerance is remarkably ameliorated by lengthy periods of regular exercise.

It has been debated whether or not exercise in itself adds years to human life span. Even if it doesn't prolong the quantity of life, it deserves strong consideration as a factor in improving the quality of life.

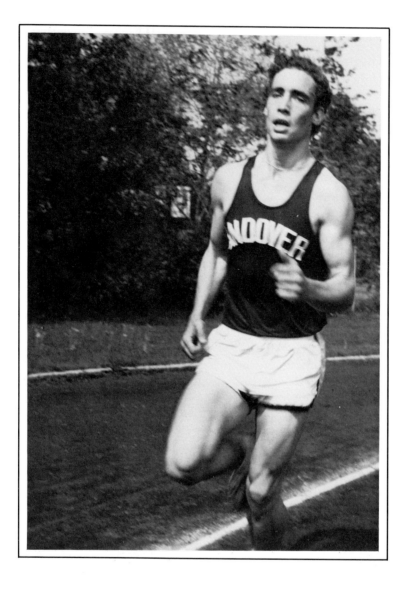

FIGURE 10-7   Endurance running. This is an excellent example of aerobic exercise. The emphasis is on distance, not speed. When speed is increased, anaerobic respiration and lactic acid formation begin to replace oxidative metabolism. (From J. W. Kimball, *Biology*, 4th ed. Reading, Mass.: Addison-Wesley, 1978.)

INJURIES FROM PHYSICAL ACTIVITY

Perhaps the most adverse aspect of strenuous exertion is the ever-present risk of trauma to the skin, muscles, tendons, ligaments, and bones. Although orthopedic problems may develop and accidents may occur in diverse activities, exercise and athletic games especially lend themselves to these risks. For example, between 1973 and 1975, injuries from skateboard accidents increased tenfold, and hospital emergency rooms treated 70,000 victims of skateboard mishaps annually during this period.

Skin

A skin problem common to active people is the development of blisters from mechanical causes such as friction from an ill-fitting shoe or from gripping the handles of racquets or bats. In any event the resulting traction on the skin tends to separate its superficial layers from the underlying dermis. This is followed by a filling of the area with exudate. The most common site of *vesiculation* is the sole of the foot, usually under the first toe or first metatarsal head. Foot blisters develop from the constant sliding of the skin on itself in running and walking, particularly when shoes and socks are not properly fitted. Once present, blisters may become infected unless precautions are exercised.

Another skin problem occurs upon receiving direct blows; the skin and underlying tissues can become bruised. The trauma is characterized by capillary rupture and an infiltrative type of bleeding that is followed by edema and inflammation. This form of injury is termed a *contusion*.

Muscles

We would expect skeletal muscle to be vulnerable to the abuse of physical exertion, particularly in the poorly conditioned individual. When leg muscles are subjected to much mechanical vibration, especially the anterior and posterior tibial ones, they undergo the painful swelling known as shin splints. The condition arises chiefly from prolonged running on hard surfaces. Muscles also are susceptible to various degrees of damage known as *strain*, which is often occasioned by overuse. Strains tend to occur at the weakest link of the muscle-tendon unit. Strains can be acute or chronic, and they are not to be taken lightly. The hamstring pull that occurs in sprinting is a muscle strain. Some strains more directly involve tendons, leading to painful tendonitis. *Lateral epicondylitis* (tennis elbow) is a tendonitis aggravated by rotating the arm while gripping an object. The popularity of tennis and racquetball has increased the frequency of this trauma. On the other hand, a common strain in those who run habitually is *Achilles tendonitis.*

Muscles are subject to cramping or spasms when there is a depletion of electrolytes such as sodium, which can result from excessive perspiration. Or muscle cramps may follow sudden changes in ambient temperature, as when a hot body is submerged into cool water. Muscle cramps also are known to occur during rest. It is thought that occurrence of some of the leg muscle cramps during the night is due to transient hypoglycemia related to the night fasting period.

Joints

Various degrees of damage to ligament fibers or their point of bone attachment are known as *sprains.* Sprains result when twisting or overstretching of a joint causes a ligament to tear or separate from its bony attachment. If the trauma is severe enough, excessive tissue fluid may accumulate, causing swelling.

A ligament is designed to permit the normal functional motion of a joint while preventing any abnormal motion. Certain ligaments bind two bones firmly together, permitting only slight rotary motion. Other ligaments reinforce a joint, and though they permit a wide excursion of motion, they prevent it in an abnormal direction. When a greater than normal force is applied that tends to cause the joint to move in an abnormal direction, the ligament begins to give at one or the other of its attachments, or perhaps at some point along the substance of the ligament. Various degrees of sprain are illustrated in Figure 10-8.

Other localized traumas of the joints include *bursitis,* an inflammatory reaction within the bursae, which are designed to facilitate motion between contiguous layers of the body. Repetitive tissue friction from violent motion of various sorts irritates and thickens the synovium, and excess fluid forms. This can result from injury, heavy exercise, or infection. Trauma to the joints may expose previously protected tissue proteins to the immune system. It is believed by some investigators that such exposure initiates the autoimmune process that appears to play a role in certain forms of arthritis.

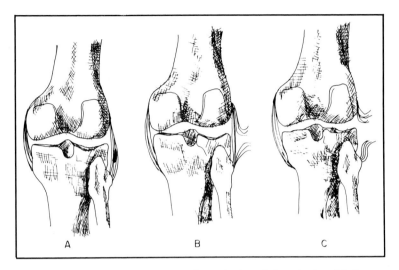

FIGURE 10-8   Various degrees of sprain in a joint. A. A mild, first-degree sprain in the ligament at right. There is a localized hematoma, but most of the fibers appear to be intact. B. A moderate, second-degree sprain. Observe the tear of the ligament, with only about half the fibers intact. C. A severe, third-degree sprain. The tear through the ligament is complete.

Bone Displacements and Fractures

The more serious injuries include dislocations (*luxations*) and bone fractures. In luxation there is an actual displacement of the opposing contiguous surfaces that make up a joint. There is usually an involvement of the ligaments as well. Dislocations vary in degree, partial ones being classified as subluxations. Sometimes the scar tissue of previously damaged ligaments cannot prevent the displacement, and the dislocation becomes chronic.

Bone fractures, of course, usually require protective casts and considerable periods of time for healing, particularly in older individuals. A unique bone trauma is called *stress fracture,* or fatigue fracture. It is not a true fracture: x-rays are usually negative for breakage. However, the metatarsal shafts of the foot may show a delayed appearance of periosteal new bone formation (Figure 10-9). A new diagnostic technique, radionuclide bone scan, will reveal the stress fracture early. Those who spend little time on their feet and are ill-equipped physically to withstand lengthy periods of excessive walking or running may experience the painful distress and tenderness of stress fracture. The best treatment for all stress fractures is rest from any activity causing pain. Most stress fractures involve bones of the feet.

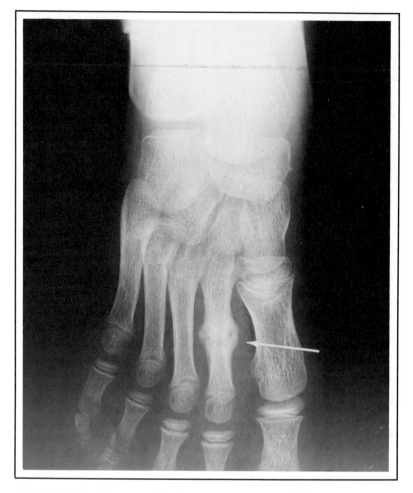

FIGURE 10-9 An x-ray showing a stress fracture. Note complete absence of a true fracture line through bone. However, there is additional bone formation of the second metatarsal shaft of the foot, indicating the primary site of the insult. (From D. H. O'Donoghue, *Treatment of injuries to athletes*, 3rd ed. Philadelphia: W. B. Saunders Co., 1976.)

Not only is acute, localized skeletal and muscular stress experienced with injuries, but the generalized stress syndrome involving the pituitary and adrenal glands also are activated when there are muscle or bone injuries. In Figure 10-10 the time course of glucocorticoid response to bone fracture is depicted.

A classification of the more common types of exercise-related injuries is presented in Table 10-5.

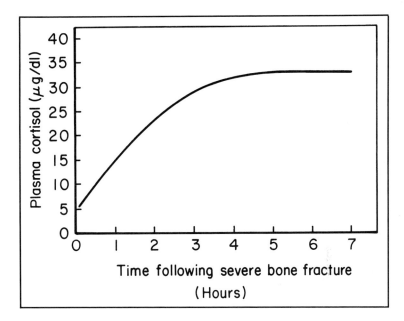

FIGURE 10-10   Time course of glucocorticoid response to bone fracture. Note that the plasma level of hormone increases sixfold in 4 hours.

OTHER PATHOLOGIC CONSEQUENCES OF STRENUOUS EXERTION

Strenuous exercise in itself can impose severe physiologic demands on the body, and the practice should be undertaken only if one is fully informed of all the proper precautions and qualifications. Individuals who do not practice some degree of moderation in exercise may unknowingly subject their bodies to eventual damage. Chronic orthopedic problems and development of osteoarthritis are foremost among the prices paid for continual rigorous use of the body in vigorous physical activities.

Extremely strong sympathoadrenal responses accompany strenuous physical performance, and when such stresses as anxiety and exposure to extreme cold coexist with exhausting exercise, high levels of systolic blood pressure may occur, which in time could become more persistent from habitual sympathetic overdrive. This effect is sometimes seen in isometric or weight-lifting forms of exertion. In other cases of severe, prolonged physical demands, there may be temporary adrenal exhaustion. Exertion in warm en-

TABLE 10-5
Common Exercise-Related Injuries

TYPE INJURY	SITE	DAMAGE
Contusion	Skin and underlying tissue	Capillary rupture and infiltrative bleeding
Strain	Skeletal muscle-tendon unit	Inflammation of tendon from overuse
Sprain	Ligaments	Ligament fibers are weakened or torn
Luxation (dislocation)	Ligaments and points of bone attachment	Displacement of contiguous surfaces comprising a joint
Stress fracture	Bone	In overuse, new periosteal bone formation is not adequately replaced
True fracture	Bone	Bone is actually separated or broken at some point along its length

vironments poses a further risk of depletion of fluid and electrolytes.

Decisions to exercise strenuously should depend upon the age, health, and weight of the participant as well as the prevailing environmental conditions. After 60 years of age it is more sensible to walk or bicycle, rather than run. An asthmatic should not run in cold air, or exert whenever ragweed pollen is rampant. A lengthy tennis exhibition under a strong sun at air temperatures of 36 to 37 C with a relative humidity of 84% may not be advisable for most of us. There are certain individuals who do not acclimate well to vigorous exertion. Indeed, there are those whose immune systems respond to this form of stress with true allergic manifestations. A choice to exercise moderately is a different matter. Walking, bicycling, golfing, and softball are activities with moderate physical demands. Even then caution is advised when other stresses are present, stresses such as extreme weather conditions, heavily polluted air, or high altitude. In addition, heavy eating and smoking, two very common stressors, do not go well with exercise. Exercise without caloric restriction will not achieve weight loss.

An underlying compulsiveness pervades some exercise regimes. This can lead to anxiety, which then becomes an associated undesirable stress. When one feels a sense of urgency and drives one's self to exercise, becoming upset and anxious when circumstances alter or prohibit the customary routine, then the physical benefits may not be worth the mental unrest associated with achieving them. Likewise, when one becomes overly conscious of competition and participates only to strive for superiority over others, then the true physiologic value of the physical activity is lessened because the mental stress takes away some benefits of an activity that should be as pleasurable and relaxed as possible. In substantiation of this point, significant ECG changes indicating decreased oxygen supply to the myocardium have been reported in individuals exercising under mental stress. The same exercise showed much less decrease in oxygen supply when performed on days when the individuals were relaxed and free of anxiety.

Though much has been made of the fact that exercise is important in preventing heart disease, once coronary artery disease has been recognized, strenuous activity is not advisable. Unfortunately this is how some individuals discover that they do have coronary vessel disease: when strenuous physical activity has actually brought on a heart attack. Such incidents are much more likely to occur in cold weather. However, with proper precaution the heart patient may benefit from moderate forms of physical activity.

Athletes undergoing a great deal of physical strain sometimes subject the kidneys to unnecessary stress. During periods of intense exercise, the redistribution of blood together with hyperventilation and sweating results in a significantly reduced renal plasma volume. This is accompanied by a marked fall in renal blood flow, promoting antidiuresis, which is additionally aggravated by increased secretion of ADH as a response to exercise. The glomerular filtration rate and urine volume are notably reduced, resulting in an elevated blood urea nitrogen (BUN) and suppressed clearance. Moreover, there is an increased specific gravity and lowered pH of the urine. The presence in the urine of albumin (proteinuria) and red blood cells (hematuria) is not uncommon in rigorous athletic activity. These effects make up a condition known as *athletic pseudonephritis*. With repeated bouts there is eventual risk of damage to the kidney.

Interestingly, professional athletes usually do not live as long as clergymen, farmers, university professors, and symphony orchestra conductors. Of course variables other than exercise may underlie these differences in life expectancy.

SUMMARY

Muscle contraction requires large amounts of adenosine triphosphate (ATP), most of which is provided by oxidative phosphorylation in the mitochondria. However, at extreme workloads the rate of ATP breakdown becomes so rapid that oxygen (O_2) can no longer be delivered fast enough to meet increased ATP demands. At this point small amounts of ATP are rapidly produced without O_2, resulting in an oxygen debt and increased production of lactic acid.

The efficiency of energy production in exercise is best assessed by measuring oxygen consumption (VO_2), and the point of maximum consumption (VO_2 max) is an index of cardiovascular fitness for exercise.

Muscle obtains more O_2 during exercise through increases in arterial blood flow and expansion of the arteriovenous O_2 difference. The major factor in increasing blood flow is the cardiac output; this is the variable that limits the VO_2 max.

Regular, reasonable exercise can play an important role in preventing cardiovascular disease and other disorders such as hypertension, depression, insomnia, gastrointestinal ulcers, obesity, and glucose intolerance.

Among undesirable stresses associated with exercise are skin blisters, strains of muscles and tendons, ligament sprains, joint dislocations, and bone fractures.

Strenuous exertion imposes a strong challenge to the sympathoadrenal responses of the body. When temperature extremes and/or anxiety habitually coexist with exercise, increases in systolic blood pressure may lead to risks of damage to the cardiovascular system.

Individuals of advanced age, or those with bronchial sensitivity, cardiac problems, and compromised renal reserve, must exercise with caution under optimal environmental conditions.

Chapter Glossary

acetate organic molecule derived from various nutrient oxidations that enters the Krebs cycle in cell mitochondria (see Chapter 12)

antidiuresis an effect resulting in decreased output of urine

bursa fluid-filled saclike structures situated in places where friction can occur from moving parts

electrolytes charged atoms or groups of atoms (ions) in solution in the body fluids. These materials function as coenzymes and serve in maintaining osmotic balance; some are indispensable in nerve and muscle function.

end-diastolic volume volume of cardiac blood present at the end of diastole, just before ventricles contract

glycolysis the cellular oxidation of glucose to pyruvic acid (without oxygen)

normoglycemia   normal levels of blood sugar
periosteal   pertaining to two layers of fibrous tissue that form an elastic lining around bones
synovium   membrane lining a joint capsule
vesiculation   the formation of blisters

For Further Reading

Apple, D. F., Jr., and Cantwell, J. D. 1979. *Medicine for sport*. Chicago: Year Book Medical Publishers, Times Mirror.

Astrand, P., and Rodahl, K. 1977. *Textbook of work physiology; physiological bases of exercise*. 2d ed. New York: McGraw-Hill Book Co.

Clarke, D. H. 1975. *Exercise physiology*. Englewood Cliffs, N. J.: Prentice-Hall, Inc.

Eliot, R. S.; Forker, A. D.; and Robertson, R. J. 1976. Aerobic exercise as a therapeutic modality in the relief of stress. In *Advances in cardiology. Physical activity and coronary heart disease*. Basel: F. Karger, Inc.

Johnson, W. R., and Buskirk, E. R., eds. 1974. *Science and medicine of exercise and sport*. 2d ed. New York: Harper & Row Pubs.

Katch, F. I., and McArdle, W. D. 1977. *Nutrition, weight control and exercise*. Boston: Houghton Mifflin Co.

Mitchell, T. H., and Blomquist, G. 1971. Maximal oxygen uptake. *N Engl J Med* 284:1018.

Morehouse, L. E., and Miller, A. T., Jr. 1976. *Physiology of exercise*. 7th ed. St. Louis: C. V. Mosby Co.

O'Donoghue, D. H. 1976. *Treatment of injuries to athletes*. 3d ed. Philadelphia: W. B. Saunders Co.

Pernow, B., and Saltin, B., eds. 1971. Muscle metabolism during exercise. In *Advances in experimental medicine and biology*. Vol. 2. New York: Plenum Press.

Ramsey, J. M., and Pipoly, S. W. 1979. Response of erythrocytic 2,3-di-phosphoglycerate to strenuous exercise. *Eur J Appl Physiol* 40: 227.

Robertshaw, D., ed. 1977. Environmental physiology II. In *International review of physiology*. Vol. 15. Baltimore: University Park Press. Chapt. 4.

Ryan, A. J., and Allman, F. L., Jr., eds. 1974. *Sports medicine*. New York: Academic Press.

Shephard, R. J. 1979. *Physical activity and aging*. Chicago: Year Book Medical Publishers, Times Mirror.

Vander, A. J.; Sherman, J. H.; and Luciano, D. S. 1980. *Human physiology: The mechanisms of body function*. 3d ed. New York: McGraw-Hill Book Co. Chapts. 10, 15.

Winder, W. W.; Hickson, R. C.; Hagberg, J. M.; et al. 1979. Training-induced changes in hormonal and metabolic responses to submaximal exercise. *J Appl Physiol* 46(4):766.

II

Malnutritive Stress and Disease

|| **Objectives:** Upon completing this chapter you should:

1. Understand the concept of nutritive balance.
2. Know the essential nutrients and recognize their importance.
3. Perceive qualitative differences among dietary carbohydrates, lipids, and proteins that pertain to chemical stress and susceptibility to disease.
4. Be acquainted with the present state of knowledge concerning the need for various vitamins and minerals.
5. Be informed about kidney disease and its relation to disturbances of body fluid regulation.

Though much popular attention is being focused upon nutrition, most individuals do not look upon what they eat, or don't eat, as being particularly stressful; yet to the nutritionist this form of stress has been, and continues to be, a matter of significant concern in most parts of the world, affecting the affluent as well as the poverty-stricken.

The 1979 surgeon general's report on health promotion and disease prevention links a diet high in sugar, fat, cholesterol, and salt, and low in dietary fiber to heart disease, high blood pressure, dental caries, and colon cancer. Furthermore, six diseases listed among the ten leading causes of death in the United States are considered to be diet-related. Of special importance among these pathologies are diabetes, cardiovascular disease, and cancer.

Although fundamental principles have been established, nutrition is far from an exact science. We know what the essential nutrients are, but establishing quantitative requirements is a different matter. Though the goal of nutrition is to establish the optimum intake for each nutrient, we cannot yet determine exactly what this optimum should be at a given time for a given nutrient in each cell. It is reasonable to assume that necessary quantities vary considerably among individuals, and at different times in the same individual. Moreover, there is the possibility that nutrients ordinarily considered desirable may not be well tolerated by certain people. Despite these variables and the questions they pose, the basic concepts underlying nutritional stress have been formulated. To understand these concepts we turn again to the principle of equilibrium.

THE CONCEPT OF NUTRITIVE BALANCE

The operations underlying nutritive balance offer an excellent example of chemical homeostasis. Body tissues require an adequate quantity of specific nutrients, which must be constantly available in the extracellular fluid. The immediate internal availability from which all needed nutrients can be directly drawn is designated as the *nutrient pool*. The maintenance of nutrient pool concentrations depends upon the balance between that which is entering the body or being synthesized, and that which is leaving the body or being catabolized. If nutrient levels exceed what is necessary for pool maintenance, they may be delegated to storage depots or incorporated into other molecular materials. Conversely, newly converted materials and storage depots can resupply the nutrient pool when necessary. The concept is diagrammed in Figure 11-1. Reference to the diagram makes it apparent that net gain to the body depends upon internal synthesis of materials as well as upon the ingestion of food and water. Likewise, net loss occurs from catabolic degradation as well as from excretion from the body. Nevertheless, total nutritive balance ultimately depends upon the rate of gain from intake proportional to the rate of loss from excretion.

When loss of a nutrient exceeds its gain, the individual is said to be in *negative balance* with regard to that nutrient. When gain exceeds loss, the individual is in *positive balance*. A relative equality between rates of gain and loss provides an equilibrium, which is considered to be the ideal outcome of homeostatic regulation. However, as with most generalizations there are exceptions to certain points of this concept. In preadult years a positive balance must be maintained for many nutrients, especially protein, calcium, and phosphate. Also, all nutrients do not have access to all the pathways shown in Figure 11-1. Minerals, for example, can be neither synthesized nor catabolized.

Any nutrient that the body cannot synthesize, at least in adequate quantities, must be supplied in the diet. Such materials are termed *essential nutrients*. Even though glucose is a high priority nutrient, it is not classified as essential because the body can synthesize all that is required. There are about 40 essential nutrients, including 8 amino acids, 3 unsaturated fatty acids, about 15 each of vitamins and minerals, and, of course, water. Most of these nutrients and imbalances among them are discussed in the following sections.

Since nutritive balance ultimately depends upon intake ver-

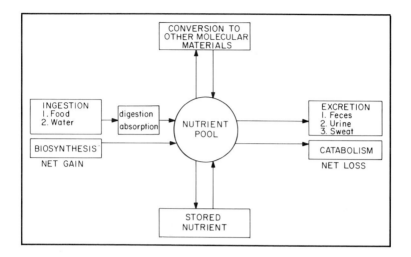

FIGURE 11-1   The principle of nutritive balance. Cells depend directly on the nutrient pool. See text for further discussion and explanation.

sus excretion, homeostasis eventually becomes impossible when the intake of any essential nutrient remains at zero. A minimal rate of excretion sets the lower limit for nutrient intake conducive to achieving balance, whereas maximum excretion sets the upper limit for intake without disrupting balance. If intake exceeds the upper limit, there is either a gain in weight, or toxic disturbances, depending upon the particular nutrients in question.

However, homeostasis does not achieve an absolute constancy; there often is a range of intake that is capable of insuring enough balance to prevent toxicity or deficiency. The extent of this range varies with different nutrients. Sodium is cited as an example. Even though the optimum intake for most young, healthy adults is considered to be about 9 grams of salt per day, a reasonable balance can be achieved at intakes ranging from 0.4 to 22.0 grams per day. When intake of salt is near either extreme, the regulatory mechanisms (primarily the kidneys) are challenged, and the sodium pool at one extreme of intake would not be quite the same as it might be at the other extreme. Nevertheless, the young, healthy adult should not experience overt problems within this range, despite the fact that excessive salt intake is a habit that should not be encouraged.

Generally speaking, the higher we ascend the evolutionary scale of organisms, the longer becomes the list of essential nutrients. Many simple organisms such as microbes and plants synthesize most of their nutrients. Since the higher animals ingest nutrients in concentrated bulk form, mutations reducing their synthesizing capability are not as crucial to survival as they otherwise might be. To have the necessary nutrients, humans are more dependent upon diet than are most other organisms. Ascorbic acid (vitamin C) affords an appropriate example. Practically all mammals can synthesize ascorbic acid from glucose, but for us (and guinea pigs) it is an essential nutrient.

Malnutrition

The meaning of the term *malnutrition* is often misconstrued. Most people associate the word with nutritional deficiencies, conjuring mental pictures of thin, semistarved children. In actuality malnutrition means that the nutrition is improper; that it is not balanced; that it is not optimum for health. The word certainly applies to nutritional deficiencies. On the other hand, malnutrition can refer as well to an excessive intake of one or more nutrients. Nutritionists customarily look upon the term as encompassing both *undernutrition* and *overnutrition;* either one promotes imbalance and is therefore stressing.

When considering either deficient or excessive nutritional intake, a distinction is made between the energy provision of the food (caloric value) and the other indispensable roles that nutrients play in maintaining cellular structure, enzyme activity, and special syntheses. The malnutrition discussed in this chapter is limited to the latter role of nutrients (essential nutrient substances). Caloric imbalance is discussed in the following chapter.

AMINO ACIDS AND PROTEIN DEFICIENCY

Proteins are synthesized from about 20 different amino acids. The amino acid pool is maintained from dietary sources plus the availability from cellular synthesis and degradation. Twelve of the amino acids can be synthesized by many body cells, but in adults the other eight are absolutely essential in the diet. The essential and nonessential amino acids are listed in Table 11-1. Proteins containing all the essential amino acids are called *complete proteins.* Complete proteins are found in meat (including poultry and fish), milk, and eggs. Incomplete proteins are lacking in one or more of the essential amino acids. Examples are the proteins from grain, legumes, vegeta-

TABLE 11-1

Essential and Nonessential Amino Acids for Adults

ESSENTIAL	NONESSENTIAL	CLASSIFICATION
Leucine	Glycine	Aliphatic and neutral
Isoleucine	Alanine	(one amino and one
Threonine	Serine	carboxyl group)
Valine		
Phenylalanine	Tyrosine	Aromatic (have ring
Tryptophan	Histidine	structure) and
	Proline	neutral
	Hydroxy proline	
Methionine	Cysteine	Sulfur-containing and
		neutral
Lysine	Arginine	Basic: two amino and
	Hydroxy lysine	one carboxyl group
	Aspartic acid	Acidic: one amino and
	Glutamic acid	two carboxyl
		groups

bles, and fruits. At this point the question of vegetarianism arises. If vegetarianism is strict enough to exclude all milk, cheese, and eggs (rather than eliminating meats only), then the practice is not recommended because there would not be enough of all the essential amino acids or of vitamin B_{12}. The matter of vitamin B_{12} deficiency is especially critical in pregnant women who practice strict vegetarianism. Breast-fed infants of these women may become comatose and die from severe anemia.

If one eats a variety of protein sources, one can make up for an amino acid that is restricted in one source, because it is likely that there is a liberal supply of that particular amino acid in one of the other many proteins. The missing amino acids in several incomplete proteins are listed in Table 11-2.

Assessment of protein balance in metabolism is usually performed by measuring the intake and excretion of nitrogen. Nitrogen equilibrium is normally expected in adults, but in growing children there is a positive nitrogen balance. Negative nitrogen balance is never desirable, especially if persistent. If there is insufficient nitrogen for synthesis of nonessential amino acids, then some of the essential ones are sacrificed for this purpose. Negative nitrogen balance may stem from an intake of incomplete proteins where needs for specific tissue replacements are not being met, or it can be associ-

TABLE 11-2

Amino Acids Missing in Incomplete Protein of Common Foods

FOOD	MISSING AMINO ACID(S)
Wheat	Lysine
Rice	Lysine and threonine
Corn	Lysine and tryptophan
Beans	Methionine
Peas	Methionine
Peanut	Several are borderline, including methionine and phenylalanine
Most vegetables	Several are missing, including threonine, phenylalanine, and tryptophan
Most fruits	Several are missing, including isoleucine, phenylalanine, tryptophan, lysine, and methionine

ated with inadequate caloric intake, which causes protein to be degraded to supply energy. When carbohydrate becomes less available as an energy source, as occurs with impaired glucose utilization in uncontrolled diabetes, tissue-wasting from negative nitrogen balance follows.

Other causes of negative nitrogen balance include extensive tissue damage, and various chronic disease processes that result in excessive tissue breakdown. Prolonged response to stress may be characterized by negative nitrogen balance because of the increased protein catabolism associated with the action of adrenocortical hormones. It must be kept in mind that the body does not store protein in the sense that fat or glycogen is stored. Once nitrogen balance becomes negative, body tissues themselves become the reserves being drawn upon. In the syndrome *kwashiorkor* (Figure 11-2), there is a noticeable wasting of the body. The condition is primarily due to protein deficiency. Other noticeable features of the syndrome include a failure to grow, edema of the abdomen, and impaired mentality.

In adults the quantity of daily protein intake necessary to prevent negative nitrogen balance is only 35 to 45 grams, providing that most energy requirements are being met by carbohydrate and fat. Deficiency in protein quantity is quite rare among people of the more advanced civilizations. Indeed, there are evidences suggesting that most Americans get too much protein. As adults, protein should comprise only 7% to 8% of our calories. Adult rats in which 25% of the diet was protein gained more weight and developed more body

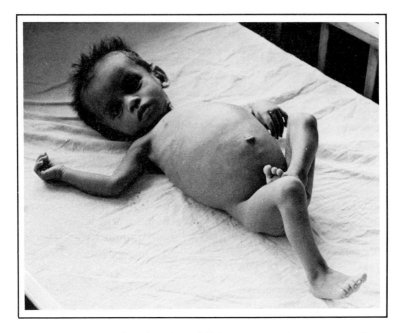

FIGURE 11-2 **Kwashiorkor in a child.** Note wasted appearance of limbs and abdominal edema. (Courtesy UNICEF Photo and Exhibit Service, N.Y.)

fat than rats on isocaloric diets in which only 5% of the diet was protein.

On the other hand, an imbalance in protein quality that fails to provide enough of the essential amino acids does sometimes occur. The result is faulty synthesis of one or more of the many key protein molecules of the body. Among such indispensable proteins are hemoglobin, the vast array of cellular enzymes, the immunoglobins that resist infection, and the majority of hormones.

Statistics have been reported that suggest an association of high protein intake with cardiovascular disease and cancer. However, one must be cautious in interpreting statistical associations. High protein intake is usually a habit of the more affluent, who often have fewer problems with infectious disease and degenerative changes earlier in life. Consequently, there may be longer life spans among these individuals, and risks of both cancer and cardiovascular disease greatly increase with age. However, high protein intake is usually associated with the intake of saturated fats, which are reputed to contribute to atherosclerosis.

LIPID AND CARBOHYDRATE

Of dietary lipid about 98% is in the form of esters of fatty acids and glycerol, known as neutral fats, or *triglycerides*. The fact that both carbohydrate and protein can be converted to lipid has prompted the idea that fats are by far the least necessary of the food components. This is not strictly the case. Certain forms of dietary lipid on a daily basis are both necessary and desirable for several reasons. Foremost among these reasons is the fact that one fatty acid, *linoleic acid*, is absolutely essential in the diet. It cannot be synthesized by the body. Moreover, *linolenic acid* and *arachidonic acid* are two additional fatty acids that may be considered semiessential; in other words they would be in short supply without an intake of dietary lipid. Linoleic acid is a precursor of much of the arachidonic acid which provides the 20-carbon skeleton from which the ubiquitous tissue hormones known as prostaglandins are derived. All three of the essential fatty acids are polyunsaturated, and each occurs as an integral part of phospholipid molecules that are necessary for cell membrane structure.

Another reason for including lipid in the diet is that it can beneficially regulate the appetite. Fats reduce the motility of the gastrointestinal tract; thus a meal containing fat remains in the stomach for a much longer time, and assimilation is delayed. The delay can significantly reduce both the frequency and intensity of hunger pangs, a gastrointestinal stability that is especially important to those prone to bouts of reactive hypoglycemia.

A point sometimes cited for excluding or restricting dietary lipid is the mistaken idea that fat intake results in much more body fat than does the eating of carbohydrate or protein. Beyond intake necessary for caloric requirements, any organic nutrient will contribute to adiposity. Most of the triglyceride in our fat cells comes from carbohydrate (glucose).

For the past 20 years much has been written concerning the dietary importance of saturated versus unsaturated fats. It has been said that a preponderance of saturated fat in the diet promotes serum elevations of the low density lipoproteins bearing cholesterol. Certain selected investigations have shown that reducing the saturated fat content of the diet can lower plasma cholesterol by 15% to 20%, yet despite such findings the need to lower serum cholesterol has been challenged recently by a number of clinical investigators. Indeed, there are statistical data that point to an association of low cholesterol with cancer.[1]

1Kolata, G. B. 1981. Data sought on low cholesterol and cancer. *Science*, 211: 1410.

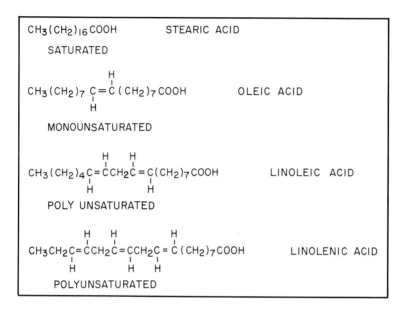

FIGURE 11-3   Fatty acids with various degrees of saturation. As indicated by the number of double-bonded carbons, each fatty acid is progressively less saturated as one reads from top to bottom.

A saturated fat is one comprised of saturated fatty acids, and saturation means that the hydrocarbon chain of the fatty acid has all the hydrogen atoms it can hold. Double bonds between carbon atoms reduce the number of hydrogens that otherwise would be present. With one double bond the fatty acid is said to be *monounsaturated,* whereas *polyunsaturation* implies that there are two or more double bonds. In Figure 11-3 four fatty acids are shown, each with a different level of saturation. The distribution of both saturated and unsaturated fatty acids in various kinds of fats is listed in Table 11-3. Oleic, palmitic, and stearic acids predominate in animal fats, whereas linoleic and linolenic acids are abundant in the polyunsaturated oils of corn, cottonseed, soybean, and safflower. The only vegetable fat that is classified as saturated is coconut oil.

Studies with dogs have indicated that the course of atherosclerosis appearing to be diet-induced can be altered by changing the source of fat in the diet. Dogs developing thromboembolic disease consumed diets in which the fat was beef tallow and coconut oil. Animals in which cottonseed oil was the dietary fat source showed no thrombosis. As a consequence of these kinds of data, diets in which the lipid intake is cholesterol-free and predominantly free from unsaturated fats have been recommended for preventing atherosclerosis. Such diets are advised also as a course of management in patients already known to have cardiovascular impairment.

As yet there are no conclusive answers on how effective these measures can be. Indeed, the Food and Nutrition Board of the National Academy of Sciences very recently stated that there is no need for the average healthy individual to be concerned about restricting dietary cholesterol and saturated fats. The board feels that there is no clear evidence that reducing serum cholesterol by dietary changes can prevent coronary heart disease. Other risk factors such as sex, heredity, hypertension, obesity, diabetes, physical inactivity, and smoking are judged to be more important. Nevertheless, the dietary precautions may be worthy of consideration, at least in men in whom low density lipoproteins are known to be elevated, as well as in individuals with the other risks of developing cardiovascular disease. Indeed, a very recent report based on a 20-year follow-up of nearly 2000 men indicates that those consuming greater quantities of saturated fats had higher serum cholesterol levels and were at greater risks of heart attacks than those on low fat diets in which the fats were predominantly unsaturated.

On the other hand, some scientists have doubts about the advisability of consuming substantial quantities of polyunsaturated fats. These investigators point out that it is the unsaturated fatty acids that are involved in the peroxidation that releases free radicals, which are known to damage cells and accelerate aging. Moreover, an intake of polyunsaturated lipids, as well as saturated fats, increases the level of bile acids in the colon, a condition favorable to colon tumorigenesis. And finally, a high intake of unsaturated fats stimulates the synthesis of prostaglandins, some of which mediate inflammatory changes and interfere with the insulin response to glucose.

In considering the role of diet in hyperlipidemia one must realize that restricting cholesterol-containing foods may not substantially reduce serum cholesterol in all cases because the endogenous synthesis of cholesterol accounts for at least 80% of that lipid in the serum. Furthermore, a reduction in dietary cholesterol tends to stimulate its endogenous production. There is a recent discovery that may explain the absence of a significant relation between diet and serum cholesterol levels in some persons. Apparently, blood cholesterol levels can be regulated by lipoprotein receptors on liver cells. Removal of cholesterol from the blood depends on these receptors. In individuals who must restrict dietary fats in order to control cholesterol levels, it is thought that receptor binding is faulty.

TABLE 11-3

Approximate Weight Percentages for Saturated and Unsaturated Fatty Acids in Some Common Foods

| Food | SATURATED | | | | |
	Capric	Lauric	Myristic	Palmitic	Stearic
Chicken	—	2	7	25	6
Egg	—	—	—	25	10
Beef	—	—	2	29	22
Butter	6	4	12	28	16
Corn	—	—	—	12	3
Peanut	—	—	—	13	4
Soybean	—	—	—	12	4
Olive	—	—	—	13	2
Coconut	8	51	20	10	3

Source: *Dietary Fat and Human Health,* Pub. 1147 National Academy of Sciences, National Research Council, 1966.

An elevation of serum triglycerides more likely stems from an excessive intake of carbohydrate rather than lipid. Triglyceridemia is often associated with glucose intolerance and obesity.

About 97% of the carbohydrate in the American diet becomes glucose in the blood. It has already been pointed out that glucose is not an essential nutrient. Moreover, there is very little carbohydrate in the structural components of the body. Does this mean that carbohydrate can be excluded from the diet? Such a practice would certainly not provide the most effective nutrition for several reasons. A primary cellular role of organic nutrient is to supply chemical energy for performing work and providing heat necessary for maintaining living tissue. Carbohydrate is ideal for this, and a diet devoid of it may not adequately spare enough of the high quality protein needed for tissue repletion. Moreover, a severe restriction of carbohydrate intake can lead to a pronounced metabolic turnover of lipid. If the rate of lipid metabolism occurs faster than the body can handle the intermediate products, the incompletely oxidized ketones promote a potentially serious acidosis. Such a state occurs in severe, uncontrolled diabetes. In this disorder the high rate of lipid turnover stems from faulty glucose utilization, which exists despite the amount of carbohydrate intake. Also, when there is an extreme restriction of dietary carbohydrate in normal individuals, the insulin response mechanism is not being adequately challenged; this in itself can result in transient intolerance to glucose (so-called starvation diabetes).

Yet another good reason for including carbohydrate in the

		UNSATURATED		
Palmitoleic	Oleic	Linoleic	Linolenic	Arachidonic
8	36	16	—	—
—	50	10	2	3
3	41	2	1	—
5	28	1	—	—
—	29	55	1	—
—	54	27	—	2
—	25	53	6	—
1	74	9	1	—
—	6	2	—	—

diet is that the coarser carbohydrate-containing foods possess indigestible polysaccharides such as cellulose, hemicellulose, and pectins. These are not nutritious, but they stimulate peristaltic movements of the gastrointestinal tract, and their absorption of water provides bulk to the intestinal contents. This facilitates elimination, a benefit that may be of importance to those predisposed to colon tumorigenesis.

Finally, it should be pointed out that severe dietary restriction of carbohydrate eventually may lead to certain chemical imbalances in the brain, since carbohydrate is needed for normal conversion of tryptophan to serotonin.

However, there are conditions, such as reactive hypoglycemia, in which the quantity of quickly absorbable carbohydrate must be restricted in the diet. Hypoglycemia is discussed at length in Chapter 12.

VITAMINS

We live in the vitamin age, meaning that many individuals have become thoroughly convinced that high intakes of various vitamin substances not only are essential to their daily well-being, but also are necessary in both preventing and curing a variety of ailments.

Except for certain circumstances, vitamin requirements probably are met by consuming a balanced diet. Exceptional circumstances include subjection to various forms of chemical stress as well as infirmity from old age, disease, or alcoholism, particularly when digestion and absorption are compromised. Yet megavitamin therapy is being advocated by a number of reputable individuals to deal with ills ranging from influenza to schizophrenia; and orthomolecular medicine, which advocates megavitamin therapy, has begun to establish a foothold among a minority of clinicians. However, it is too early to announce a verdict in the controversy pervading megavitamin benefits, despite reports of promising indications in some usages of the water-soluble vitamins.

Although given amounts of certain vitamins can be synthesized in the body by colon bacteria, or formed from precursor substances, we consider the vitamins to be essential nutrients. Dietary requirements ordinarily amount to extremely minute quantities. Vitamin substances are conveniently divided into those which are primarily lipid-soluble and those which are water-soluble. The distinction is significant in determining how vitamins are absorbed and distributed in tissues, as well as how long they persist in the body. Lipid-soluble vitamins tend to accumulate in fatty tissues, which means that they are cleared much more slowly than water-soluble substances. For this reason daily intake of water-soluble vitamins is more crucial.

Lipid-soluble vitamins are known popularly by the letter designations, A, D, E, and K. Water-soluble vitamins include ascorbic acid (vitamin C) and the group known as the B complex. A special Food and Nutrition Board of the National Academy of Sciences has established *recommended dietary allowances* (RDA) for the daily intake of vitamins. The allowances change from time to time, and obviously are not magic numbers upon which even the experts agree. At best they are arbitrary guidelines. A complete list of RDA values for vitamins is presented in Table 11-4. Note that allowances for the lipid-soluble vitamins are given in international units (IU), whereas the water-soluble substances are given in milligrams (mg) or micrograms (μg). An IU represents a given amount of biologic activity. Though subclinical vitamin deficiencies are recognized from time to time, true vitamin deficiency diseases are no longer common among most people of the more advanced, industrial nations.

Lipid-Soluble Vitamins

The most active form of vitamin A is *retinol* (Figure 11-4). Most of its requirement is met through the ingestion of plant carotenes. In an adult, liver reserves of retinol can last for several months without replenishment. Like most lipid-soluble substances, absorption of ret-

TABLE 11-4

Recommended Daily Allowances for Vitamins in Adults

VITAMIN	RDA
Retinol (vitamin A)	5000 IU
Cholecalciferol (vitamin D)	400 IU
Tocopherols (vitamin E)	30 IU
Vitamin K	90 μg
Thiamine (B$_1$)	1.5 mg
Riboflavin (B$_2$)	1.7 mg
Niacin	18.0 mg
Pyridoxine (B$_6$)	2.0 mg
Pantothenic acid	7.0 mg
Cobalamin (B$_{12}$)	3.0 μg
Folic acid	0.4 mg
Choline	not established
Ascorbic acid (vitamin C)	60.0 mg

Source: Food and Nutrition Board, National Academy of Sciences, National Research Council Revised Recommendations, 1980.

inol is enhanced by bile secretion, but impaired by the presence of mineral oil. In addition to the well-established roles of vitamin A, animal experiments within the past few years have suggested that the vitamin and its derivatives (retinoids) can interfere with the cellular transformation of metabolites brought about by carcinogens. Thus some believe that retinol deficiency may heighten carcinogenic changes. Also, there has been some success with use of vitamin A in treating acne.

Vitamin A deficiency is not often a problem among adults except for alcoholics. The dehydrogenase enzyme necessary for metabolizing ethanol to acetaldehyde is the same one required in converting beta carotene to retinol. Thus the presence of ethanol blocks the synthesis of retinol. Excessive levels of vitamin A are probably more frequent than deficiencies of the vitamin. A daily intake exceeding 50,000 IU produces toxicity within a few weeks, resulting in pain in the bones and joints, loss of hair, skin desquamation, and anorexia. In some individuals such symptoms have prompted the idea that they need more vitamins! There are over 4000 *reported* cases each year of poisonings from vitamins A and D.

The physiologic role of vitamin D (cholecalciferol) was discussed in Chapter 6 in relation to its synthesis in the skin from exposure to ultraviolet radiation. Because of the widespread incorporation of vitamin D in milk and other foods, there may be a greater risk of vitamin D excess than vitamin D deficiency. The toxicity from

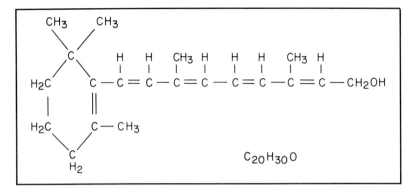

FIGURE 11-4 **Chemical structure of retinol (vitamin A).** Two molecules of this substance are produced by the oxidation of a molecule of carotene ($C_{40}H_{56}$).

excessive vitamin D produces similar effects and symptoms as are found in hypervitaminosis A.

Vitamin E substances (*tocopherols*) are resistant to high temperature and acids, but are readily oxidized; therefore they tend to prevent molecular oxygen from combining with other molecules. The potent antioxidant capability of alpha tocopherol underlies its principal function as a vitamin. For example, vitamin E helps to prevent the oxidation of vitamin A. Therefore, its presence spares this vitamin. Tocopherols also suppress the oxidation of polyunsaturated fatty acids.

The RDA of 15 to 30 IU for vitamin E was not established until a few years ago, and there is much controversy and disagreement concerning the requirement. With greater intakes of polyunsaturated fats, as has been recommended for the prevention of atherosclerosis, the requirement for vitamin E is increased. Also, in regions of heavy air pollution, where the levels of ozone and other atmospheric oxidants are formidable, it would appear that high dosages of vitamin E can help protect the lungs from tissue damage. No toxicity to large amounts of the vitamin has ever been shown.

For the past 20 years the tocopherols have been claimed by some to be miraculously effective in treating a variety of disorders, and many individuals faithfully consume vitamin E supplements in order to prevent and alleviate a number of vascular problems. Yet in truth the use of the vitamin in cardiovascular disorders appears to be based primarily on hope and speculation. Despite the paucity of positive effects from clinical use, in vitro studies and experiments with animals have indicated that vitamin E, because of its antioxidant properties, may be capable of slowing the rate of the aging process. As far as humans are concerned, there is as yet no striking evidence that high doses of vitamin E retard changes associated with aging, although there are claims that extremely high dosages are helpful in promoting repair of tissue damaged from burns.

The RDA for vitamin K is only recently established. Fortunately, dietary deficiency is seldom a problem. Much of the vitamin is synthesized by normal colon bacteria. Deficiencies of vitamin K infrequently occur among the newborn and the elderly. Newborns have less intestinal flora and therefore synthesize the vitamin less readily. For this reason vitamin K injections are frequently given, particularly to premature newborns. In elderly persons, deficiencies of vitamin K may result from liver disease, biliary insufficiency, and uremia, or from the use of drugs such as blood anticoagulants (dicumarol), aspirin, and certain antibiotics. Antibiotics destroy the synthesizing bacteria in the colon.

Water-Soluble Vitamins

Without frequent replacement the tissues may become depleted of water-soluble vitamins, particularly during stress. This fact has prompted the designation *antistress vitamins* for ascorbic acid and substances of the B complex. Daily requirements probably are significantly increased in a stressed individual.

Many of the substances grouped together as B complex vitamins share an interrelated role as essential factors in the oxidative enzyme systems of all cells. A food plentiful in one B vitamin is often a reliable source for some of the other B complex vitamins. With the advent of flour-refining, concern developed over potential deficiencies in B vitamins. As a consequence, practically all breads and cereals today are fortified with at least thiamine, riboflavin, and niacin.

Several of the B vitamins are synthesized by bacteria in the colon. When the metabolic rate of the body is elevated, as occurs with increases in thyroid output, the requirement for B vitamins becomes substantially greater. The requirement is also much greater when the diet is high in calories. When the intake of B vitamins exceeds their utilization, they are excreted with little delay. Indeed, the determination of the level of any water-soluble vitamin in a urine sample can offer some measure of whether or not the individual may be getting too much or too little.

Thiamine (B_1), riboflavin (B_2), and niacin are essential coenzymes in the oxidative dehydrogenations and decarboxylations

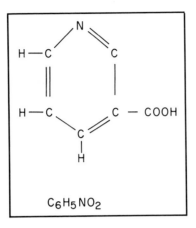

$C_6H_5NO_2$

FIGURE 11-5   Molecular structure of nicotinic acid (niacin). This substance forms an essential part of nicotinamide adenine dinucleotide, a necessary coenzyme in the respiratory chain of all cells.

characterizing cellular respiration, whereas pantothenic acid forms an integral part of coenzyme A, so vital in introducing acetate to the Krebs cycle (see Chapter 12). A clinical deficiency of thiamine is termed *polyneuritis* (in Asia the disease is called *beri-beri*). Niacin (Figure 11-5) has the highest RDA of any B vitamin, and since it can be synthesized from tryptophan, deficiencies of niacin are associated with protein malnutrition. A clinical deficiency of niacin is called *pellagra*, which once was frequently encountered in the backward areas of southeastern United States, where corn was the chief dietary staple. Megadoses of niacin are being employed clinically for treating schizophrenia, alleviating cerebral vasoconstriction, and lowering serum cholesterol. Despite some optimistic claims, a number of individuals so treated have not been able to maintain striking benefits over prolonged periods of time. High dosages of niacin can produce palpitations and flushing of the skin.

Other B vitamins are pyridoxine (B_6), choline, cobalamin (B_{12}), and folic acid. The latter two substances are mentioned in Chapter 9 as essential in preventing anemia.

Like vitamin E, ascorbic acid (vitamin C) has had lavish claims made in its behalf in regard to prevention and cure of disease. Megadoses of ascorbic acid have been purported to both prevent and cure colds and influenza. In addition, vitamin C has been said to lower blood levels of cholesterol and glucose, alleviate arthritis, and counteract numerous effects of stress. The fact that the vitamin is concentrated in the adrenal glands has excited speculation that it is some sort of antistress substance. Despite these notions it has yet to be resolved whether or not vitamin C does indeed prevent upper respiratory infections or effectively reduce their severity or duration. The other claims are also controversial.

It is well established that ascorbic acid is essential for the hydroxylation of two amino acids (proline and lysine), which are important constituents of collagen, the protein so necessary for wound-healing and the repair of injury to connective tissue. However, only 15 to 30 mg of vitamin C per day prevents *scurvy*, the clinical deficiency of vitamin C. The same amount of the substance replenishes metabolic turnover in ordinary instances, and taking more than 100 mg per day will not appreciably increase the blood level of ascorbic acid. This is not to say that intake beyond 100 mg will not enhance cellular utilization of the vitamin by certain tissues.

Even though moderate doses of ascorbic acid are nontoxic, an intake exceeding 3 to 4 grams per day has been known to interfere with action of vitamin B_{12} and dispose the urinary system to stone formation. Diarrhea and urinary irritation also have resulted from extremely high doses. However, ascorbic acid (Figure 11-6) is a strong chemical-reducing substance, theoretically capable of suppressing formation of many toxins and other organics such as nitrosamines, which are formed from food additives and are reputedly carcinogenic. In vitro studies are showing that ascorbic acid indeed can perform as an anticarcinogen.

MINERAL IMBALANCE

There does not appear to be quite the same degree of popular obsession with dietary minerals as there is with vitamins. Yet, minerals are just as essential. Certain ones such as calcium, phosphorus, magnesium, sodium, potassium, and chloride are required in relatively large amounts (> 100 mg per day). Sodium, potassium, and chloride are discussed as electrolytes along with water in the next section. Practically speaking, phosphorus warrants little comment since deficiencies of this element are rare.

Only a few micrograms per day are needed for most mineral substances; nevertheless they are very important. Physicians interested in preventive medicine have adopted a procedure of having hair samples from their patients analyzed in order to determine the level and balance of trace minerals. It has been found that deficien-

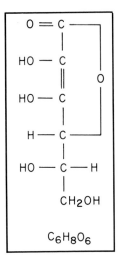

FIGURE 11-6 **Molecular structure of ascorbic acid (vitamin C).** This controversial substance is capable of participating in many cellular reduction-oxidation reactions. It has a structural similarity to glucose.

cies of calcium, magnesium, iron, and iodine are not infrequent. According to the 1979 surgeon general's report, iron is the most common nutrient deficiency in America. The RDA values for minerals are listed in Table 11-5.

The body regulation of the calcium pool maintains the blood level of this mineral at about 9 to 11 mg/dl. A number of interactions are involved in calcium regulation; these are displayed in Figure 11-7. The absorption of calcium from food can vary from 10% to 40%. Other dietary ingredients such as oxalic acid, phytic acid, excessive fat, and excessive phosphate reduce the absorption of calcium. Many adults would experience improved mineral balance with additional calcium intake. However, calcium supplements do not dramatically correct the osteoporosis found in elderly women. In these cases the significant deficiency is not calcium content alone, but involves an underproduction of estrogens, which influence calcium deposition. In normal cases, excessive calcium intake is not a problem since it is excreted within a short time. Actually, excessive intake is quite uncommon.

About 80% of the iron pool is incorporated into hemoglobin, and the remainder is utilized in the synthesis of myoglobin and mitochondrial cytochrome. The body's utilization of iron is depicted in Figure 11-8.

In healthy men there is a combined iron reserve in the liver,

TABLE 11-5

Recommended Daily Allowances for Minerals in Adults

MINERAL		RDA
Calcium		1.0 g
Phosphorus		1.0 g
Magnesium		400.00 mg
Sodium	usually considered	3–9 g
Chlorine	together (NaCl)	
Potassium		2–5 g
Iron		women 20 mg; men 15 mg
Iodine		women 150 ug; men 150 ug
Manganese		3–5 mg
Copper		2–3 mg
Zinc		15 mg
Fluorine		2.5 mg
Selenium		0.1 mg
Chromium		0.1 mg
Sulfur		not established; adequate with normal protein intake

Source: Food and Nutrition Board, National Academy of Sciences, National Research Council Revised Recommendations, 1980.

spleen, and bone marrow of about 1000 mg, compared to about 300 mg in premenopausal women, a surprising portion of whom experience borderline anemia.

Within a 24-hour period the turnover of iron in the body amounts to about 27 mg, of which the average absorption from food is only 10%. The degree of absorption can vary considerably. Indeed, it is the absorption rate that is the primary regulator of the iron pool. An acidic medium which reduces ferric iron to the ferrous form stimulates absorption. Excessive intake of iron supplements can irritate the gastrointestinal mucosa. Moreover, this practice is wasteful in that absorption eventually becomes suppressed, leading to excretion of practically all the iron. Along with iron, the trace minerals, cobalt, manganese, and copper are important in hemoglobin synthesis.

Iodine is required for the iodination of the amino acid tyrosine in the thyroid gland. When thyroid hormones are utilized, iodine is released into the circulation, and about one-third of it can be reincorporated into hormones. The remainder is excreted. A significant insufficiency of dietary iodine results in simple goiter. Only a minute quantity of iodine is required, but most foods are poor iodine sources and not all salt is iodized.

In recent years nutritionists have begun to express concern

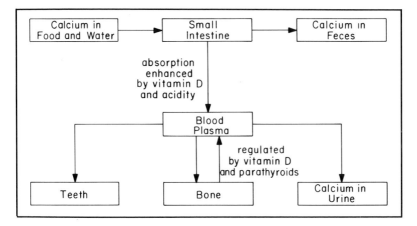

FIGURE 11-7   Regulation of the body's calcium pool. Regulation is aimed at maintaining a stable blood level of the mineral.

with the needs for several trace minerals, notably fluorine, zinc, chromium, and possibly selenium. The fluoride salts of calcium are less readily mobilized from bones and teeth than is calcium phosphate; hence, fluorides stabilize the mineral content of these structures. Zinc is an essential constituent of several important enzymes, notably carbonic anhydrase, whereas chromium appears to be associated with a normal insulin response in glucose tolerance. In fact, a chromium-containing glucose tolerance factor (GTF) has now been recognized.

As with all essential nutrients, the key to optimum mineral utilization in the body is an appropriate balance among them. For example, when calcium intake is high, zinc is poorly absorbed. More attention is being given to mineral imbalance as a factor associated with susceptibility to several chronic ailments, among which are irregular cardiac rhythms, anemia, glucose intolerance, infertility, and neuromuscular weakness. The cations are especially important. Magnesium, for example, is a highly significant anabolic cofactor in sparking many cell reactions.

WATER, ELECTROLYTES, AND RENAL IMPAIRMENT

As stated in Chapter 3, the interchange of materials that constantly occurs between cells and the internal environment is dependent upon a fluid medium that is precisely regulated in both volume and

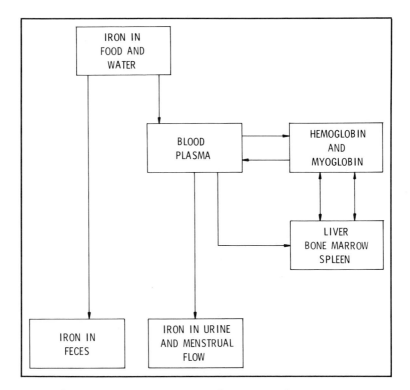

FIGURE 11-8   Regulation of iron in the body. Observe the interaction existing between the blood and reservoirs such as the liver, bone marrow, and spleen. A considerable amount of iron from hemoglobin and myoglobin decomposition can rejoin the iron pool in the plasma.

composition. The need for water intake is a significant component in the regulation. One may survive for weeks without food, but death occurs after several days of water deprivation; even a 15% loss of body water can be critical. Obligatory losses of water in the feces, from the lungs, and through insensible perspiration occur regardless of fluid intake. The amount of obligatory water loss from the kidneys depends upon how much urea and sodium chloride must be dissolved and excreted. It is estimated that there should be around 1 milliliter of water intake per calorie of food ingested. Diets with substantial quantities of protein have higher water requirements because there is a greater production of urea. The balance of water intake and water excretion is shown in Table 11-6.

Under normal circumstances the amount of water in the body is controlled by the amount of sodium we retain, and body sodium content is regulated primarily by the kidney. Thus an impairment in kidney function resulting in faulty filtration and/or increased so-

TABLE 11-6
Balance of Water in the Body

DAILY AVAILABILITY		DAILY EXCRETION	
Water intake (fluids)	1000–1200 ml	Urine volume	900–1100 ml
Water intake in food	800–1000 ml	Water in feces	100– 300 ml
Water from oxidation	100– 300 ml	Water vapor from skin	500– 700 ml
		Water vapor from lungs	400– 500 ml
	1900–2500 ml		1900–2600 ml

dium resorption risks hypervolemia and a consequent elevation in blood pressure. This subject is pursued at greater length in the next subsection.

It is recalled that various stresses promote aldosterone secretion, which increases the renal resorption of sodium. Excessive dietary intake of salt has become a strongly ingrained habit among many people. By the time these individuals reach middle age, a number of them may have become hypertensive. Diuretics are then prescribed to reduce sodium resorption and stimulate loss of excess fluid.

In fasting, or the elimination of dietary carbohydrate, the kidneys are not as effective in bringing about retention of sodium. The consequent loss of body water suddenly reduces body weight. However, there is no fat removal. Weight loss due to fluid reduction is brief.

In addition to sodium, other electrolytes are potassium and chloride. There is rarely a deficiency of chloride, and even though potassium deficiencies occur, they ordinarily are not of dietary origin, but are often associated with drug therapies. The body regulation of sodium and potassium shows an inverse relationship. The hormone aldosterone increases potassium excretion while decreasing sodium excretion. Most potassium deficiencies are associated with the administration of drugs used as diuretics that restrict renal resorption of potassium as well as sodium. Potassium deficiency (hypokalemia) is characterized by fatigue, weakness, and tachycardia. The ECG may show alterations. In fact, potassium depletion can produce serious irregularities in the cardiac cycle as well as induce behavioral aberrations.

Dehydration can become a serious problem when there is excessive sweating, prolonged fever, and persistent diarrhea or vomiting. Another condition in which the fluid balance becomes deranged is *diabetes insipidus.* In this disorder there is a deficiency of

TABLE 11-7
Conditions That May Lead to Progressive Kidney Failure

Infections

Inflammatory processes

Widespread vascular disease

Connective tissue disorders

Metabolic abnormalities (diabetes mellitus)

Toxicity

Obstructions

Congenital disorders

Hypertension, particularly the malignant form

---

antidiuretic hormone (ADH) from the posterior pituitary, resulting in excessive thirst and the excretion of unusually large volumes of urine.

Renal Impairment

Imbalances in the volume and composition of body fluids and electrolytes typically result from faulty operation of the kidney, the major organ responsible for this homeostasis. There are various types of conditions that can lead to progressive kidney failure. Some of these are listed in Table 11-7. In malignant hypertension renal damage progresses rapidly (Figure 11-9).

The most encountered form of kidney pathology is *glomerulonephritis*, which can be acute or chronic. Acute inflammation classically follows a streptococcal infection, and the glomerular damage is brought about by the body's immune reaction to beta-hemolytic streptococcus. In chronic glomerulonephritis the onset is insidious, and the condition may not be discovered until late in the course. The causes of chronic glomerulonephritis are variable. Hypertension is often involved, but it is not always clear whether this is a cause or an effect of the nephritis. Immune complexes from various parts of the body may become trapped in the glomeruli, where they produce inflammation. Long-standing cases of diabetes mellitus also may be associated with progressive glomerular pathology (Figure 5-10). Some of the specific conditions that can lead to chronic glomerulonephritis are presented in Table 11-8.

The course of chronic renal failure can be monitored by denoting changes in glomerular function. Such changes are assessed

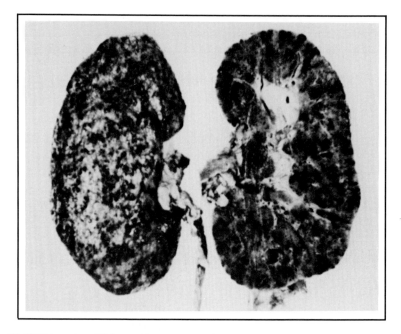

FIGURE 11-9   Kidney disease brought about by malignant hypertension. The gross pathology reveals much mottling and discoloration, due to microscopic hemorrhages. (From W. Boyd and H. Sheldon, *An introduction to the study of disease*, 7th ed. Philadelphia: Lea & Febiger, 1977.)

through measurement of the glomerular filtration rate (GFR) by means of such methods as creatinine clearance or inulin clearance. Blood urea nitrogen (BUN) levels are measured also, but BUN values may vary considerably in relation to the amount of dietary protein and fluid intake. Administration of diuretics raises BUN levels. Serum creatinine values may be more reliably interpreted than BUN. This is because creatinine levels are more stable and less subject to variation. Normal values for several assessments of renal function are presented in Table 11-9.

In the first stages of progressive kidney failure there are insidious decreases in renal reserve, though the values for serum creatinine and BUN may appear normal unless severe demands are being imposed on the kidney. By the second stage of impairment the GFR is at least 25% less than normal, and the BUN is somewhat elevated. At this point the condition is characterized by *azotemia* (nitrogen retention). Nocturia and polyuria may become frequent during this stage, and there may be transient edema of the lower legs.

TABLE 11-8
Disturbances Leading to Chronic Glomerulonephritis

Hypertension
Repeated infections with hemolytic streptococcus
Systemic lupus erythematosus
Diabetes mellitus
Gout
Lead toxicity
Overuse of phenacetin (an analgesic)
Renal arteriosclerosis

TABLE 11-9
Normal Values for Renal Function Tests

Glomerular filtration rate (GFR)	110 ml/min–140 ml/min
Blood urea nitrogen (BUN)	7–25 mg/dl
Blood creatinine	0.7–1.5 mg/dl
Blood uric acid	3.5–7.5 mg/dl
Urinalysis (pH)	5.0–7.5
Urinalysis (specific gravity)	1.02
Urinalysis	Absence of proteinuria and hematuria

The final stage of progressive renal failure is *uremia.* The GFR is only 10% of normal, and the creatinine clearance may be as low as 10 ml per minute. It is apparent that fluid and electrolyte homeostasis has failed. The urine becomes iso-osmotic with the plasma at a fixed specific gravity of 1.01, and the urine output per day diminishes to less than 500 ml. Azotemia markedly increases, and BUN values may exceed 75 mg/dl.

Before the point of severe uremia is reached, the patient should resort to treatment of periodic hemodialysis (Figure 11-10), or a kidney transplant. A newer, and even more effective therapy is called *continuous ambulatory peritoneal dialysis* (CAPD). At the start of therapy, a special cleansing solution is injected into the peritoneal cavity of the patient's abdomen. This space serves as a reservoir for the cleansing fluid, which attracts impurities from the blood through the walls of the blood vessels by diffusion. Four times daily

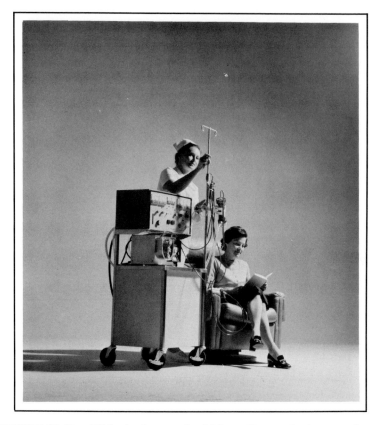

FIGURE 11-10   Dialysis therapy for kidney disease. In the procedure, blood withdrawn from an artery of the patient enters the dialysis machine (artificial kidney) at the top. After passing through dialysis membranes, purified blood leaves the machine and is returned to a vein of the patient's arm. (Courtesy of Cordis Corporation.)

the patient empties the fluid into a throw-away plastic bag and instills a fresh solution through a permanently implanted catheter. This treatment is far superior to conventional dialysis: it is less time-consuming, is more convenient, is free of pain, eliminates restriction in diet and fluid intake, and is less expensive. It does seem to make more sense to put the washing solution into the body rather than take the blood out of the body and expose it externally to a cleansing solution.

The uremic syndrome is characterized by a severe metabolic acidosis associated with hyperkalemia, which in turn has a critical

TABLE 11-10
Abnormal Body Effects Associated with Uremia

Metabolic acidosis
Azotemia (nitrogen retention)
Hyperkalemia (excessive serum potassium)
Proteinuria
Hypertension
Congestive heart failure
Anemia
Anorexia
Muscle wasting
Weakness
Lethargy
Hypocalcemia
Restlessness and confusion

influence on the electrical conductance of the heart. Indeed, the overall breakdown of fluid and electrolyte regulation imposes serious changes throughout the body. The major complications of uremia are listed in Table 11-10. When the pH of the blood remains below 7.0, death occurs within a short time.

SUMMARY

To avoid nutritive stress, an adequate pool for each nutrient must be maintained. Pool input that exceeds output produces positive nutritive balance, whereas excessive output promotes negative balance, both of which can eventually lead to disease.

An essential nutrient is one whose requirement cannot be fulfilled by synthesis alone. Water, vitamins, and minerals are essential. So are eight amino acids and three fatty acids.

Only 35 to 45 grams of protein per day are normally needed to prevent negative nitrogen balance. Diets deficient in complete proteins are much more frequent than those deficient in protein quantity. One or more of the essential amino acids is missing in incomplete proteins.

It is thought by some researchers that liberal intake of saturated fats promotes cholesterolemia, which can lead to atherosclerosis, at least in predisposed persons. Diets high in any form of fat are believed to play a role in the development of colon tumors.

Thus far, the claims of health benefits from megavitamin usage have not been unequivocally substantiated. On the other hand, there are thousands of cases each year in which there are adverse effects from hypervitaminosis. Except for instances of infirmity and prolonged subjection to stress, most vitamin requirements can be fulfilled by consuming an adequate diet.

Minerals are essential in the diet, and deficiencies in calcium, magnesium, and iron are not infrequent, particularly iron in premenopausal women.

The major variable underlying water balance in the body is sodium regulation, performed primarily by the kidney. Thus renal impairment favors fluid retention and consequent hypertension. A common dietary stressor of importance in this regard is an unrestricted salt intake.

The most frequently encountered form of renal pathology is chronic glomerulonephritis, in which filtration becomes progressively impaired. The impairment results in azotemia (nitrogen retention) and eventually the nephritis leads to uremia, a condition in which the kidneys have failed.

Chapter Glossary

adiposity   storage of body fat

antioxidant   a substance interfering with oxygen's combining with other materials

cation   atom or group of atoms with positive charge; e.g. Na^+, K^+

creatinine   a nitrogenous derivative of creatine phosphate that is excreted in the urine

hyperkalemia   excessive levels of potassium in the body fluids

isotosmotic   osmotic equilibrium; the osmolar concentrations on each side of a cell membrane are equal

ketones   compounds containing the $C=O$ group that are usually acid-producing

nocturia   the need to urinate during the night

polyuria   frequent, excessive urination

precursor   a preceding chemical stage or substrate

reactive hypoglycemia   a reduction in postprandial blood glucose that is significantly greater than usual

For Further Reading

Cameron, J. S. 1972. Natural history of glomerulonephritis. In D. A. K. Black, ed., *Renal disease.* 3rd ed. London: Blackwell Pub.

Draper, H. H., ed. 1979. *Advances in nutritional research.* Vol. 2. New York: Plenum Press.

Fernstrom, J. D., and Wurtmen, R. J. February, 1974. Nutrition and the brain. *Sci Am* 230:84.

Freeland, R. A., and Briggs, S. 1977. *A biochemical approach to nutrition.* New York: John Wiley and Sons.

Guyton, A. C. 1971. *Medical physiology.* 4th ed. Philadelphia: W. B. Saunders Co. Part 10, Chaps. 68, 69, 73.

Hodges, R. E., ed. 1979. Nutrition: Metabolic and clinical applications. In *Human nutrition: A comprehensive treatise.* Vol. 4. New York: Plenum Press.

Hunt, S. 1980. *Nutrition: Principles and clinical practice.* New York: John Wiley and Sons.

Kurtzman, N. A., ed. 1977. *Pathophysiology of the kidney.* Springfield, Ill.: Charles C Thomas Pubs.

Lamb, L. E. 1974. *Metabolics: Putting your food energy to work.* New York: Harper & Row Pubs.

Levy, J. V., and Bach-y-Rita, P. 1976. *Vitamins: Their use and abuse.* New York: Liveright Publishing Corp.

Overton, M. H., and Lukert, B. P. 1979. *Clinical nutrition: A physiologic approach.* Chicago: Year Book Medical Publishers. Times Mirror.

Phillips, M., and Baetz, A., eds. 1981. Diet and resistance to disease. In *Advances in experimental medicine and biology.* Vol. 135. New York: Plenum Press.

Robinson, C. H. 1972. *Normal and therapeutic nutrition.* 14th ed. New York: Macmillan Publishing Co.

Roche, A. F., and Falkner, F. 1974. *Nutrition and malnutrition: Identification and measurement.* New York: Plenum Press.

Roe, D. A. 1979. *Clinical nutrition for the health scientist.* Boca Raton, Fla.: CRC Press, Inc.

Schier, R., ed. 1976. *Renal and electrolyte disorders.* Boston: Little, Brown & Co.

Taylor, T. G. 1978. *Principles of human nutrition.* London: Edward Arnold Publishers.

Thiele, V. 1977. *Clinical nutrition.* St. Louis: C. V. Mosby Co.

Vander, A. J. 1976. In Introduction to *Human physiology and the environment in health and disease.* San Francisco: W. H. Freeman and Co. Part 1, Articles 1, 2, 3.

Vander, A. J.; Sherman, J. H.; and Luciano, D. S. 1980. *Human physiology: The mechanisms of body function.* 3rd ed. New York: McGraw-Hill Book Co. Chaps. 7, 15.

Weldy, N. J. 1976. *Body fluids and electrolytes.* 2d ed. St. Louis: C. V. Mosby Co.

12

Caloric Imbalance and Food Intolerance

Excessive Calories and Obesity
Energy Metabolism
Formation of Fat
The Problem of Overeating
Glucose Intolerance
Insulin Resistance
Hypoglycemia and Glucose Tolerance
Lactose Intolerance
Food Sensitivity

‖ **Objectives:** Upon completing this chapter you should:

1. Recognize the causes and pathologic consequences of excessive caloric intake, probably today's most serious stress on the body.
2. Understand how energy metabolism becomes deranged from overeating and physical inactivity.
3. Be fully informed about the nature, causes, and correction of glucose intolerance in adult-onset diabetes.
4. Know how a relative deficiency of lactase leads to intolerance of lactose (milk sugar).
5. Be acquainted with the occurrence and nature of chronic sensitivity to foods.

The preceding chapter treats the principle of nutritive balance: in this chapter that principle is applied to calories. Concepts are emerging that provide new and exciting insight into the relationship of nutritive intake to metabolic stress, obesity, diabetes, and adverse reactions to foods. Excessive caloric intake and poor tolerance of various food ingredients are combined here because in certain respects they appear to be interrelated.

The reality of what is sometimes termed *chemical addiction,* though poorly understood, appears to be applicable to food, as well as to alcohol, tobacco, and various drugs. Whatever the nature of chemical addiction, it has much to do with the stress and health impairment discussed in this chapter. When we feel jittery, restless, tired, depressed, or tense in social situations, we often feel compelled to partake of something. For many people the something is often food. The practice frequently leads to an established habit of indiscriminate eating. There is reason to believe that in many of us the hunger drive has become altered, and food is being relied upon to satisfy psychologic needs, or needs rooted in biochemical disturbances within the body. What one does not eat may promote health as well as what one does ingest.

EXCESSIVE CALORIES AND OBESITY

Without question the major malnutritive problem in most industrialized regions of the world is excessive caloric intake, resulting from an overindulgence in sugars, fats, and protein. This is especially true in the United States, according to a report of the Senate Committee on Nutrition and Human Needs.

The direct consequence of hypercaloric stress is excessive weight. Obesity is the most common disease in America—and the precursor of other diseases. Indeed, nearly one-third of the nation's population is obese, and an additional one-third is considered to be above normal weight much of the time. Furthermore, the incidence shows no sign of improving. Based upon a comparison of figures from the 1960s with those from the 1970s, it is apparent that the incidence of obesity is increasing.

It must be understood that what constitutes ideal weight is not an objective standard uniformly agreed upon. Nevertheless, recommended weights for all adult ages are being revised downward. A recent weight chart indicative of this downward trend is presented in Table 12-1.

Excessive weight is *strongly* associated with cardiovascular and renal diseases, diabetes, and hypertension. It also greatly aggravates degenerative arthritis, gout, gallbladder disease, and hyperlipidemia. Moreover, excessive weight appears to intensify susceptibility to cancer. How does one accumulate excessive weight?

Living cells must continually supply chemical energy in order to create the oxygen-phosphate bonds that make adenosine triphosphate from adenosine diphosphate. ATP is the energy currency of all tissue. The heat necessary for optimum biochemical activity and the electron energy trapped and coupled to ATP synthesis both are derived from the cellular oxidation of organic nutrient. The major form of nutrient that is oxidized is carbohydrate, but fat, protein, and alcohol serve just as well; in fact, fat supplies 9 kilocalories per gram, whereas carbohydrate and protein each supply 4 kcal per gram, and alcohol 7 kcal per gram. The principal reason for the higher energy of fats is that fatty acids are highly reduced compounds (in other words, they have much hydrogen). In addition, fats have a much lower water content than other nutrients, and water has no calories. Points like this are important to remember in preparing diets. Over 70% of the weight of raw, lean steak is water, whereas the water in butter and some salad dressings is less than 20%. Eating vegetables, fruits, and cereals with indigestible fibrous matter also means less body calories per gram ingested.

Of course, physical activity is an important variable in determining whether caloric intake becomes energy or additional body weight. In a study of obese high school girls it was shown that they consumed less food than a group of normal weight girls. However, the obese girls had much less physical activity than those with normal weight. Indeed, many overweight persons express the fact that they are often tired and seem to have little energy.

TABLE 12-1

Desirable Weights for Optimum Health in Adults

	MEN (NUDE)	
Height (in)	Weight (lb)	(kg)
62	112–130	51–59
63	115–134	52–61
64	118–137	54–62
65	121–140	55–64
66	124–144	56–66
67	128–148	58–67
68	132–153	60–69
69	136–157	62–71
70	140–161	64–73
71	144–166	65–75
72	148–171	67–77
73	152–176	69–80
74	156–181	71–82
75	160–186	73–84
76	164–191	75–86
	WOMEN (NUDE)	
58	92–108	42–49
59	94–111	43–50
60	96–114	44–52
61	99–117	45–53
62	102–120	46–55
63	105–123	48–56
64	108–127	49–58
65	111–131	50–60
66	114–136	52–62
67	118–140	54–64
68	122–144	55–65
69	126–148	57–67
70	130–152	59–69
71	134–156	61–71
72	138–160	63–73

Source: Modified from charts of the Metropolitan Life Insurance Company. The modification is based upon the recent concept that the individual should weigh no more than the ideal weight at age 21.

Yet the interesting and somewhat surprising discovery has been made that reduced levels of physical activity can cause an increase in food intake. Studies of both rats and humans have confirmed that low levels of activity do not reduce food intake but actually stimulate eating. These results appear contrary to the example described in the previous paragraph. Such a discrepancy can be explained by the principle of metabolic shifting described in a later subsection of this chapter. As will be explained in the following section, an inactive individual may secrete excessive insulin, which can lead to hypoglycemia and a consequent craving for food. As a beginning in understanding how people become overweight, let us briefly examine what happens to the carbohydrate, fat, protein, and alcohol we consume.

Energy Metabolism

All digested carbohydrate becomes glucose, all protein becomes the various amino acids, and fat becomes fatty acids and glycerol. Once inside cells, each molecule of glucose becomes 2 molecules of 3-carbon pyruvic acid through a series of steps called glycolysis which occur in the cell cytoplasm. Pyruvic acid then permeates mitochondria, where CO_2 is removed, leaving a 2-carbon acetate molecule. Activated acetate is the main metabolic intersection that brings together several biochemical pathways in the cell. In this sense acetate represents the hub of the pathways linking the metabolism of carbohydrate, fat, protein, and alcohol. About two-thirds of the ATP from carbohydrate, oxidation is realized when activated acetate is channeled through the *Krebs cycle*[1], located in the mitochondria. The major points in the oxidation of glucose are summarized in Figure 12-1.

What happens to the fatty acids and glycerol from the fats we eat? Glycerol is a 3-carbon alcohol that is readily converted to phosphoglyceraldehyde, which then becomes pyruvic acid, and its fate from that point is the same as if it originally had been carbohydrate. The carbon chain of fatty acids is decomposed into 2-carbon fragments, each of which is actually 2-carbon acetate which can enter the Krebs cycle. The process of degrading fatty acids to acetate is know as *beta oxidation.* There is an energy yield from the degradation itself, in addition to the energy potentially available after the acetate enters the Krebs cycle.

Before undergoing oxidation, amino acids first must lose the amino NH_2 radical (deamination), and become what are known as *keto acids,* many of which are 2-carbon compounds directly convertible to acetate, which is then available to the Krebs cycle. A few keto acids have 3-carbons and are converted to pyruvic acid, and a few others directly enter various stages of the Krebs cycle.

---

[1]The Krebs cycle is a cyclic series of oxidations that creates most of the ATP energy in the aerobic respiration of all cells of the body. It is named after Sir Hans Krebs, who discovered these reactions.

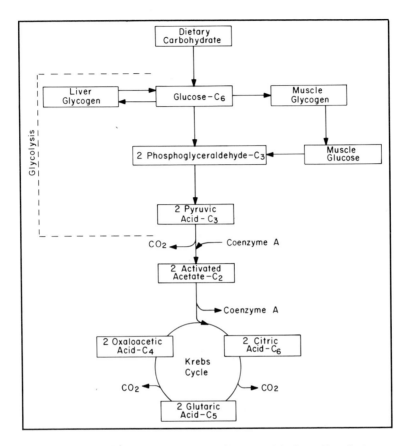

FIGURE 12-1   Pathways of cellular glucose oxidation. Glycolysis occurs in the cytoplasm and does not require oxygen. However, it yields very little energy. The remainder of the process takes place in the mitochondria and yields most of the energy from the original glucose. See text for additional details.

Ethyl alcohol is a 2-carbon molecule, and as one might expect, it also is readily converted to acetate. Millions of people each day consume many calories as alcohol. A standard cocktail contains 100 calories or more from the alcohol alone, exclusive of such additives as fruit juice, sugar, or olives. The relationship among carbohydrates, fats, proteins, and alcohol as energy sources is depicted in Figure 12-2.

Formation of Fat

Acetate, the chemical common denominator of most of our food intake, has fates other than entering the Krebs cycle and generating

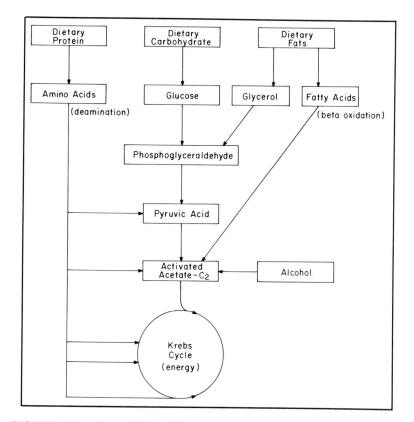

FIGURE 12-2   Interrelationships among the various foodstuffs as energy sources. Regardless of whether the organic nutrient is carbohydrate, fat, protein, or alcohol, practically all of it becomes acetate. See text for further explanation.

ATP and heat. Just as acetate can be derived from fatty acids, so can molecules of acetate be resynthesized to fatty acids, which then combine with glycerol to form fats in cells. However, fat formation is not simply a reversal of fat degradation. The breakdown of fatty acids to acetate is an oxidation. Oxygen in the mitochondria is required to receive the removed hydrogen. On the other hand, the formation of fatty acids from acetate requires no oxygen. No energy is produced; rather energy is consumed. Therefore, when acetate pursues this pathway, fat is being produced, and at the same time energy is being utilized rather than being generated. Thus people gaining weight generate less energy. This may partially explain their inclination to be sedentary.

The synthesis of cholesterol also is from acetate. Hence the essence of the whole energy picture is that all food, whether it be

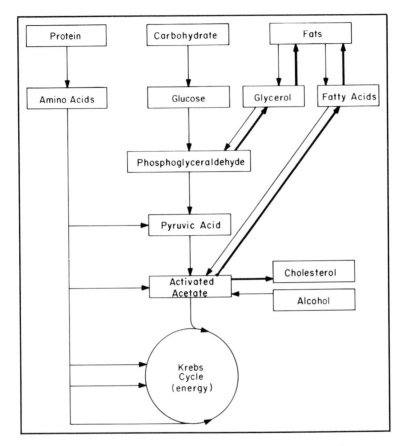

FIGURE 12-3   Dual fate of acetate in metabolism. Activated acetate either generates energy or becomes fat. Which pathway is predominant depends upon the amount of caloric intake in proportion to how much acetate the Krebs cycle can handle. In referring to the diagram it becomes clear why dietary carbohydrate, protein, and alcohol can make a person fat.

carbohydrate, fat, protein, or alcohol, can be converted to energy, fat, and cholesterol. This is what happens to most of the food eaten by adults. The essential features of these metabolic interactions are diagrammed in Figure 12-3.

The practical question arising at this point asks what prompts the body to favor the synthesis of fat over the generation of energy. Why does acetate follow the "fat path" rather than the "energy path"? The major determinant of which pathway is favored at a given time is the amount of calories eaten at that time. It has been stated repeatedly and simply that when the number of calories eaten exceeds those being expended, there will be a gain in weight. When the metabolic mill is overloaded, only a restricted amount of traffic can revolve around the Krebs cycle, which represents the primary energy-producing pathway of the cells. An overflow of acetate must become fat and cholesterol. When an excessive amount of food enters the body, it must be channeled in some direction and metabolized accordingly. When the Krebs cycle is saturated, the remaining acetate has to be pushed into alternate pathways. Normally, a moderately active individual needs only about 15 kcal per day per pound to maintain a desirable weight.

There are individuals, however, who question the simple arithmetic of the relationship of caloric intake to body weight. Such doubts arise from observations of persons who appear to eat generously but never gain weight. For example, a lean farmer may consume his share of hot biscuits, butter, jam, fat pork, and apple pie. In some way he appears to direct more acetate to the energy path than to the fat path. Can the capacity of the Krebs cycle be expanded? How? One possibility is to increase the amount of oxygen reaching the mitochondria. Additional oxygen accepts more hydrogen so that more energy is generated, thereby allowing additional acetate to enter the Krebs cycle. Remember also that the degrading of fatty acids requires oxygen, and the synthesis of fat does not. More oxygen entering the cell would tend to favor the degradative pathway through the principle of mass action. How can more oxygen be supplied? The answer is by increasing the effectiveness of blood circulation and lung ventilation, both of which are vastly improved by the demands of exercise. In all likelihood the lean farmer is physically active. It would appear that many individuals supply their cells with too many calories, while at the same time these cells do not get enough oxygen. The result is formation of fat within the adipose tissue.

A second variable determining the capacity of the Krebs cycle is the availability of B complex vitamins. Many of the coenzymes and carrier molecules operating in the respiratory chain of the mitochondria are derived from thiamine, riboflavin, niacin, pantothenic acid, and others. A regular, balanced supply of these substances can improve the reserve of the Krebs cycle. However, the foremost regulator of Krebs cycle capacity is thyroid secretion. Thyroid hormones stimulate all reactions of the respiratory chain in the mitochondria. The lean farmer may have a somewhat higher than average output of T_3 and T_4.

An additional factor contributing to fat formation, discussed at further length in the following section, is the amount of circulating insulin. Fat synthesis is significantly facilitated by insulin; thus individuals showing excessive insulin secretion eventually tend to have excess weight.

When one becomes significantly overweight, body metabolism attunes to this state, and as a rule the weight tends to be easily maintained. Indeed, once an individual is in this condition, additional weight may accumulate despite what may appear to be negligible, or at least minimal, increases in food intake. Conversely, when heavy persons lose weight to the point of normality, they often find that they eventually can eat more than usual without regaining weight. Apparently their metabolism has shifted toward a predominance of energy production as opposed to fat formation.

The Problem of Overeating

Obesity is a consequence of some sort of failure in controlling the intake of food. Why do people overeat? First let us examine what is known of the physiologic control mechanisms. In studies with animals it was demonstrated that injury to the ventromedial region of the hypothalamus induced profound hyperphagia (overeating) and obesity. On the other hand, damage to nuclei in the lateral hypothalamus inhibited food intake. The theory then developed that the lateral hypothalamic appetite center tends to operate continually, and eating proceeds unless the ventromedial satiety center is stimulated by some signal. According to this idea we begin eating because we have stopped being satiated, not because we become hungry.

However, recent investigations do not fully support this concept. The hypothalamus may be involved, but other areas of the brain are as important. Leastwise, regardless of where regulatory centers are located, there must be some form of stimulatory or inhibitory signals to these centers. What constitutes the inhibitory signals?

There are glucose receptors in the limbic portions of the brain, including the hypothalamus. Apparently these are sensitive in some way to glucose *utilization*, not just blood glucose levels, since in diabetes mellitus there is increased appetite despite elevated glucose in the plasma.

Other physiologists think that temperature elevation of the blood is a satiety signal. Eating does increase metabolism (specific dynamic action of food), and we do eat more under colder conditions. Still other investigators consider that the ideal indicator of the need to inhibit food intake would be a substance released from adipose cells. A positive energy balance that promotes storage in

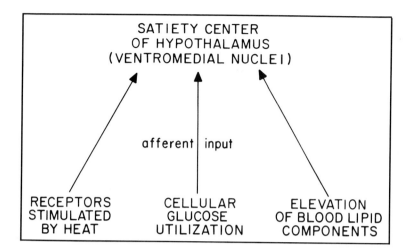

FIGURE 12-4   Signals believed to stimulate the hypothalamic satiety center.

adipose cells would signify that it is time for satiety. Recently this idea has received support from experimental data. An elevation in blood concentration of glycerol (a lipid component) led to hypophagia and weight loss in rats injected daily with glycerol solutions. Termination of injections was followed by hyperphagia and weight gain. Can the blood glycerol concentration be a significant satiety signal? Glucose utilization, temperature elevation, and shifts in plasma lipid components all may contribute to the promotion of satiety.

Still other evidence points to concentrations of hormones in regulating appetite. Rising insulin levels are known to suppress hunger, whereas elevated glucagon stimulates appetite. Another investigation with rats has indicated that receptors sensitive to intragastric pressure from a full stomach fire impulses to noradrenergic neurons in the hypothalamus. In addition, it has been shown that a naturally occurring opiate, *beta-endorphin*, found in the pituitary, enhances appetite in stressed animals and leads to the obesity syndrome. A summary of some of the satiety signals thought to be operative and their relation to the hypothalamus is depicted in Figure 12-4.

Much has been written about the role of psychologic and social factors as causes of overeating. Undoubtedly these factors are important. Are psychologic influences merely superimposed upon innate physiologic mechanisms, or are they capable of overriding basic physiologic control? It is of interest that obese animals do not maintain their hyperphagia indefinitely. Eventually their food intake gradually tapers, and their weight, though excessive, stabilizes. Thus there is a regaining of caloric regulation, but the regulation is being operated from higher than normal values of body weight and caloric requirement. More significant is the fact that after this state is attained, the weight-stabilized animal can be launched again into a later bout of overeating by what may appear to be subtle environmental changes, such as increasing the amount of sweetener in the food or reducing the ambient temperature. Apparently, basic physiologic regulation can be strongly influenced or even altered by the reinforcement (positively and negatively) of many sensory and psychologic stimuli such as smell, taste, and former associations. Such psychologic factors, though having little to do with energy balances within the body, nevertheless are of very great significance in causing and maintaining obesity; and emotional drives must be considered a strong part of any theory relating to control of food intake.

Overeating in humans appears to be related in principle to what has been termed chemical addiction pertaining to such substances as alcohol, tobacco, caffeine, and drugs. Though the mechanisms underlying chemical addiction as it relates to food intake are not well understood, a few enlightening points are considered later in the chapter.

Does an individual instinctively seek foods that his or her body badly needs? This is true as far as water, sodium, and a minimum of calories from nonspecific food sources are concerned, but beyond this the idea cannot be supported. Food selection in humans is based primarily on habit, psychologic associations, and sociocultural influences.

GLUCOSE INTOLERANCE

When the ingestion of carbohydrate results in blood levels of glucose that regularly exceed 170 to 180 mg/dl, and the postprandial elevation in glucose is slow in diminishing, the individual is said to show intolerance to glucose. This is the basis for the diagnosis of diabetes mellitus.

It was stated in Chapter 4 that over three-fourths of all diabetics have a comparatively mild form of glucose intolerance (Type II diabetes) that usually does not appear until after about 40 years of age. It is this form of the disorder that warrants our attention here, and it is especially this form that is increasing in incidence each year. It has been speculated that the increasing incidence of adult-

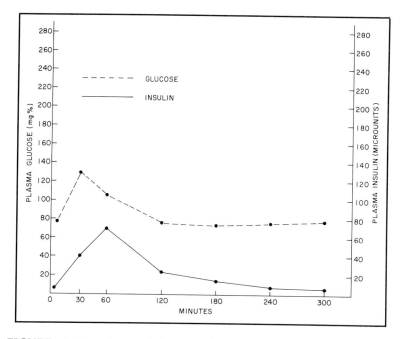

FIGURE 12-5 A.   Normal glucose tolerance. Circulating insulin was measured along with glucose at the same time intervals. Note that glucose had returned to the fasting level in 2 hours. Observe also that there are fewer than 50 microunits of insulin at all times except the 1-hour period.

onset diabetes during the past half century is related to the popular habit of hypercaloric intake leading to excessive body weight. During past centuries the consumption of concentrated sugars together with sedentary habits was not commonplace as it is today; therefore, individuals in the past with a genetic predisposition to glucose intolerance were not as likely to show glycosuria or other clinical manifestations of diabetes. Metabolic stress from hyperphagia is indeed necessary to reveal that there is an inherited predisposition to glucose intolerance. According to this view, the genetic predisposition may have always had a much higher incidence than realized. Some physiologists question the practicality of using as much as 100 g of concentrated glucose in tolerance tests.[2] Such a high dose certainly will reveal whether or not an individual possesses remarkable insulin reserve. On the other hand, it is doubtful if our forebears in

[2]In a glucose tolerance test, the subject is given a concentrated solution of glucose to drink rapidly. Blood and urine samples are taken immediately before glucose administration and again at 30, 60, 120, and 180 minutes after administration. Blood glucose is measured each time and a tolerance curve constructed from the prints (see Figure 12-5).

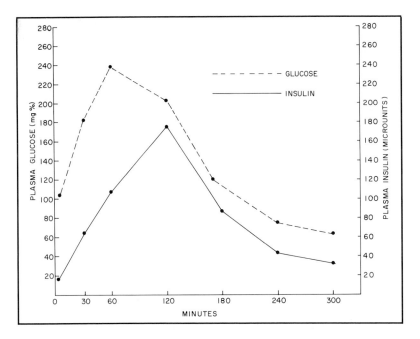

FIGURE 12-5 B.   Glucose tolerance in adult-onset diabetes. Mild intolerance in an overweight 50-year-old patient. Note the hyperglycemia within the first 2 hours, followed by a drastic plunge of the glucose level to values that are significantly below the fasting level. Observe also the great amount of insulin secretion, which remains above 50 microunits for most of the period, and reaches 170 microunits at 2 hours. (Both records courtesy of Ultrachem Biomedical Laboratories, Inc., Dayton, Ohio.)

their everyday life ever consumed such a high glucose concentration all at once.

Some 90% of adult- or maturity-onset, diabetics are significantly overweight at the time of onset, and there is evidence that the glucose intolerance is not from direct beta cell damage but instead is somehow related to a progressive functional imbalance, in which metabolic regulations have become maladaptive for the existing eating habits, body weight, and hormonal responses to stress. A major revelation supporting this concept appeared when the measurement of circulating insulin by radioimmunoassay became a realization. Most adult-onset diabetics not only show no insulin deficiency, but they apparently have excessive quantities of circulating insulin! Many of the same individuals also show an excess of glucagon, and the failure of postprandial glucagon to decrease may be the result of a partial loss of glucose-sensing by pancreatic alpha cells. At the same time, the secretion of glucagon often accompanies activity of the sympathetic nervous system; thus many nonspecific stresses are known to elevate plasma glucagon.

The discovery of an abundance of circulating insulin in adult-onset diabetes has led to the recent concept that for some reason these individuals appear to require larger quantities of insulin than usual. It has been shown that persistently elevated plasma insulin induces a loss of insulin receptors, thus reducing target cell reactivity to the high hormone concentration. Excessive body weight and the presence of insulin antagonists also are thought to be involved in some way. At any rate, an examination that reveals excessive insulin levels, even without evidence of glucose intolerance, marks that individual as at risk in eventually developing glucose intolerance. It is desirable to measure insulin along with glucose when glucose tolerance tests are performed.

In Figure 12-5, values for both insulin and glucose are given for a normal glucose tolerance test (A), and also for a test (B) which clearly reveals mild glucose intolerance. These are 5-hour tests. Note that in curve B the intolerance occurs within 2 hours, indicating a delay in the insulin response. Yet once the insulin response is under way, the glucose level plummets due to the excessive insulin.

What is responsible for this common form of glucose intolerance? The fact that it tends to occur later in life suggests that chronic stresses of some sort could be implicated. Long-term stressing of the insulin response mechanism and the glucose-regulating devices in the liver as a consequence of overnutrition, excessive weight, and emotional strain certainly contribute. Some investigators think that inhibition of the output of hypothalamic somatostatin, brought on by chronic stress, is involved, as was pointed out in Chapter 4. Somatostatin inhibition may explain the excessive insulin. At the same time, the associated elevation in glucagon secretion would tend to maintain hyperglycemia despite the presence of insulin.

Insulin Resistance

When cellular glucose utilization becomes impaired despite adequate or even excessive quantities of circulating insulin, the designation *insulin resistance* is employed. Some investigators insist that insulin resistance, whatever its causes, contributes to the genesis of adult-onset diabetes. In insulin resistance there is usually some degree of fasting hyperglycemia, although this is not invariably true. There also may be a tendency to postprandial hypoglycemia, especially in those who are overweight. Apparently there can be several different factors related to the development of insulin resistance. These may combine to contribute to the development of the condition. Without question the foremost factor is obesity. However, insulin resistance may be associated also with persistent elevations of the diabetogenic hormones, epinephrine, glucagon, cortisol, and growth hormone. There are yet other instances in which neither obesity nor hormonal stress is apparent.

In the cases of resistance associated with cortisol and growth hormone, it has been shown that diminished binding of insulin to cell membrane receptors of the liver and adipose tissue underlies the reduction of glucose transport into these cells. Along similar lines it has been found that erythrocytes and monocytes from adult-onset diabetics of normal weight appear to have a lesser number of insulin-binding sites than are present in the blood cells of those with normal glucose tolerance.

In overweight individuals it is well known that the adipose cells become enlarged. Such enlarged cells then become resistant to insulin action. The resistance in turn prompts the manufacture and secretion of excessive insulin in order to overcome the difficulty. Even the overweight nondiabetic shows insulin resistance and resulting hyperinsulinemia, but apparently is spared extreme hyperglycemia either by a quicker insulin response to glucose, or a better beta cell reserve. Or perhaps there is less antagonism from glucagon and other diabetogenic secretions. Defective receptor-binding does not appear to be involved in glucose intolerance associated with many cases of obesity, although diminished binding has been induced when the carbohydrate proportion of the diet exceeds 45%, and when there is little or no exercise. Exercise increases receptor-binding of insulin. A recent concept of why glucose intolerance occurs in cases with normal receptor-binding is that there is interference with the transport protein thought to be involved with moving glucose through the cell membrane.

It has been theorized that the problem of glucose intolerance in obesity may center around a limitation of reactions in glycolysis imposed by enzyme-overloading once the glucose is in the cell. Since the cell can metabolize only so much glucose at a time, overnutrition and possibly excessive glucagon secretion tend to maintain a level of blood glucose above what can be metabolized intracellularly. This would eventually retard insulin action, resulting in a sustained elevation of glucose in the blood despite the presence of insulin. Furthermore, the persistent elevation of glucose would continue to stimulate a pancreatic release of insulin, which could account for the hyperinsulinemia and would impose a stress on the beta cells.

Could a genetically conditioned limitation of intracellular enzyme capacity be the inheritance factor that has been postulated for overweight adult-onset diabetics? It is not really surprising, when hypercaloric intake and excessive body weight are maintained, that glucose intolerance eventually makes its appearance in many individuals. Each additional pound of weight requires a larger volume of insulin, and a greater output of insulin tends to compound the problem by promoting an additional gain in weight.

The only practical measure available to adult-onset diabetic patients is to forego eating habits that lead to excessive weight and eventually bring on the predicament of glucose intolerance. This is especially true in respect to carbohydrate intake, particularly the quickly absorbable sugars. Indeed, the majority of adult-onset diabetics who keep weight at a minimum, and maintain appropriate dietary and exercise regimes, are able to reduce their blood levels of glucose to normal, even in tolerance tests. Even in so-called normal subjects, significant weight gain tends to promote carbohydrate intolerance, higher insulin levels, and insensitivity of muscle and fat tissue to insulin action. Weight loss alone corrects all this, and the metabolic derangements disappear. Thus clinical adult-onset diabetes can become subclinical when body weight is normalized.

Of course, stressors other than nutritive ones can also be important if they persistently provoke increases in blood glucose, thereby imposing greater demands on the insulin response mechanism. In this regard certain individuals may inherit a tendency toward labile hypothalamic responses to many stresses. Hypothalamic activity in turn would promote frequent release of the diabetogenic hormones, epinephrine, cortisol, growth hormone, and glucagon.

It is obvious that in most cases of adult-onset diabetes, insulin injections are unnecessary. The administration of sulfonylureas (oral antidiabetic drugs) to these patients merely stimulates additional insulin production from a pancreas that may already be producing excessive amounts. Moreover, sulfonylurea therapy, by stimulating an even greater release of insulin, promotes a gain in weight, and there has been evidence of several dangerous side effects of the drug, foremost of which is heart damage (see Chapter 14).

Although there is general agreement that weight loss, caloric restriction, and regular exercise constitute the primary therapeutic measures for most cases of maturity-onset diabetes, there is some disagreement concerning quality of the diet. Some specialists urge restrictions on the amount of carbohydrate in the diet, with emphasis on a greater proportion of calories from protein and fat. There is evidence that a dietary regime of this kind controls hyperglycemia, as well as prevents elevated blood levels of insulin and triglycerides. Others advise a high carbohydrate diet as long as the carbohydrates are starches, not sugars, especially starches with much indigestable fiber, such as bran. This would retard the rate of absorption into the blood. Advocates of a lower protein–higher carbohydrate intake point to the fact that glucagon secretion is stimulated by plasma amino acids but not by glucose. It is desirable to avoid such an occurrence in view of the hyperglycemic action of glucagon.

Apparently it is very difficult for those predisposed to adult-onset diabetes to appropriately control their eating habits and prevent weight accumulation. In a reversal of the common notion of cause and effect, it has been stated that the individual may be fat because of being diabetic, rather than diabetic because of being fat. This view is sound in that liberal quantities of insulin are required to promote fat synthesis, and as previously stated, the milder form of glucose intolerance is often characterized by excessive secretion of insulin. In fact, there is reason to suspect that chronic hyperinsulinism could be a significant factor in the eventual occurrence of glucose intolerance, as we shall see in the next subsection.

Hypoglycemia and Glucose Tolerance

It was noted in the diabetic tolerance curve shown in Figure 12-5B that there is a surge of insulin release that results in a reduction of blood glucose to levels that are surprisingly low at 4 and 5 hours. If glucose tolerance tests were performed over a 6-hour period rather than the traditional 3 hours, the tolerance curves of many adult-onset diabetics would show this "hypoglycemic tail." Oddly enough, relative degrees of hypoglycemia and hyperglycemia may exist in the same individual. It is now recognized that many individuals with tendencies to reactive hypoglycemia (low blood glucose) are risks for eventually developing glucose intolerance. The hypoglycemic of today becomes the diabetic of tomorrow.

Much has been written about reactive hypoglycemia within the past 20 years amid a certain amount of controversy. However, several points are becoming clear. In certain individuals a rapid elevation in the level of blood glucose from substantial amounts of quickly absorbable carbohydrate does stimulate exaggerated insulin responses which lower blood sugar to unusual levels within 3 to 5 hours following the ingestion. Moreover, various stresses may aggravate the hypoglycemia through facilitating release of a pituitary peptide, beta-endorphin, known to stimulate insulin secretions. Caffeine and allergic reactions also aggravate hypoglycemia.

When blood sugar levels are low, hunger pangs and jittery feelings prompt the craving for food, especially carbohydrate. Eating will provide immediate relief, but not for long. After 3 hours the nervousness, palpitations, and feelings of faintness begin to return, typifying a positive feedback cycle. Most of these symptoms are due to the release of epinephrine, which stimulates glucose production from glycogen. Indeed, repeated bouts of hypoglycemia promote output of all the stress hormones, epinephrine, glucagon, cortisol, and growth hormone. Habitual elevation of these substances can lead to insulin resistance.

There is clinical evidence that years of cyclic hypoglycemia tend to favor two outcomes in certain types of individuals. One is excessive weight and the other is a dullness of the glucose stimulus in initiating insulin release from the pancreatic beta cells. The immediate beta cell response is known as *first phase insulin secretion*, and in Figure 12-5B it appears to be faulty. It is not surprising to find that the hypoglycemic eats a great deal of carbohydrate, and glucose in excess of that needed for energy requirements becomes added weight, especially with an abundance of insulin to promote fat synthesis. Just how the initial insulin response to the glucose stimulus becomes dull is not clear. However, excessive carbohydrate intake over the years could certainly stress the insulin response mechanism, perhaps through impaired glucose-binding to beta cell receptors. At least there appears to be defective glucose recognition by the beta cell. There is evidence that first phase insulin secretion can become inhibited by chronic alpha adrenergic activity and certain prostaglandins such as PGE_2. An alpha receptor blocker such as phentolamine, and PGE_2 antagonists such as sodium salicylate have been shown to improve first phase insulin secretion. Once again we can see how stress is associated with the development of pathology.

There is no drug therapy for hypoglycemia, so those showing the tendency must follow a set of dietary rules if they are to stabilize their blood sugar levels and possibly prevent eventual intolerance to glucose. The same dietary policies apply to many adult-onset diabetics. These are:

1. Restrict the overall quantity of dietary
   carbohydrate to no more than 20 grams per meal,
   and completely eliminate concentrated forms
   such as sugars and any sweetened foods or
   beverages. Choose carbohydrates with bulk and

fiber (whole grain and vegetables). Fresh fruit should be eaten sparingly and last at a meal, after the stomach is partially filled.

2. Proportionately increase the amount of dietary protein and fat, and eat these foods first at a meal. Fats retard digestion and absorption. Unsaturated fats are probably preferable.

3. Eat small quantities of food often, 4 to 6 feedings per day if possible. Studies with both laboratory animals and humans have clearly shown that frequent nibbling, when compared with 2 or 3 large meals a day, results in less body fat, achieves more normal, stable levels of blood glucose, and is associated with less serum cholesterol and triglycerides, despite the fact that the total calories per day may be the same in each case. Consuming a large meal stresses the liver, the insulin response mechanism, and redirects metabolism to favor the fat path over the energy path.

4. Avoid caffeine. It stimulates insulin secretion and thereby promotes hypoglycemia (see Chapter 14).

Fortunately it appears that the later vascular complications of diabetes are not as likely to develop unless there is an actual deficiency in insulin *production.* This conclusion is based upon an 18-year follow-up of 334 "diabetic" patients with no insulin deficiency conducted at the Diabetes Center at St. Francis Hospital in Milwaukee, Wisconsin.[3]

The particular conditions and their interactions that are believed to lead to the glucose intolerance characterizing adult-onset diabetes are summarized in Figure 12-6.

LACTOSE INTOLERANCE

More and more adults are discovering that the reason they suffer periodic bouts of intestinal upset and discomfort is that they have a poor tolerance for milk sugar (*lactose*). The symptoms of the intolerance include flatulence, abdominal cramping, and diarrhea. Some

---

[3]R. W. Turkington and H. K. Weindling: personal communication.

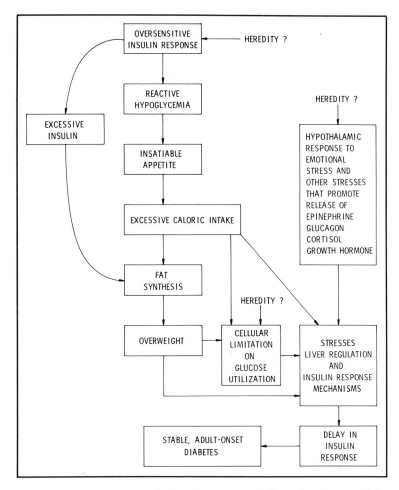

FIGURE 12-6   Proposed chain of causes and effects leading to adult-onset diabetes. As indicated in the figure, it is not known exactly at which point(s) heredity is influential.

individuals also experience stubborn constipation. All ethnic groups are susceptible to lactose intolerance, yet the percentage (50% to 75%) in Orientals, blacks, Eskimos, Jews, Hindus, and American Indians is appreciably higher than that found in those of European descent (10% to 25%). However, practically all humans show some reduction in the quantity of the lactase enzyme after three years of age. This is true of all mammals. After weaning, milk may not be as desirable a food as we are led to believe.

Lactose is a disaccharide found in milk. Lactase is the enzyme

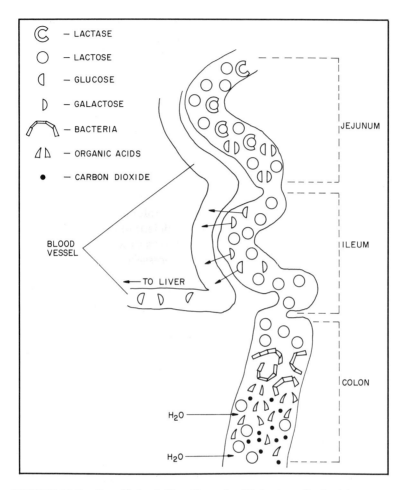

FIGURE 12-7   Insufficient digestion of milk lactose. In the jejunum the lactose molecules are broken down by lactase to glucose and galactase, which enter the bloodstream. When there is insufficient lactase, some lactose will enter the colon from the ileum, where it is fermented by bacteria, resulting in discomfort from the resulting acids and gas (CO_2). Because of an excessive number of particles in the colon material, water is absorbed, disposing the subject to diarrhea.

secreted by mucosal cells of the jejunum that catalyzes the hydrolysis of lactose to its two component monosaccharides, glucose and galactose. Investigators have been unable to distinguish any qualitative chemical difference in this enzyme among infants, lactose-tolerant adults, and lactose-intolerant adults. The difference is quantitative. Adults with lactose intolerance have very little lactase. When the amount of lactose ingested exceeds the capacity of the available lactase, some of the lactose will not be hydrolyzed. Though small amounts of the undigested sugar may be taken into the blood and excreted in urine, most of it moves into the colon, where it is fermented by bacteria, generating organic acids and carbon dioxide, which promote various degrees of bloating, belching, and cramping. Lactose in the colon also increases the particle content there, leading to osmotic action that tends to draw water into the colon from tissue. It is this mechanism that contributes to diarrhea. The principal points of the entire intestinal action are diagrammed in simplified fashion in Figure 12-7.

Deficiencies of the lactase enzyme in adults vary considerably. Persons with a mild deficiency may tolerate small quantities of milk, but there are other individuals deficient to the point of having to exclude from the diet all milk or products in which lactose is present. For these people label-reading is necessary, since milk is added to many processed foods, even some breads. Yogurt may be tolerated because the lactose has already been converted to lactic acid by the bacterial culture. Butter and some cheeses have negligible lactose, but ice cream may have a considerable quantity of the sugar.

Although the symptoms can be similar, lactose intolerance is not to be confused with milk allergy. The latter condition stems from sensitivity to specific milk proteins; thus, adverse reactions would extend as well to cheese and yogurt. If, for example, the individual reacts to cow's milk but tolerates goat's milk, the problem is allergy to proteins in cow's milk, not lactose intolerance. Milk from most mammals has lactose; in fact, cow's milk has less than many of the others.

How do we know for sure that intestinal symptoms are due to lactose intolerance? Can lactose breakdown be reliably measured? If a test dose of 2 grams of lactose per kilogram of body weight is ingested following a fast, the occurrence of symptoms within 2 to 3 hours is rather convincing. However, a more refined approach to quantify lactase activity involves the measurement of blood glucose 15 minutes following the ingestion of the test dose of lactose. If the elevation in blood glucose is less than 20 mg/dl, the lactose was not completely digested.

What can be done for the adult with lactose intolerance? The idea that regular ingestion of milk will progressively stimulate the production of lactase has not been experimentally supported. On the contrary there are findings indicating that the predisposition to lactose intolerance is rather fixed and transmitted genetically through a dominant gene. Recently, there has been some success with providing lactase preparations for intolerant individuals to take with their milk. This and avoidance are the only present solutions to the problem.

FOOD SENSITIVITY

For a number of years there has been a growing body of evidence indicating that many individuals suffer from reactions to what they eat, yet fail to recognize the association. It appears that the reactions are allergic in nature, although in many instances it is not easy to demonstrate antibody production. The matter is not nearly so simple as classic inhalant allergy to pollen, for example. A more comprehensive consideration of allergic disease as a deviation in immune response is reserved for Chapter 15; however, the topic of sensitivity to food is receiving so much attention today amid considerable controversy and conflicting viewpoints, that a discussion of the major points rightfully belongs with the coverage of nutritive stress and disease.

A certain amount of what may appear to be food sensitivity could be a reaction to myriad food additives, to antibiotics and hormones with which butchered animals had been treated, to the many sprays used on fruits and vegetables, to contaminants such as molds, or even to chemicals such as phenolic resins found in the lining of metal cans. Many of these nonfood materials are discussed as polluting ingestants in Chapter 13. In question here is the actual sensitivity to certain foods.

The point is well taken that of all exogenous materials and conditions to which we adapt and maladapt, none may be more significant than food, in view of its complex chemistry, sheer bulk, and the frequency, intimacy, and duration of exposure. As necessary as food is, maladaptation to it is to be expected, and unfavorable cellular reactions to specific food ingredients do develop. The nature of many of these reactions is cytotoxic, resembling a cellular immune response more than a humoral immune reaction. One of the questions asked throughout the clinical community has to do with just how widespread the phenomenon of food allergy is, particularly among adults.[4] More controversial yet is the question of the sig-

---

[4]Food allergy is more expected among infants and younger children where the digestive processes are less mature. Protein materials that are not completely digested may become allergenic in easily sensitized individuals.

nificance of food reactions as a basis for alleged symptoms. At one end of the spectrum is the view that food sensitivity is capable of eliciting practically every known symptom. Proponents of this view claim that a history of chronic stress from food abuse can result in mental illness, rheumatoid arthritis, ulcerative colitis, thyroid imbalance, hypoglycemia leading to glucose intolerance, gastrointestinal ulcers, spastic colitis, obesity, alcoholism, migraine headaches, hyperkinesis in children, and nephritic syndromes. At the opposite end of the spectrum are those who look upon the subject of chronic illness from food sensitivity as some sort of myth.

A major factor contributing to the dilemma enshrouding food allergy is the problem of diagnosis. How can the association of a specific food with a specific reaction be objectively demonstrated? Clinical symptoms are probably derived from cellular reactions to degraded by-products of the original food, and virtually nothing is known of the actual chemical configuration of these products. Therefore, skin-testing with natural food ingredients has no reliability. Several other testing procedures are employed, but none really circumvent the problem mentioned above.

Symptoms of food sensitivity can be enormously varied, taking place in almost any body system. Headache, gastrointestinal discomfort, rhinitis, various neural disturbances, and depression are the complaints most frequently reported. Moreover, a milk sensitivity may produce diarrhea in one individual, but headache in another. The body structure most prone to symptoms in an individual has come to be known as the *shock organ*. A tension-fatigue syndrome, neural in origin, is commonly experienced as a result of chronic exposure to foods to which sensitivity has developed. The individual is always tired yet cannot relax and rest.

A person can be sensitized to any food. However, the 20 foods that are most commonly incriminated are listed in approximate descending order in Table 12-2. Note that most of these items are staples that are consumed on a daily basis. The mechanism by which foods produce reactions is thought to work in two ways. In one of these there is direct contact of food allergens with IgE antibodies in the gastrointestinal system, resulting in a swift reaction that is potent in its effects. IgE antibodies are the immunoglobulins mobilized in typical allergic reactions (see Chapter 15). Only a very small amount of the food is required, and the sensitivity is always there regardless of the interval between exposures. Tolerance does not develop. This form of reaction is termed *fixed* allergy, and it is effective in about 5% to 10% of all food sensitivity.

In the other mechanism the allergens are thought to be de-

TABLE 12-2
Foods Suspected of Producing Allergic Symptoms
(Approximate Reported Frequency)

Cow's milk (all forms, including cheese)

Corn

Wheat

Egg

Yeast

Coffee

Chocolate

Peanut

Tomato

Fish

Citrus Fruit

Nuts

Cabbage

Strawberry

Soybean

Beef

Cane sugar

Banana

Pork

---

graded substances that are absorbed into the blood, resulting in cellular reactions there or in various organs. In this case, a greater quantity of the food is required to elicit symptoms, and the reaction is neither as rapid nor as explosive as it is in fixed allergy. In this form of reaction, low-grade symptoms may persist as long as the food remains in the body, by which time the same thing may have been eaten again, resulting in chronic discomfort that tends to mask the true relationship of specific food with specific effect. However, in chronic forms of food reaction, intervals without exposure tend to promote tolerance, and the best way to combat the problem is to vary the diet each day by rotating various foods. This form of sensitivity has been designated *cyclic* food allergy, and it is by far the more common type. However, the condition can be unbelievably elusive and frustratingly difficult to diagnose. In addition, the expression of cyclic food allergy depends considerably upon many

TABLE 12-3
Factors Exacerbating Cyclic Food Allergy

Inhalant allergy

Psychologic stress

Nutritive imbalances (particularly mineral and vitamin)

Physical stressors (weather changes)

Infections

Fatigue

Compromise in gastrointestinal function

Constipation

Food additives

Drugs and medications

Chronic alcoholism

Smoking

---

other conditions, a major one being compromised digestion, in which peptides from incompletely digested protein tend to be absorbed into the blood, where they become antigenic. Several factors known to enhance the effects of cyclic food allergy are listed in Table 12-3.

Of particular interest in respect to cyclic food allergy is the theory that people actually become addicted to the foods to which they are sensitive. Not only does the victim crave the allergenic food, but even may derive immediate but brief relief from eating this food. However, symptoms may be experienced later, some time after feeling relief. The entire matter of chemical addiction is undergoing much investigation. Whether the chemical comes from food, tobacco, alcohol, or prescribed medication, the bodies of those seemingly predisposed to addiction tend to become physiologically dependent. Apparently the predisposition lies in the manner in which particular cellular materials respond to specific chemicals and chemical change. According to advocates of the theory of addiction in food sensitivity, the more reactability to a food becomes established, the more craving for the food, until the situation grows upon itself in the typical fashion of positive feedback. Could this process explain how a pattern of addictive eating is established and becomes seemingly uncontrollable?

A relationship between cyclic food allergy and reactive hypoglycemia has been postulated. Indeed, many alcoholics experience periodic hypoglycemia, and recent studies have begun to reveal that numerous alcoholics, in addition to their sensitivity to alcohol, also have multiple food sensitivities.

‖ SUMMARY

The foremost malnutritive problem in advanced, affluent cultures is the excessive intake of calories, which is often combined with physical inactivity. This leads to obesity, which poses a substantial risk of developing cardiovascular and renal disease, hypertension, and diabetes.

Most of the carbohydrate, fat, protein, and alcohol we ingest eventually becomes acetate, which can either produce energy by entering the Krebs cycle, or become body fat and cholesterol. The primary variable determining which pathway acetate takes is the amount of food consumed at a given time.

Overeating is evidence of some degree of failure or alteration in the physiologic mechanisms regulating food intake. Either certain brain centers are not responding normally to afferent signals, or the reception of signals is being overridden by input from higher brain centers.

In most adults with mild to moderate glucose intolerance, there are excessive amounts of circulating insulin. Despite this, there is resistance to insulin action in promoting additional cellular utilization of glucose. This form of glucose intolerance often evolves from tendencies to reactive hypoglycemia. Appropriate weight loss, caloric restrictions, and exercise restore normal blood glucose levels.

An insufficient amount of lactase enzyme in lactose-intolerant adults produces bloating, abdominal cramping, and diarrhea, caused by the action of bacteria on undigested milk sugar in the colon.

There is a growing awareness that a variety of chronic symptoms may be due to allergic reactions to ingested foods. Usually, rapid and potent reactions indicate a fixed allergy. However, cyclic food allergy is difficult to diagnose. In addition to being dependent upon the frequency of intake of the particular food, the expression of the cyclic allergy is significantly influenced by other stresses.

Chapter Glossary

allergenic   capable of initiating an allergic reaction
amino radical (NH_2)   a portion of all amino acids, the building blocks of proteins

cytotoxic chemical material or antibody capable of deranging or damaging cellular organization

diabetogenic capable of significantly elevating blood levels of glucose

flatulence distention of the gastrointestinal tract with gas

hyperinsulinemia excessive levels of circulating insulin

hyperkinesis abnormally increased motor activity

hypophagia significantly decreased intake of food (opposite of hyperphagia)

Krebs cycle a cyclic series of oxidations in cell mitochondria that creates most of the ATP energy

opiate any substance having a sedative effect like opium

postprandial after a meal

respiratory chain series of substrates and enzymes in the mitochondria that transports electrons to oxygen

For Further Reading

Bajaj, J. S., ed. 1977. *Insulin and metabolism.* New York: Excerpta Medica.

Brothers, M. J. 1976. *Diabetes: The new approach.* New York: Grosset & Dunlap.

Camerini, R. A., and Hanover, B., eds. 1979. Early treatment of diabetes. In *Advances in experimental medicine and biology.* New York: Plenum Press.

Cheraskin, E.; Ringsdorf, W. M.; and Clark, J. W. 1970. *Diet and disease.* Emmaus, Pa.: Rodale Books.

Deutsch, J. A.; Young, W. G.; and Kalogeris, T. J. 1978. The stomach signals satiety. *Science* 201:165.

Dickey, L. D., ed. 1976. *Clinical ecology.* Springfield, Ill: Charles C Thomas Pubs.

Frazier, C. A. 1974. *Coping with food allergy.* New York: Quadrangle/New York Times Book Co.

Herman, R. H.; Cohn, R. M.; and McNamara, P. D., eds. 1980. *Principles of metabolic control in mammalian systems.* New York: Plenum Press.

Katch, F. I., and McArdle, W. D. 1977. *Nutrition, weight control and exercise.* Boston: Houghton Mifflin Co.

Katzen, H. M., and Mahler, R. J., eds. 1978. *Diabetes, obesity, and vascular disease: Metabolic and molecular interrelationships.* Parts 1, 2. New York: Halsted Press.

Kolata, G. A. 1977. Obesity, a growing problem. *Science* 198:905

Kraft, J. R. 1975. Detection of diabetes mellitus in situ (occult diabetes). *Lab Med* 6:10.

Lamb, L. E. 1974. *Metabolics: Putting your food energy to work.* New York: Harper & Row Pubs.

Lockwood, D. H.; Livingston, J. N.; and Amatruda, J. M. 1975. Relation of insulin receptors to insulin resistance. *Fed Proc* 34:1564.

Maugh, T. H., II. 1977. Drug-free therapy for diabetics. *The Sciences* 17:16.

Misbin, R. I.; O'Leary, J. P.; and Pulkkinen, A. 1979. Insulin receptor binding in obesity: A reassessment. *Science* 205:1003.

Morley, J. E., and Levine, A. S. 1980. Stress-induced eating is mediated through endogenous opiates. *Science* 209:1259.

Myers, R. D., and McCaleb, M. L. 1980. Feeding: Satiety signal from intestine triggers brain's noradrenergic mechanism. *Science* 209:1035.

Overton, M. H., and Lukert, B. P. 1979. *Clinical nutrition: A physiologic approach.* Chicago: Year Book Medical Publishers. Times Mirror.

Robinson, C. H. 1972. *Normal and therapeutic nutrition.* 14th ed. New York: Macmillan Publishing Co.

Roe, D. A. 1979. *Clinical nutrition for the health scientist.* Boca Raton, Fla.: CRC Press, Inc.

Rowe, A. H., and Rowe, A., Jr. 1972. *Food allergy, its manifestations and control, and the elimination diets—A compendium.* Springfield, Ill.: Charles C Thomas Pubs.

Silverstone, T., ed. 1976. *Appetite and food intake.* Berlin: Life Sciences Research Report, no. 2.

Unger, R. H.; Dobbs, R. E.; and Orci, L. 1978. Insulin, glucagon, and somatostatin secretion in the regulation of metabolism. *Ann Rev Physiol* 40:307.

Vander, A. J. 1976. In Introduction to *Human physiology and the environment in health and disease.* San Francisco: W. H. Freeman and Co. Part 1, article 5.

Vander, A. J.; Sherman, J. H.; and Luciano, D. S. 1980. *Human physiology: The mechanisms of body function.* 3rd ed. New York: McGraw-Hill Book Co. Chapt. 15.

Wirtshafter, D., and Davis, J. D. 1977. Body weight: Reduction by long-term glycerol treatment. *Science* 198:1271.

PART FOUR

STRESS AND DISEASE FROM MAN-MADE CHEMICAL STRESSORS

CHAPTER 13
Health Effects of Environmental Pollution

CHAPTER 14
Tobacco, Alcohol, and Drugs

Part Four considers the stress and pathologic changes resulting from exposures to chemical substances that the body does not require. The chemicals are either generated as by-products of our modern industrialization, or are intentionally prepared for direct human consumption.

Health Effects of Environmental Pollution

|| Objectives: Upon completing this chapter you should:

1. Be better able to evaluate the overall risk of potential pathology from exposure to environmental pollutants.
2. Be familiar with individual air pollutants, their sources, and their health effects.
3. Be well informed of the presence of specific toxins and carcinogens in our food and water.
4. Understand the mechanisms of disease-producing action of the major chemical pollutants.
5. Recognize the paucity of the body's defensive measures against pollutant exposure.

Over three-fourths of the United States population inhabits urban and suburban centers where the degree of industrialization and mechanized transportation has skyrocketed to heights that might strike our forebears as pure fantasy. Since World War II, more and more of the country has rapidly become a densely populated habitat of concrete and steel enveloped in an atmosphere of toxic gases and particles. Lakes and streams have become outlets for chemical disposal, and our food is laden with chemical additives.

Since 1960 considerable time and expense have been devoted to studying the problem of environmental pollution and proposing solutions. Despite remedial efforts, progress has not been overwhelming. Some streams have become cleaner and some cities are now less smog-ridden. Electrical power plants and many industries have been forced to spend huge sums for pollution abatement. On the other hand, there has yet to be a very strong, realistic confrontation with the automobile, which is without question the primary source of most environmental pollution. Moreover, the energy crisis already has been cited as justification for renouncing many of the established pollution controls.

Regardless of how insulting environmental pollution may be to our senses and esthetic values, the important question is whether it significantly stresses our bodies and leads to illness. This is a matter that can only be indirectly attacked. On one hand we can investigate effects on animals from controlled laboratory exposures, which of course are not real situations, and on the other hand, we can collect health statistics of people living in heavily polluted areas. The latter type of study is unavoidably cluttered with numerous variables, making a cause and effect relationship difficult to determine. Despite these obstacles, there are indications that chronic exposure to certain pollutants imposes significant chemical stress on our bodies which ultimately can lead to disease processes. However, before health effects are discussed, let us identify the polluting chemicals and determine whence they come.

IDENTIFICATION OF POLLUTANTS AND THEIR SOURCES

Unlike the question of health effects, there is no uncertainty concerning our knowledge of the quality and quantity of pollutants in the environment. Moreover, the sources of these materials are well known. Chemical engineers have been studying the nonbiologic aspects of air and water pollution for a quarter of a century. Daily monitoring of pollutant levels has become a well-established practice.

Pollutants often are considered in respect to their means of entering the body. Thus we speak of *inhalants* from the atmosphere, and *ingestants* from food and water. Some pollutants, such as lead and fluoride, are both inhaled and ingested. This chapter does not include all of the myriad chemicals to which individuals are exposed in special industrial occupations, nor does it include radioactive isotopes (radioactive materials were discussed in Chapter 6).

Atmospheric Pollutants

Inhalants are usually divided into two categories: aerosols and gases. Aerosols are microscopic particles (either solid or liquid) dispersed in the air. Although particles may be referred to as soot, dust, fly ash, and mist, they are frequently considered in collective fashion as *suspended particulates.* The range of particle size is enormous, some attaining dimensions approaching visibility without magnification ($> 100\mu$), whereas others may be less than 0.01μ. Larger particles are filterable, but the very smallest ones are difficult to filter. Suspended particulates are usually measured in micrograms per cubic meter of air ($\mu g/m^3$). Substantial levels of these materials are produced by many large-scale combustion processes such as those undergone in electrical power plants and numerous industrial concerns. Particulates are emitted also by motor vehicles, incinerators, and construction operations.

The list of gaseous atmospheric pollutants is quite lengthy. The major ones are carbon monoxide, ozone, peroxyacetyl nitrate (PAN), and a variety of hydrocarbons, nitrogen oxides, and sulfur

TABLE 13-1

Major Air Pollutants

POLLUTANT	PRIMARY SOURCE	EMISSION STANDARD*	AVERAGE ANNUAL EMISSION (TONS $\times$ 10^6)
Carbon monoxide	Automobiles	9.0 ppm (8 hr aver.)	155
Sulfur oxides	Electrical power plants	0.14 ppm (24 hr aver.)	35
Nitrogen oxides	Automobiles	0.05 ppm (annual aver.)	25
Hydrocarbons	Automobiles	160.0 $\mu g/m^3$ (3 hr aver.)	38
Photochemical oxidants	Automobiles	0.08 ppm (1 hr aver.)	†
Suspended particulates	Industry and power plants	75.0 $\mu g/m^3$ (annual aver.)	26

Source: Environmental Protection Agency, 1976.

*Expressed as either ppm (parts per million) or $\mu g/m^3$ (micrograms per cubic meter of air).

†These are not emitted in oxidant form. They result from chemical reactions of hydrocarbons with nitrogen oxides.

oxides. Gaseous inhalants lesser in incidence include ammonia, fluoride, chlorine, hydrogen sulfide, organic acids, and lead compounds. Gaseous pollutants are of molecular dimensions, and unless they are bound to particles, they cannot be filtered, even with electrostatic precipitators. Gas concentrations have been expressed in various units, but the most frequently encountered measurement is parts per million (ppm). The primary source of all the major gaseous pollutants, except the sulfur oxides, is the internal combustion engine. Over 90% of the carbon monoxide, and about 70% of the hydrocarbons, ozone, and PAN, come from automotive emissions. A list of the most important air pollutants, along with their sources, their federal standards, and the nationwide annual emission of them, is provided in Table 13-1.

The major variable determining the concentrations of atmospheric pollutants is the volume being emitted into the air. Meteorologic conditions and topography are the next two variables in importance. Stable atmospheres with little air turbulence restrict dispersion, resulting in greater pollution concentrations, while rain washes pollutants out of the atmosphere.[1] Also, it is well known that pollutants tend to concentrate in low valleys surrounded by hills.

[1]In one manner rain creates pollution. Pollutant gases such as sulfur dioxide and nitrogen dioxide become hydrated by water droplets to produce sulfuric and nitric acids; hence "acid rain."

A striking atmospheric condition that concentrates air pollutants is a *thermal inversion*. On dry sunny days the solar rays warm the air near the ground, and by noon this air begins to rise to considerable heights, taking pollutants with it. However, after sundown, especially on chilly nights (as in autumn), the air near the surface cools, resulting in a trapped stable layer of cooler air beneath a warmer layer. Thus there is no vertical dispersion of pollutants until the radiation of the following day has had time to warm the surface once more. This is why air pollutants are most concentrated during morning hours. The principle is illustrated in Figure 13-1.

Sunshine plays another significant role in air pollution. When nitrogen oxides are released into the atmosphere along with various hydrocarbon molecules, they absorb solar rays, which induce photodissociation of these materials, creating highly reactive peroxy radicals. Such radicals initiate long chains of oxidizing reactions, resulting in a fantastic array of chemical garbage collectively termed *photochemical oxidants*. The major oxidant is ozone (O_3), which is also the simplest chemically. Many others such as PAN are organic, nitrogen-bearing oxidants. Together these substances present an atmospheric condition commonly called *photochemical smog* (Figure 13-2). This is why the dry, sunny, windless cities, formerly so attractive in climate, are now so uncomfortable and unhealthy. Los Angeles, Denver, and Phoenix are prime examples.

Pollutants in Drinking Water

Drinking water affords a much less frequent entry of pollutants into the body than is the case with inhalants. Furthermore, a number of pollutants found in water can also be inhaled from the atmosphere or ingested with food. Several important water pollutants are not industrial chemicals but biologic entities such as bacteria, viruses, and algae, some of which may be pathogenic. The pathogens most frequently transmitted in drinking water are those responsible for infections of the intestinal tract; indeed, the method commonly used to assess bacterial contamination of water is the enumeration of coliform bacteria. These bacteria are usually benign organisms abundant in feces; however, if such bacteria are thriving in water samples, then pathogenic intestinal forms could be present also. In any instance in which there is risk of sewage contamination of water supplies, the means exists of conveying coliform bacteria to drinking water.

A widespread treatment for preventing bacterial contamination of water is the application of chlorine as a disinfectant. City drinking water is rather strongly chlorinated for this reason. In re-

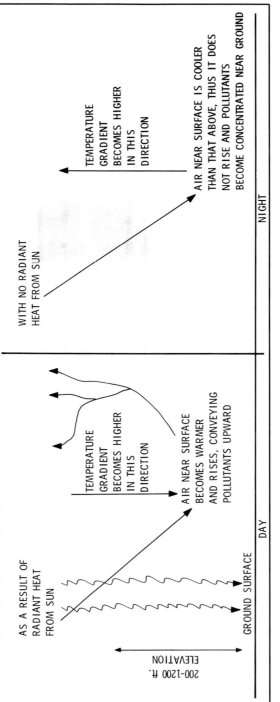

FIGURE 13-1   The principle of thermal inversion. When the air nearer the ground is cooler than that above, pollutants become concentrated within a few hundred feet of the surface.

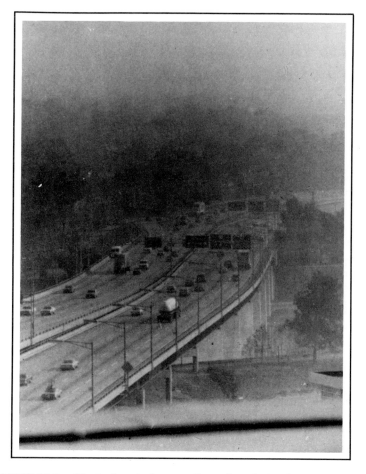

FIGURE 13-2   Photochemical smog. Even though the day is cloudless, visibility is extremely poor, requiring some vehicles to use headlights during the day. (Courtesy Regional Air Pollution Control Agency, Dayton and Montgomery Counties, Ohio.)

cent years it has become evident that the added chlorine can react with many soluble organic substances present in sources of drinking water. Chlorinated hydrocarbons such as chloroform are produced in this way, and many of these materials have been shown to be carcinogenic.

Heavy metals that find their way to water supplies from the effusion of many kinds of industrial operations can become serious pollution threats. Mercury, lead, and cadmium are of foremost concern, but arsenic, chromium, and nickel are also worthy of mention.

TABLE 13-2
Important Water Pollutants

POLLUTANT	PRIMARY SOURCE	LIMITS FOR POTABLE WATER
Coliform bacteria	Sewage	<200/liter
Chlorine	Water treatment	250 mg/liter
Nitrates	Fertilizers	10 mg/liter
Fluoride	Industrial waste, intentionally added	1.5　mg/liter
Chlordane	Organochlorine pesticide	0.003 mg/liter
Heptachlor	Organochlorine pesticide	0.018 mg/liter
DDT	Organochlorine pesticide	0.042 mg/liter
Malathion	Organophosphorus pesticide	0.10　mg/liter
Mercury	Industrial waste, pesticides	0.03　mg/liter
Lead	Industrial waste, plumbing	0.05　mg/liter
Cadmium	Industrial waste	0.01　mg/liter
Arsenic	Industrial waste, pesticides	0.05　mg/liter
Chromium	Industrial waste	0.05　mg/liter
Cyanide	Industrial waste	0.2　mg/liter

Source: U.S. Public Health Service Reports.

Among the organic pollutants found in water are the various pesticides used to control insects and weeds. Included are chlorinated hydrocarbon insecticides, organophosphorus insecticides, and herbicides. When soil contaminated with pesticides erodes and washes into lakes and streams or the water table, there may be risks of contaminating drinking supplies. The more important water pollutants, their sources, and the current health limits are listed in Table 13-2.

Food Contaminants and Additives

Although food pollution is not a traditional expression, more artificial chemicals enter the body with food than they do with water. Some of these substances are inadvertent contaminants, whereas others, classified as additives, are included in food intentionally.

Among nonintentional food contaminants are the pesticides just referred to. Toxicity from heavy metals, particularly mercury, lead, and cadmium, also can be a consequence of food contamination as well as water contamination.

In recent years much attention has been given to the contamination of food with organic industrial chemicals, of which the

TABLE 13-3
Common Chemical Contaminants of Food

CONTAMINANT	MAJOR FOOD SOURCES	PRIMARY TOXICITY
Heptachlor	Meat fat, milk, eggs	Nervous system depressant
DDT	Meat fat, milk, eggs	Nervous system depressant
Malathion	Fruits and vegetables	Inhibits cholinesterase
Mercury	Fish and sea food	Damage to brain and nervous system
Lead	Fruits, vegetables, grain	Anemia and neural impairment
Cadmium	Grains, coffee, tea	Renal damage
PCBs	Fish, poultry, milk	Liver damage
PBBs	Fish, poultry, milk	Liver damage

polychlorinated biphenyls (PCBs) and polybrominated biphenyls (PBBs) have prompted deep concern because of both their toxicity and their voluminous industrial production. These substances are extremely persistent in living organisms because of their lipid solubility. They have been found in fish and milk, as well as in chickens and eggs when fish meal was used in poultry feed. PCBs and PBBs are stable compounds that may contaminate water used by such animals as fish and cattle. A list of the pesticides, heavy metals, and biphenyls most commonly found in foods is presented in Table 13-3.

There are two ways chemicals are intentionally added to food. One is indirect, when the additive is fed to the animals we eat. It is estimated that 80% of the meat, milk, and eggs consumed in this country comes from animals fed medicated feed. Foremost among indirect additives are antibiotics, arsenicals, and steroid growth promoters. A list of such additives is provided in Table 13-4.

The number of additives incorporated directly into foods processed for human consumption is astonishing. Hundreds of chemicals are being used regularly in this way. Some of these substances are pH buffers, bleaching agents, flavorings, and nonnutritive sweeteners, whereas others are coloring agents, preservatives, antioxidants, and propellants. Still other additives are surface-active agents, mold inhibitors, and nutrient supplements. A listing of 52 ingredients appearing on a single packaged food item is shown in Figure 13-3.

It is true that certain chemical additives are necessary to prevent spoilage and putrefaction of perishable foods. However, ar-

TABLE 13-4

Major Drugs Added to Animal Feed

TYPE OF DRUG	NAME
Antibiotic	Penicillin
	Erythromycin
	Tetracycline
	Sulfonamide
	Nitrofuran
Antiparasite (protozoan and helminth)	Sulfanitran
	Piperazine
Hormonal growth promoter	Diethylstilbestrol
	Estradiol
	Progesterone
	Testosterone
Arsenical growth promoter	Arsanilic acid
	Nitarsone

tificial colors, flavor enhancers, nonnutritive sweeteners, and nutrient supplements do not serve much chemical advantage. Major types of food additives are listed in Table 13-5.

TOXIN, ALLERGEN, IRRITANT, OR CARCINOGEN?

Before the pathologic implications of individual environmental pollutants are presented, it may be helpful to classify the four types of effects that these materials are known to have on the body. Chemicals that induce injury by altering cellular metabolism through enzyme defects, or by combining chemically with specific cell constituents are termed *toxins.* Mercury and arsenic, for example, attach to the active site of certain cellular enzymes, thereby altering their configuration, which then blocks their activity as enzymes (enzyme inhibition). Some metal pollutants compete with the metal components of certain enzymes. For example, cadmium inactivates carbonic anhydrase by replacing zinc, whereas lead tends to replace calcium and magnesium, which function as cofactors for certain enzymes. In some instances the toxin forms chemical combinations with key molecules of certain cells. The association of carbon monoxide with the hemoglobin of red blood cells is a prime example.

Certain organic and inorganic toxins are known to combine

```
┌─────────────────────────────────────────┐
│        NUTRITION INFORMATION             │
│             PER SERVING                  │
│ SERVING SIZE                  2 BARS     │
│ SERVINGS PER CONTAINER          4        │
│    CALORIES                    380       │
│    PROTEIN, GRAMS               12       │
│    CARBOHYDRATE, GRAMS          45       │
│    FAT, GRAMS                   17       │
│                                          │
│   PERCENTAGE OF U.S. RECOMMENDED         │
│      DAILY ALLOWANCES (U.S. RDA)         │
│ PROTEIN      25   VITAMIN D      25      │
│ VITAMIN A    25   VITAMIN E      25      │
│ VITAMIN C    25   VITAMIN B6     25      │
│ THIAMIN      25   FOLIC ACID     25      │
│ RIBOFLAVIN   25   VITAMIN B12    25      │
│ NIACIN       25   PHOSPHORUS     25      │
│ CALCIUM      25   IODINE         25      │
│ IRON         25   MAGNESIUM      25      │
│                                          │
│ INGREDIENTS: SUGAR, VEGETABLE SHORTENING │
│ (CONTAINS ONE OR MORE OF THE FOLLOWING   │
│ PARTIALLY HYDROGENATED OILS: SOYBEAN,    │
│ COTTONSEED, PALM, PALM KERNEL, AND/OR    │
│ PEANUT OIL), FLOUR BLEACHED, SORBITOL,   │
│ ISOLATED SOY PROTEIN, DRIED MILK PROTEIN,│
│ PEANUT BUTTER, BROWN SUGAR SYRUP, EGG    │
│ WHITE, MONO AND DIGLYCERIDES, COCOA,     │
│ SALT, CORN STARCH, ARTIFICIAL AND        │
│ NATURAL FLAVORS, DEXTROSE, MAGNESIUM     │
│ CARBONATE, ARTIFICIAL COLOR, DICALCIUM   │
│ PHOSPHATE, SOY LECITHIN, BAKING SODA,    │
│ SODIUM ALUMINUM PHOSPHATE, DRIED YEAST,  │
│ CALCIUM SULFATE, CALCIUM CHLORIDE,       │
│ CALCIUM CARBONATE, PROPYLENE GLYCOL      │
│ MONOESTERS, SODIUM ASCORBATE (VITAMIN C),│
│ MONOCALCIUM PHOSPHATE, ALPHA TOCOPHEROL  │
│ ACETATE (VITAMIN E), TRICALCIUM PHOS-    │
│ PHATE, NIACIN (a B VITAMIN), ALUMINUM    │
│ SULFATE, SPICE, IRON, VITAMIN A          │
│ PALMITATE, PYRIDOXINE HYDROCHLORIDE      │
│ (VITAMIN B6), RIBOFLAVIN (VITAMIN B2),   │
│ THIAMIN MONONITRATE (VITAMIN B1), FOLIC  │
│ ACID, POTASSIUM IODIDE, VITAMIN D2,      │
│ CYANOCOBALAMIN (VITAMIN B12). FRESHNESS  │
│ PRESERVED BY SODIUM PROPIONATE, BHA,     │
│ CITRIC ACID, BHT, AND PROPYL GALLATE.    │
└─────────────────────────────────────────┘
```

FIGURE 13-3 An example of the many additives in a single food item.

with metals normally occurring in the blood and tissues, a process called *chelation.* In this way some biologically active metals can be removed from the system. Though toxic effects may be localized, they can become widespread throughout the body when the pollutant gains access to the bloodstream from either the lungs or the gastrointestinal tract.

When a pollutant directly or indirectly induces connective tissue (mast cells) to release stressing mediators such as histamine, serotonin, and bradykinin, the pollutant is considered an *allergen.* Lymphocytes and immunoglobulin are often involved as intermediates in what essentially may be a typical immune response. Some pollutants are capable of producing a direct effect on mediator release without antibody involvement. Allergic effects may be localized or spread throughout the body. For example, toluene diisocyanate (TDI), a constituent of polyurethane plastic, is a potent occupational allergen which causes constriction of the bronchial airways.

Some pollutant chemicals disturb the pH of exposed tissue or alter the oxidation-reduction balance through chemical reactions with cell membranes. Such pollutants are classified as *irritants.* Inhal-

TABLE 13-5
Common Food Additives

ADDITIVE PURPOSE	MATERIAL	SAFETY
Bleaching agents	Benzoyl peroxide	Inconclusive
Flavor enhancers	Monosodium glutamate	Produces allergic reactions
Coloring	Red dye no. 3 Red dye no. 40 Yellow dye no. 5	All may be carcinogenic
Nutrient supplements	Amino acids Iodide Vitamins Minerals	Safe but unnecessary
Nonnutritive sweetener	Saccharin	Appears to be carcinogenic
Preservatives	Sodium benzoate Sorbic acid Propionates	Inconclusive, poorly tested
	Nitrates Nitrites	Carcinogenic in nitrosamine form
Antioxidants	Butylated hydroxyanisole (BHA) Butylated hydroxytoluene (BHT)	Poorly tested at present
Surface-active agents	Monoglycerides Diglycerides	Safe
	Vegetable gums Carrageenan Acacia	Appear to be safe, but poorly tested

ants such as sulfur dioxide, ozone, chlorine, and ammonia are good examples of irritants. Their effects are usually localized in the body.

It is pointed out in Chapter 5 that our environment is teeming with chemicals that under conducive conditions are capable of promoting the development of cancer. These pollutants are classified as *carcinogens*. Prime examples are polynuclear hydrocarbons and nitrosamines, discussed later.

There are pollutants that do not produce any of the four types of effects mentioned above. On the other hand, a single pollutant may fall into more than one of the four categories. For example, nickel and chromium are irritants as well as carcinogens.

A specific form of stress from pollutants, such as toxicity, can be associated also with generalized stress responses mediated through the pituitary and adrenal cortex. This is especially true when exposures are prolonged. For example, plasma corticosterone levels have been shown to increase sharply in rats given PCBs in their food over a period of days.

INGESTED POLLUTANTS AND DISEASE

When an environmental pollutant gains entrance to the body, the severity of its effects is determined largely by five variables. These are: (a) chemical nature of the pollutant; (b) its concentration; (c) duration of exposure to it; (d) presence of other pollutants or other stressors; (e) the individual variation in susceptibility, which is based primarily on age, nutritional state, and general health.

Unintentional Ingestants

Systemic toxicity results from the ingestion of metals such as mercury, lead, and cadmium. These substances tend to accumulate in the body, where they eventually produce pathologic changes that develop slowly and insidiously.

The major risk of mercury poisoning is from eating fish caught in fresh and coastal waters near industrial sites in parts of the United States, Canada, and Europe. Pickerel caught in Lake St. Clair (near Detroit, Michigan) have contained as much as 5 ppm of methyl mercury. A lesser means of food contamination with mercury is through the application of mercurial fungicides to grain, which is then fed to animals whose flesh we eat.

Ingested mercury is likely to be in organic form, which is water-soluble and circulates in the bloodstream attached to red blood cells. Whole blood levels of 0.2 to 0.5 ppm are associated with toxic symptoms (Table 13-6). Organic mercury diffuses across the blood-brain barrier. Thus it will eventually become responsible for observable neurologic symptoms. In mercury poisoning the first symptoms are numbness in the fingers, lips, and tongue, followed shortly by slurred speech and ataxia.

Lead is ingested in larger quantities than any other poisonous heavy metal. Indeed, the average daily diet provides about 0.3 mg of inorganic lead. We also inhale the metal in organic form from the tetraethyl lead incorporated as an antiknock additive in gasoline. Among the primary sources of ingested lead are fruits, vegetables,

TABLE 13-6

Blood Levels of Mercury and Toxic Symptoms

SYMPTOMS	WHOLE BLOOD (PPB)*	RED BLOOD CELLS (PPB)
Average normal level	5	10
Maximum asymptomatic level	50– 100	100– 200
Numbness in fingers, lips, and tongue	150– 500	250–1000
Slurred speech, blurred vision	350– 800	700–1400
Weakness, ataxia, mental confusion	700–1200	1400–2000
Inability to sit or stand; usually fatal	1300	2400

Source: U.S. Water Pollution Control Federation.
*Parts per billion.

and grain grown along heavily traveled highways. Contamination from water pipes, cooking vessels, and some types of dishware is not infrequent; and many small children experience lead toxicity from ingesting flaking paint.

Ingested lead circulates in the blood, and within a short time it is responsible for several effects. It retards the maturation of red blood cells in the bone marrow and inhibits the synthesis of hemoglobin. Lead also replaces calcium, which means that it accumulates in bones (Figure 13-4). Interestingly, the lead content of human bones today is over ten times the amount found in ancient human bones. An inevitable consequence of lead toxicity is anemia. In advanced cases the kidneys are affected and the nervous system becomes involved, leading to brain damage and convulsions.

Cadmium can be toxic to all systems of the body, but it especially accumulates in the kidneys. The metal inhibits enzymes containing sulfhydryl groups, which are dependent on the presence of zinc, cobalt, and other metals. Cadmium has been incriminated as a factor promoting hypertension. Indeed, some people with arterial hypertension have been known to excrete 40 times more urinary cadmium than individuals with normal blood pressure. Apparently this effect is somehow related to an increased ratio of cadmium to zinc in the kidneys.

Although fluoride is not a metal, it is a potent systemic toxin because of its strong affinity for magnesium, manganese, and other metals that play strategic roles in enzyme systems. Chronic fluoride poisoning (fluorosis) results in excessive calcification around joint

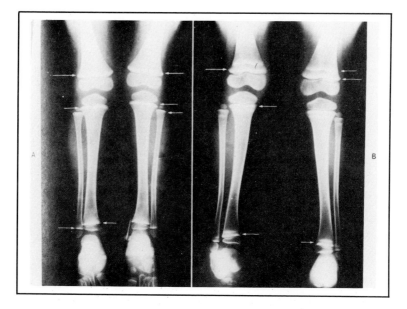

FIGURE 13-4   Skeletal accumulation of ingested lead. The roentgenograms are of the legs of a 3-year-old girl showing typical lead lines, *arrows*. Double lines appear in photo B, indicating a second lead exposure. (From G. L. Waldbott, *Health effects of environmental pollutants.*)

ligaments, thereby causing arthritic symptoms. Peculiar skin lesions called *Chizzola maculae* occur in many cases of fluorosis (Figure 13-5). Tea, wine, seafood, and drinking water are some of the ingestants containing minute quantities of fluoride. That fluoride is added to drinking water in an effort to reduce incidence of dental caries is well known. Although there has been controversy surrounding this practice, the amounts used are considerably below toxic levels.

The most likely food sources of PCBs and PBBs are milk, poultry, and fish. These pollutants have been shown to interfere with functioning of a variety of hepatic enzymes, leading to jaundice and liver injury.

Among pesticides, the chlorinated hydrocarbon group, represented by DDT, dieldrin, and chlordane, is considered the most toxic. Damage to liver and kidney is a common consequence of chronic exposure to chlorinated hydrocarbons. In higher concentrations these materials depress the central nervous system. The organophosphorus insecticides such as malathion and parathion inhibit the enzyme cholinesterase, which is indispensable in regulating nerve pathways. The action of these insecticides is somewhat similar to that of strychnine.

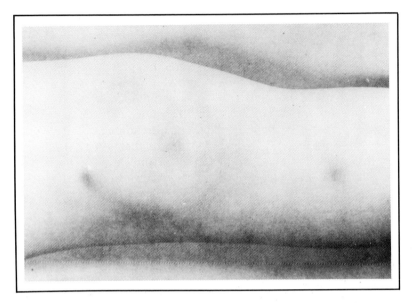

FIGURE 13-5   Chizzola maculae from exposure to fluoride. The darkened spots are reddish-brown in color and mimic bruises. This is the leg of a 3-year-old boy living near an area in Detroit where fluoride was emitted into the atmosphere. (From G. L. Waldbott, *Health effects of environmental pollutants.*)

There is not a great deal known about the toxic potential of some of the herbicides, although a few, such as paraquat, can produce irreversible lung damage. Such an effect would occur more often from inhalation than ingestion.

Intentional Ingestants

As pointed out earlier, most of our meat, milk, and eggs contain additives that were included originally in animal feed. The ingestion of antibiotic residues from this source constitutes a health hazard in two respects. First, habitual intake may induce progressive hypersensitivity to the drug in those with allergic dispositions, and second, the persistent presence of antibiotic in the system may promote the development of antibiotic-resistant strains of pathogenic microorganisms among the human microflora. Levels of tetracycline exceeding 3 ppm have been found in a small percentage of meat products. Moreover, in recent years over 4% of hog liver samples have been shown to exceed the 2 ppm tolerance level of arsenic.

There has been much popular interest in additives directly incorporated into processed foods. The greatest concern has been directed toward those materials with potential carcinogenicity, foremost of which are the nitrites, used as both a preservative and color enhancer in packaged meats, such as bacon, wieners, and bologna. It has been shown without question that sodium nitrite can react with secondary amines such as diethylamine under conditions of gastric acidity to form a variety of carcinogenic nitrosamines. More recently it has been demonstrated that the nitrites themselves may be directly carcinogenic. This has led the Food and Drug Administration (FDA) to consider phasing out the use of nitrites in meat preservation. There has been a similar issue in regard to the nonnutritive sweeteners, cyclamates and saccharin. Experimental evidence indicates that there is risk of tumorigenesis in long-term use of both substances. A number of dyes used as artificial coloring agents also are potentially carcinogenic and mutagenic.

Another concern with food additives is derived from the fact that there are pronounced individual sensitivities to some of them. Indeed, what is often construed as an allergy to a food may be a reaction to an additive in the food. Products of corn, yeast, and soya are added to a great variety of processed foods. Recall that these three materials are high on the list of food allergens (Table 12-2). Practically all B vitamins that are added for enrichment of processed foods are derived from yeast.

One of the more raging controversies has centered around a theory introduced by pediatric allergist B. F. Feingold, who contends that the hyperkinetic syndrome in children is caused by sensitivity to ingestants, food additives in particular. In the Feingold diet all artificial colors, artificial flavors, the antioxidants BHA and BHT, and a number of natural salicylates are completely eliminated. The diet is also high in protein and low in carbohydrate, since hyperirritability and hyperactivity are often associated with hypoglycemia.

It has been claimed that numerous children have benefited from the Feingold diet. In other cases the results have not been positive, prompting many clinicians to be skeptical concerning the scientific basis of the matter. However, others who have recently reexamined the problem are beginning to support Feingold's contention. New studies show that food dyes can act as toxic drugs in young children, definitely impairing various behavioral performances in children who are labeled hyperactive. Moreover, in animals it has been demonstrated that a food dye produces an increase in the release of neurotransmitters in the brain.

EFFECTS OF INHALED POLLUTANTS

The stress effects of several inhaled pollutants (lead, fluoride, carbon monoxide, and pesticides) have already been discussed in previous sections. It should be pointed out that substantial concentrations of some molecular materials are not always inhaled in free gaseous form. More frequently gaseous molecules enter the respiratory tract adsorbed to the surfaces of particles. In this manner greater concentrations of molecular pollutants are inhaled, and lung deposition is more assured. This is why there is so much concern about suspended particulates in the air. Particles convey the molecular pollutants into the respiratory tract.

Suspended Particulates

Much of the airborne particulate matter in itself is chemically innocuous. However, specific types of particles such as silica granules, asbestos fibers, and mica dust can progressively damage lung tissue; and asbestos is carcinogenic. The Department of Health and Human Services estimates that more than half the 4.5 million people who worked with asbestos in naval shipyards in World War II carry strong risks of developing lung cancer, particularly when other conducive factors such as smoking are present.

It is primarily silicon dioxide that scars the lungs of miners or anyone else exposed chronically to coal dust. Long-term exposure inevitably leads to pulmonary fibrosis, the essential feature of *pneumoconiosis* (Figure 13-6). The size of inhaled particles is especially important. Particles greater than 5μ in diameter do not reach the alveoli. They are trapped in the upper respiratory tract, whence they are soon cleared. This is not to imply that they are not troublesome. Before removal they can be irritating, or they may initiate allergic responses. On the other hand, particles deposited deep within the lungs can remain for months, or even years. Furthermore, it has been shown that the dangerous gaseous materials that adhere to aerosols tend to predominate in the smallest range of particle size. It is this size particle that is deposited in the lung and retained there. Lead, cadmium, sulfate, and benzo[a]pyrene, a potent carcinogen, tend to adhere to particles less than 1μ in diameter. However, there is a way in which the larger inhaled particles can convey chemicals to the deeper recesses of the body. They can be cleared to the throat region, whence they are swallowed. At that point they become ingestants.

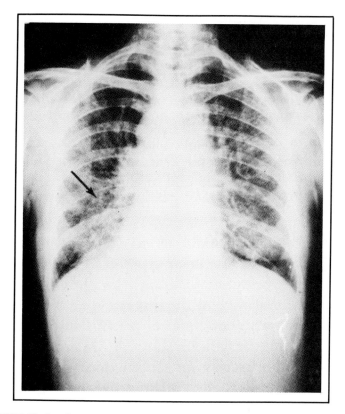

FIGURE 13-6   A roentgenogram showing pneumoconiosis. The roentgenogram is of the lungs of a former coal miner. In long-term exposure to silica, many small nodules develop, (around arrow.) Also note the two large shadows in the upper portion of each lung, indicating progressive deposition of silica. This condition can develop among nonminers residing near mines. (From G. L. Waldbott, *Health effects of environmental pollutants.*)

Gaseous Inhalants

Nitrogen oxides (NO_2) and sulfur oxides (SO_2) are common gaseous pollutants that strongly irritate the respiratory epithelium. The former group abounds in automotive exhaust, whereas the SO_2 group is emitted primarily by coal combustion. Both NO_2 and SO_2 become hydrated in the moisture of the respiratory tract to form nitric and sulfuric acids. Eye, nose, and throat irritation is experienced in exposures to 5 to 10 ppm of either gas. Of the two, sulfur dioxide has the greater water solubility, which means that the irritation and damage it produces are more confined to the upper respiratory regions. On the other hand, chronic inhalation of NO_2, which is also abundant in tobacco smoke, eventually damages the lungs. The initial effect of NO_2 is an edematous inflammation of bronchial epithelium, which in time may lead to chronic bronchitis, pulmonary fibrosis, and emphysema.

A wide variety of hydrocarbons are being discharged into the air from combustion processes and evaporation. Vapors of aromatic hydrocarbons such as benzene, toluene, and xylene are irritants of the mucous membranes. Chronic inhalation of these substances can affect the blood-forming tissues and result in anemia and leucopenia. Some of the worst forms of tissue irritation are produced by the aldehydes (acrolein and formaldehyde). Certain individuals are especially sensitive to their effects, some of which are allergic in nature. A burning sensation in the eyes, nose, and throat is a common aldehyde reaction. Other people may experience asthmatic wheezing, coughing, and headaches.

Without question the most dangerous organic inhalants are the polynuclear aromatic hydrocarbons (PAH), which are potent carcinogens. Benzo[a]pyrene and benzanthracene are the best-known examples. The primary air pollution source of PAH is vehicle exhaust. These materials are also found in tobacco smoke.

As threatening as hydrocarbon pollutants may be in themselves, they play a still greater role in air pollution by reacting with nitrogen oxides on sunny days to form photochemical oxidants. The foremost oxidant is ozone, potentially the most hazardous gaseous pollutant in ambient air. Ozone is an extremely active free radical, capable of interfering with innumerable intracellular metabolic processes. It destroys sulfhydryl-containing molecules, and produces additional free radicals in the process. The carbon-carbon double bonds of unsaturated fatty acids are particularly vulnerable to the oxidative attack of O_3.

Brief exposures to ozone irritate the eyes, nose, and throat. The gas impairs the function of pulmonary macrophages, thus facilitating susceptibility to respiratory infections. In long-term exposures to O_3, pulmonary congestion and edema develop, accompanied by chest pain and cough. There is reason to believe that chronic oxidant exposures contribute to the development of emphysema and hasten the aging process.

THE BODY'S DEFENSE AGAINST POLLUTANTS

Exposure to chemical pollutants is a relatively recent event in human history. Therefore it is not surprising that we have not had time to evolve effective defenses against many of them. The upper respiratory tract, liver, and kidneys offer the major means of protection. However, these regions must be healthy if they are to be at all effective. Obviously those with chronic illnesses, the very young, and the elderly are least tolerant of pollutant exposures. In fact, there are many groups that are especially susceptible to pollutants and thus are considered high risk groups. For example, people with cardiovascular impairment are particularly susceptible to carbon monoxide and the quality of drinking water, whereas those with bronchial and lung problems are vulnerable to exposures to inhalants such as ozone, nitrogen oxides, and sulfur oxides.

Acute toxicity and allergy from environmental chemicals can activate the pituitary-adrenal system and promote secretions of glucocorticoids. Indeed, those individuals who poorly mobilize adrenal and thyroid reserves are especially sensitive to the chemical environment.

Many so-called foreign chemicals are metabolized in the healthy liver. A restricted number of chemical reaction types are involved. Some are oxidations or reductions, while others are hydrolyses and conjugations. In many instances the liver converts fat-soluble compounds to hydrophilic materials that can be removed from the blood by the kidneys. However, it must be emphasized that the enzyme systems catalyzing these reactions were evolved originally to metabolize small quantities of such endogenous substrates as cholesterol and steroid hormones. Hence the capacity of the system becomes overtaxed when it is overwhelmed by barrages of new chemicals from the environment. Likewise, the delicate mechanisms of the kidney are adversely stressed when constantly confronted with water-soluble toxins.

It has been well established that nutritional intake is a significant variable in the body's defense against pollutants. Alpha-tocopherol (vitamin E) and ascorbic acid (vitamin C) both possess antioxidant action. Therefore they can be safeguards against the oxidant effects of photochemical inhalants. Likewise, an increasing number of investigations indicate that ascorbic acid subdues carcinogenic activity in animals fed certain carcinogens such as nitrites. Vitamin A likewise appears to have anticarcinogenic action. Along the same lines it has been shown that individuals deficient in calcium and magnesium are much more susceptible to toxicity from lead, zinc, and fluoride when exposed to these materials. Once again we must emphasize the point that a stressor is much more damaging when there are other preexisting stresses.

‖ SUMMARY

In the modern urban environment we are perpetually exposed to pollutants that enter the body with air, food, and water. Many of these materials are capable of producing toxicity, allergic reactions, irritations, and cancer. They may be ingested or inhaled.

Inhalation of silica particles can damage the lungs, and asbestos fibers are carcinogenic. Although all microscopic particles can convey concentrated molecular pollutants into the lower respiratory tract, those of the smallest size are most likely to do so.

The foremost gaseous air pollutants are carbon monoxide, photochemical oxidants (such as ozone, which is a strong respiratory irritant), and various hydrocarbons. Chronic exposure to oxidants can irreversibly damage the lungs, whereas inhalation of polynuclear hydrocarbons, such as benzo[*a*]pyrene, produces cancer.

Lead, the most ubiquitous of the toxic ingestants, suppresses the maturation of red blood cells, inhibits hemoglobin synthesis, and replaces calcium in the skeleton.

Ingestion of organic mercury produces neurologic disturbances, whereas cadmium toxicity is associated with kidney damage and hypertension.

Fluoride is a systemic toxin that combines with metals such as magnesium, which performs as an important coenzyme in cellular chemical reactions.

The antibiotics and hormones used in livestock feed plus the enormous array of chemicals added to processed foods are important intentional food contaminants. Among chemical additives are the nitrites, certain coloring dyes, and a nonnutritive sweetener, all of which possess carcinogenic capability.

The body does not possess highly effective defenses against most chemical pollutants, particularly when chronic illness and/or nutritional deficiencies exist.

Chapter Glossary

arsenicals   compounds containing arsenic

chelation   the combining or sequestering of a metallic ion into a ring form

coliform   bacteria resembling the common intestinal inhabitant *Escherichia coli*

heavy metal   metals such as lead, mercury, and cadmium that have high atomic weights

hydrophilic   substances attracted to water; water-soluble

photodissociation   chemical decomposition of substances due to solar radiation

pneumoconiosis   a lung condition characterized by chronic fibrous reaction to inhalation of dust

sulfhydryl groups   a sulfur-hydrogen bonding, principally found in the amino acid cysteine, essential for function in some enzymes

tetracycline   a broad-spectrum antibiotic

For Further Reading

Augustine, G. J., Jr., and Levitan, H. 1980. Neurotransmitter release from a vertebrate neuromuscular synapse affected by a food dye. *Science* 207: 1489.

Bailey, R. A.; Clark, H. M.; Ferris, J. P.; et al. 1978. *Chemistry of the environment.* New York: Academic Press.

Calabrese, E. J. 1978. *Pollutants and high-risk groups. The biological basis of increased human susceptibility to environmental and occupational pollutants.* New York: John Wiley and Sons.

Deichmann, W. B., ed. 1973. *Pesticides and the environment: A continuing controversy.* New York: Intercontinental Medical Book Corp.

Duffus, J. H. 1980. *Environmental toxicology.* New York: Halsted, a division of Wiley.

Feingold, B. F. 1975. *Why your child is hyperactive.* New York: Random House.

Holland, W. W., ed. 1972. *Air pollution and respiratory disease.* Westport, Conn.: Technomic Publishing Co.

Lave, L. B., and Seskin, E. P. 1977. *Air pollution and human health.* Baltimore: Johns Hopkins University Press.

Lee, D. H. K., ed. 1977. *Biochemical effects of environmental pollutants.* Ann Arbor, Mich.: Ann Arbor Science Pubs.

———, ed. 1977. Reactions to environmental agents. In *Handbook of physiology.* Bethesda, Md.: American Physiological Society. Section 9, Chapts. 9, 10, 11.

Marquardt, H.; Rufino, F.; and Weisberger, J. H. 1977. Mutagenic activity of nitrate-treated foods: Human stomach cancer may be related to dietary factors. *Science* 196:1000.

Natusch, D. F. S., and Wallace, J. R. 1974. Urban aerosol toxicity: The influence of particle size. *Science* 186:695.

Pettyjohn, W. A. 1972. *Water quality in a stressed environment: Readings in environmental hydrology.* Minneapolis: Burgess Publishing Co.

Purdom, P. W., ed. 1971. *Environmental health.* New York: Academic Press.

Randolph, T. 1967. *Human ecology and susceptibility to the chemical environment.* Springfield, Ill.: Charles C Thomas Pubs.

Slonim, N. B., ed. 1974. *Environmental physiology.* St. Louis: C. V. Mosby Co. Chapt. 13.

Swanson, J. M., and Kinsbourne, M. 1980. Food dyes impair performance of hyperactive children on a laboratory learning test. *Science* 207:1485.

Taub, H. J. 1974. *Keeping healthy in a polluted world.* New York: Harper & Row Pubs.

Vander, A. J. 1976. In Introduction to *Human physiology and the environment in health and disease.* San Francisco: W. H. Freeman and Co. Part 2.

Waldbott, G. L. 1978. *Health effects of environmental pollutants.* 2d ed. St. Louis: C. V. Mosby Co.

Tobacco, Alcohol, and Drugs

Tobacco Smoke and Disease Processes
    Smoke Constituents
    Health Effects of Smoking: An Overview
    Action of Nicotine
    Effects of Carbon Monoxide
    Carcinogens
    Chronic Obstructive Pulmonary Disease (COPD)

Toxicity and Damage from Ethanol
    Ethanol Metabolism
    Neural Effects
    Cirrhosis and Liver Damage
    Alcoholism

Caffeine and Salicylates
    Caffeine
    Salicylates

Adverse Effects of Prescribed Pharmaceuticals
    Hypnotic Depressants
    Stimulants and Antidepressants
    Major and Minor Tranquilizers
    Antibiotics
    Drugs for Hypertension
    Hypoglycemic Agents
    Steroids

Physiologic Implications of Illegal Drugs
    Opiate Narcotics
    Neural Stimulants
    Hallucinogens
    Marijuana

|| Objectives: Upon completing this chapter you should:

1. Be able to associate specific forms of self-inflicted body damage with individual constituents of tobacco smoke.
2. Understand the toxic qualities of ethyl alcohol and its metabolites, as well as appreciate the role of alcohol usage in causing behavioral disorders, liver disease, and chronic alcoholism.
3. Be informed about the health risks in overuse of caffeine and aspirin.
4. Be aware of the abuse of drug-prescribing, particularly the psychoactive ones such as barbiturates, amphetamines, and tranquilizers.
5. Be acquainted with the mode of action that underlies the body derangements and addiction resulting from use of illegal drugs.

The most devastating forms of disease from manufactured chemicals are those produced by tobacco smoke, ethyl alcohol, and drugs. With environmental pollution we usually have little choice about being exposed. However, with smoking, drinking, and drug use, there is a choice, at least in the beginning. Moreover, in the use of these materials, an intake of substantial concentrations is virtually ensured because the ingredients are being personally directed into the body.

A pertinent question in the use of any drug is personal control. Is the consumer in control, or is the drug controlling the consumer? This point returns us to the matter of chemical addiction mentioned in Chapter 12. Addiction can be accurately described, but the underlying biochemical mechanisms are poorly understood at present. It has been theorized that there is an inherent predisposition to chemical addiction in which chemical imbalances easily develop within the body, particularly with stress. Addicts may be victims of labile neuroendocrine responses, and they may be plagued with hypoglycemic reactions and nutritive deficiencies even before addiction. Individuals showing addiction to one material, nicotine for example, are also likely to become addicted to additional chemicals such as caffeine and sugar.

Psychologic dependency upon tobacco, alcohol, and many sorts of drugs appears to be associated in some way with primitive pleasure-seeking as a relief or escape from the unpleasantness of threatening stress, particularly mental conflict and boredom. Experiments with animals support this idea; indeed, dogs have been conditioned to happily anticipate their cigarette-smoking, and monkeys have discovered solace in alcohol.

TOBACCO SMOKE AND DISEASE PROCESSES

Tobacco is largely an American contribution to the world. When Sir Walter Raleigh first lighted his new pipe upon his return to England from Virginia, his aides threw water on him, thinking he was on fire. However, by 1978 over 57 million people in the United States had developed the smoking habit to the point of burning about 600 million cigarettes per year. In barely 400 years, use of tobacco had become the most widespread addictive habit in human history. Worse is the fact that more and more young people continue to adopt the habit. The number of teenage girls who smoke has doubled in the past 10 years.

Dried leaves of the tobacco plant are burned in cigarettes at temperatures exceeding 870 C, yielding trillions of separate microscopic particles and nearly 1000 different combinations of chemical compounds. One cigarette produces about 1/50 of an ounce of this mixture, and when the smoke is inhaled, at least 75% of the particulate is deposited in the lungs.

Smoke Constituents

Over 80% of tobacco smoke by weight consists of the molecular gases nitrogen, carbon dioxide, and oxygen, which are relatively harmless. About half of the remaining weight is comprised of particles, and the other half is water and a mixture of toxic gases. Nicotine and the hydrocarbon-containing tars tend to form particles that enhance their deposition in the lungs. Carcinogenic materials such as nitrosamines, beta-naphthylamine, radioactive polonium 210, and metallic nickel also are conveyed with particles. Cadmium, lead, and fluoride are other inorganic ingredients that are particle-borne, whereas compounds such as carbon monoxide, nitrogen dioxide, formaldehyde, hydrogen sulfide, ammonia, hydrogen cyanide, and acrolein enter the body as free gases. A listing of some of the principal ingredients in tobacco smoke is presented in Table 14-1.

The number of cigarettes, cigars, or pipefuls smoked per day is all-important, and so is the smoking technique. Practically all cigarette smokers inhale the smoke, a practice that ensures the same lung exposure from four cigarettes that one would get from merely puffing two whole packs. In addition, cigarette smokers usually smoke more tobacco than do pipe and cigar smokers. One reason for this is that cigarette-smoking tends to be much more addictive and uncontrollable than the other smoking habits.

TABLE 14-1

Principal Ingredients in Tobacco Smoke

COMPOUND	AMOUNT* (MG/CIGARETTE)
Particulates (no. per cigarette)	1.05×10^{12}
(Particulate Phase)	
Tars	20.8
Nicotine	0.92
Benzo[a]pyrene	3.5×10^{-5}
Benzanthracene	2.6×10^{-5}
Pyrene	13.0×10^{-5}
Cadmium	12.5×10^{-5}
Total phenols	0.228
(Gases)	
Water vapor	7.5
Ammonia	0.16
Carbon monoxide	31.4
Carbon dioxide	63.5
Nitrogen oxides	0.02
Aldehydes	0.08

Source: U.S. Department of Health, Education, and Welfare Public Health Service Report, 1975.
*Figures are for mainstream smoke only, which is the smoke that is drawn through during puffing. Sidestream smoke rises from the burning cone of the tobacco between puffs. It has an abundance of water and carbon monoxide.

Health Effects of Smoking: An Overview

Before discussing specific chemical stress on the body from individual tobacco ingredients, the overall seriousness of smoking in the development of disease deserves comment. The health implications of tobacco-smoking are now positively identified and can be clearly ascribed to explicit biochemical mechanisms rather than to the mere recitation of statistical associations. Nevertheless, the statistics in themselves are convincing. A comparison of mortality risks from a number of diseases in smokers and nonsmokers is shown in Figure 14-1. The National Commission on Smoking and Public Policy estimates that each year 350,000 deaths in the United States are linked to cigarette-smoking. The death rate alone exceeds the number of fatalities attributed to highway accidents, wars, and all other types of accidents combined.

The most significant single health consequence of cigarette-

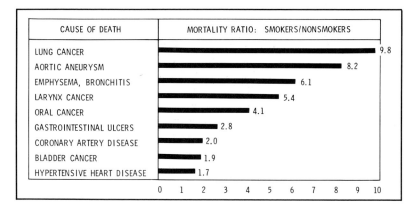

CAUSE OF DEATH	MORTALITY RATIO: SMOKERS/NONSMOKERS
LUNG CANCER	9.8
AORTIC ANEURYSM	8.2
EMPHYSEMA, BRONCHITIS	6.1
LARYNX CANCER	5.4
ORAL CANCER	4.1
GASTROINTESTINAL ULCERS	2.8
CORONARY ARTERY DISEASE	2.0
BLADDER CANCER	1.9
HYPERTENSIVE HEART DISEASE	1.7

FIGURE 14-1   Smokers to nonsmokers ratio for death from nine major diseases. The figures speak for themselves. In each disease the value significantly exceeds the balanced ratio of 1. (From Public Health Service Report, 1975. U.S. Department of Health, Education, and Welfare.)

smoking in terms of the number of people affected is the development of premature coronary heart disease. Smoking has been shown to be one of the major independent risk factors in promoting coronary atherosclerosis. Autopsy records clearly reveal that persons who smoked cigarettes have a much greater degree of coronary atherosclerosis than do nonsmokers.

A second major health consequence of smoking is malignant tumors. The risk of developing lung cancer increases with the number of cigarettes smoked per day and the number of years the habit has been sustained. However, the lung is not the only susceptible organ. Smokers have significantly higher incidences of cancer of the mouth, larynx, esophagus, pancreas, and urinary bladder than do nonsmokers. The death rate from lung cancer in women has increased by 263.3% during the past 25 years, reflecting the increasing number of women smokers since 1950. Nearly 26 million females over age 17 smoke. The surgeon general predicts that by 1983, lung cancer will kill more American women than breast cancer.

Nonmalignant respiratory disease is the third pathologic consequence of smoking. This form of morbidity is represented chiefly by the diseases emphysema and chronic bronchitis. Smoking has been shown to be the primary factor in the etiology of these conditions. Autopsy records reveal that smokers are much more likely than nonsmokers to show the macroscopic lung changes characterizing emphysema.

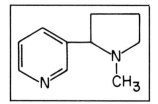

FIGURE 14-2   Chemical structure of nicotine. The active site is believed to be associated with each nitrogen atom, but particularly the one of the pyrrole ring at right.

Action of Nicotine

Nicotine is one of the most potent toxins known (Figure 14-2). A blood level of 60 mg is fatal within a few minutes. There is enough nicotine for two lethal doses in a cigar were it to be taken into the blood all at once. The nicotine in one typical filter cigarette amounts to over 20 mg, about 12% of which reaches the bloodstream of a smoker. After reaching the bloodstream, the drug is slowly deactivated in the liver.

Although nicotine is considered to be a nervous system stimulant, it is a unique one in that it produces both adrenergic and cholinergic effects. Nicotine mimics acetylcholine at certain nerve synapses, thereby stimulating salivation and gastric secretion, while inhibiting the release of bicarbonate from the pancreas and liver. Both these effects aggravate the disposition to gastrointestinal ulcers. However, nicotine's major effects center around the activation of sympathetic pathways and the release of catecholamines from the adrenal medullae. Consequences of these actions include an increase in heart rate and stroke volume, pronounced peripheral vasoconstriction that elevates blood pressure, increase in platelet aggregation favoring thrombus formation, and elevation of serum lipids and glucose. These combined effects stress the cardiovascular system, providing some of the explanation for the relationship of smoking to hypertensive heart disease.

The effect of nicotine on peripheral vasoconstriction is especially striking. When 0.5 mg of nicotine is injected into an albino laboratory rabbit, the red blood vessels, so prominently observable in the ear, practically disappear. An additional mechanism underlying the vasoconstriction is the release of pituitary vasopressin prompted by nicotine.

Nicotine also affects higher brain centers, enhancing catecholamine action in the reticular activating system (RAS) and the cerebral cortex. There is an increase in the frequency of cerebral electrical activity which shifts the electroencephalogram (EEG) toward an arousal pattern, which often accompanies an elevation of mood. A binding site for nicotine has been detected on rat brain membranes. Apparently these sites serve as nicotinic cholinergic receptors. It is primarily nicotine that is the addictive substance in tobacco smoke, and it is probably its effects in the brain that has much to do with the chemical addiction to smoking. The withdrawal symptoms from nicotine addiction include nervousness, depression, insomnia, and gastrointestinal distress. In some cases these effects can become severe.

Effects of Carbon Monoxide

There is much carbon monoxide in tobacco smoke. An extensive account of the physiologic action of this gas is presented in Chapter 9. As indicated therein, carbon monoxide is not a respiratory irritant, but is a potent asphyxiant, responsible for various degrees of anemic hypoxia which, along with nicotine, increases the risk of coronary heart disease.

Carcinogens

A number of tumor initiators, promoters, or accelerators have been identified in cigarette smoke. The majority of tumor initiators enter the body in the particulate phase of the smoke. This is particularly true of the polynuclear aromatic hydrocarbons, which pose the greatest cancer risks. However, a nitrosamine, N-nitrosonornicotine, has been found in concentrations of 1.9 to 6.6 micrograms per gram of unburned tobacco. This is the highest concentration of an environmental nitrosamine yet identified. Concentrations of nitrosamines in food and drink rarely exceed 0.1 microgram per gram.

Several organic constituents in tobacco smoke are thought to be tumor accelerators rather than initiators. In addition, some carcinogens in tobacco smoke are known to act synergistically with other environmental inhalants in inducing cancer. For example, chrysotile asbestos has a high adsorption activity for benzo[a]pyrene, and the combination has been shown to increase lung carcinogenicity nearly 60% above that due to benzo[a]pyrene alone. The roles played in carcinogenesis by several tobacco smoke ingredients are outlined in Table 14-2.

Some of tobacco smoke is deposited in the mouth, throat, and larynx. Also, a gaseous portion of that reaching the lungs diffuses into the blood, which accounts for the increased incidence of cancer

TABLE 14-2

Role in Carcinogenesis of Tobacco Smoke Ingredients

COMPOUND	ROLE IN TUMORIGENESIS
Benzo[a]pyrene	Initiator
Benzanthracene	Initiator
Alkyl pyrenes	Initiators
N-nitrosonornicotine	Initiator
Trans-4, 4-dichlorostilbene	Accelerator
N-alkyl indoles	Accelerators
N-alkyl carbazoles	Accelerators

Source: U.S. Department of Health and Human Services.

in regions of the body other than the respiratory tract. The urinary bladder is particularly vulnerable to blood-borne carcinogens because it stores kidney filtrate for extended periods of time. The longer any carcinogen lingers anywhere in the body, the greater the probability of tumorigenesis.

Chronic Obstructive Pulmonary Disease (COPD)

The chronic nonneoplastic lung diseases (emphysema and chronic bronchitis) are the major causes of permanent and temporary disability in the United States. Though a detailed account of these disorders appears in Chapter 9, the relationship of cigarette-smoking to these pathologies warrants special mention. A dose-related effect of cigarette-smoking on the severity of pathologic changes characterizing emphysema has been clearly demonstrated. Rupture of alveolar septa, thickening of bronchial epithelium, and hypertrophy of mucous glands are a few of the alterations. Smokers invariably have impaired ciliary action within the respiratory passages. In addition, they have a decreased number of pulmonary macrophages. This means less resistance to respiratory infections that recurrently plague sufferers of chronic bronchitis.

Chronic exposure to substantial concentrations of irritant gases is believed to be responsible for COPD. Nitrogen dioxide, acetaldehyde, and acrolein are foremost among these gases. The respiratory epithelium becomes inflamed and edematous, and incessant smoking denies the opportunity for healing. Consequently, the chronic inflammation progresses to degenerative damage (Figure 14-3). The same group of gases are responsible for the eye, nose, and throat irritation produced by cigarette smoke.

In regard to emphysema, it has been shown that ingredients

in tobacco smoke suppress activity of alpha-antitrypsin, the enzyme that normally counteracts the damaging effects of alveolar elastase. Just which ingredients has not been resolved, but nitrogen oxides are strongly suspected.

Certain air pollutants act synergistically with the irritants of tobacco smoke in producing and aggravating COPD. However, smoking is usually considered the more responsible of the two stressors.

TOXICITY AND DAMAGE FROM ETHANOL

Ethyl alcohol (ethanol) may be the oldest drug known to humanity, yet some authorities believe that if it were discovered today, it would never be approved by the Food and Drug Administration, even as a prescription drug. Despite this acknowledgment of its potential toxicity, 80% of adults living in urban areas of the United States use alcoholic beverages, and of these 80 million drinkers, over 7% are labeled as alcoholics. Interestingly, less than 50% of rural inhabitants drink, suggesting that social or urban stress somehow may be implicated in promoting usage. Of special concern is that 25% of the present population has a family problem related to alcohol. The figure in 1974 was only 12%.

Ethanol is our most popular tranquilizer and has long been our major means of escape from reality. It is unquestionably the most abused drug of all. Yet when consumed in small quantities, ethanol can be a beneficial relaxant and innocuous nutrient. Exactly when it becomes toxic varies considerably under different conditions and with different individuals. Generally, when the consumption of ethanol approaches the upper limit of the biochemical mechanisms responsible for its metabolism and elimination, the alcohol becomes a potent drug. When used to excess it is capable of producing psychomotor impairment, mental derangement, and eventual damage to liver tissue and brain cells. For a better understanding of how ethanol can become a chemical stressor, let us inspect the manner in which it is metabolized in the body.

Ethanol Metabolism

Alcohol requires no digestion since it is quickly absorbed unchanged from the stomach and small intestine. Protein and fats in the stomach help to delay absorption. From the bloodstream alcohol

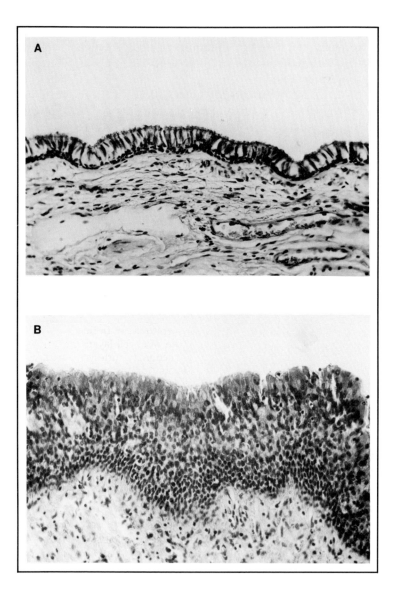

FIGURE 14-3   Progressive pathology in chronic obstructive pulmonary disease. A. Normal bronchial epithelium, characterized by an intact row of columnar cells with hairlike cilia projecting into the lumen. Dark-staining cells at the bases of the columns are basal cells. B. Chronic inflammation resulting in damage to columnar cells and their cilia, making invasion through them more accessible. Note expansive edema brought on by widespread proliferation of basal cells, which promotes obstruction of air flow. C. Columnar epithelium and its cilia virtually nonexistent, taking

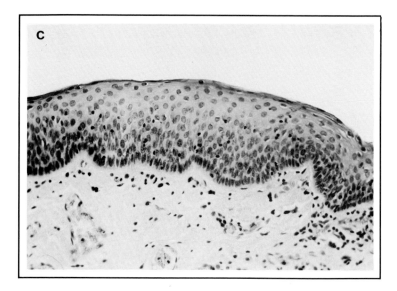

FIGURE 14-3   *(continued)*

on the appearance of a layer of squamous epithelium. In this stage degenerative changes occur throughout the basal cell layers, culminating in susceptibility to disorganization and destruction. (Courtesy of Dr. Oscar Auerbach, Distinguished Physician, Veterans Administration Medical Center, East Orange, N.J.)

passes immediately to the liver, where the enzyme *alcohol dehydrogenase* oxidizes it to acetaldehyde, which is further oxidized by a second enzyme (aldehyde dehydrogenase) to form acetic acid (Figure 14-4). More than 75% of the oxidation to acetate occurs in the liver at a rather slow, consistent rate of about 0.33 ounce per hour. Thus it is apparent why individuals with liver impairment are especially susceptible to ethanol toxicity. If the rate of alcohol intake exceeds the oxidation rate, the blood levels of the drug are forced to increase. If, for any reason, the first metabolite, acetaldehyde, is not oxidized rapidly enough, it becomes progressively toxic as it accumulates in the system.

Some physiologists have attributed several hangover symptoms such as headache, dizziness, and nausea to delayed reactions from acetaldehyde, whereas other scientists think that tissue dehydration may in some way be responsible for these symptoms. Ethanol is a dehydrating agent, and thirst ofter follows its consumption. In addition, as blood levels of alcohol rise, it acts as a diuretic by depressing the hypothalamic region responsible for the output of antidiuretic hormone (ADH).

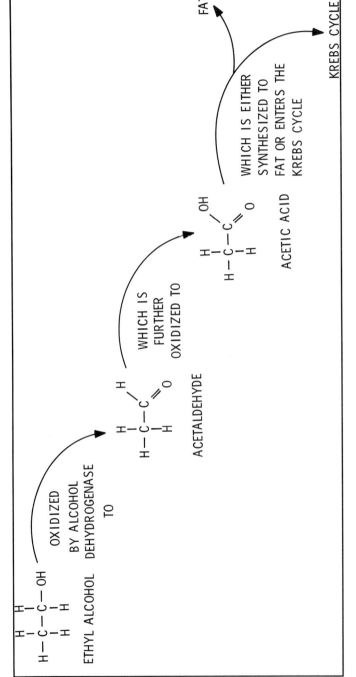

FIGURE 14-4   Metabolism of alcohol. When blood levels of alcohol exceed the capacity of this pathway, the substance behaves as a toxic drug.

Physiologists measure blood levels of ethanol in milligrams per 100 milliliters of blood (mg/dl). On the other hand, in law enforcement agencies concentrations are usually expressed as percentage by volume; thus, 100 mg/dl equals a 0.10% concentration of alcohol in the blood. At blood levels of less than 20 mg/dl (0.020%), most individuals experience no noticeable effects. Beyond this level functional neural impairment becomes observable.

Neural Effects

The major short-term effect of ethanol on the body is a depressed action throughout the central nervous system (CNS). Alcohol crosses the blood-brain barrier easily, and the rich blood supply to the brain can establish peak levels of ethanol there as blood concentrations of the drug continue to rise. Like other anesthetics, alcohol first begins to depress the *reticular activating system* (RAS) at the lowest effective blood level (about 20 mg/dl). The RAS regulates the cerebral cortex and is responsible for certain integrated relays between the cortex and other parts of the CNS. The relation of the RAS to the rest of the brain is depicted diagrammatically in Figure 14-5. There is further reference to this system in Chapter 16.

It has been shown that ethanol's mechanism of action on nerve tissue is directed at the fiber membrane and not at synapses. The electrochemical impulses along individual fibers become slowed. Apparently there is an interference with the membrane transport of sodium and potassium resulting from an inhibition of the enzyme adenosine triphosphatase.

The general sequence of progressive behavioral deviation is the same with alcohol as with most neural depressants. The more recently acquired, complex mental responses are the first to be disrupted at the lower blood levels of alcohol. As blood concentrations of the drug rise, the better learned, simpler patterns are affected. Contrary to popular notion, ethanol is not a stimulant. It may appear so because it reduces inhibitory action throughout the cerebral cortex, which may lead to aggressive, belligerent responses. However, individual behavioral changes accompanying ethanol intake are highly unpredictable. The essential danger in intoxication is that both judgment and psychomotor performance are impaired, while at the same time the drinker is lulled into a false sense of assurance and confidence in everything he or she attempts. One tragic consequence of the drinking habit is that at least half of the 50,000 fatal automobile accidents each year involve ethanol consumption. The

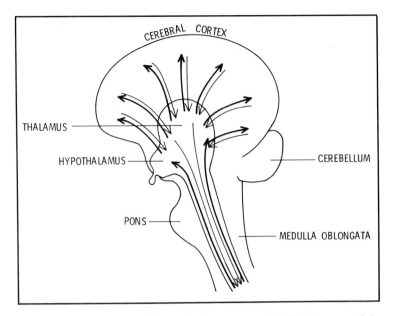

FIGURE 14-5   The reticular activating system (RAS). The core of the system is within the curved line surrounding the thalamus and continues through the hypothalamus, brain stem, and cord. Observe, however, that prominent fibers extend into the cerebral cortex. When pathways of the system are stimulated, excitation spreads through practically all of the brain, particularly arousing and regulating cortical activity. Note potential two-way traffic of the impulses indicated by the arrows, which implies that the system can be activated from a multitude of points, although the thicker arrows indicate the more likely direction of impulses.

mental and neural effects of progressively higher blood levels of ethanol are presented in Table 14-3.

The neural intoxication from an intake of alcohol is not permanent. When the blood is completely cleared of the drug, recovery gradually occurs within a few hours. However, a sober physical and mental depression may linger for an additional number of hours. The depression is often accompanied by the aforementioned hangover.

The dangers of taking ethanol concurrently with other nervous system depressants are well known. For example, the toxicity of barbiturates is insidiously increased in persons consuming alcoholic beverages; in fact, a combination of the two drugs can be fatal. This is because alcohol and barbiturates compete for the same hepatic microsomal enzyme system, resulting in a decreased rate of catabolism of

TABLE 14-3
Mental and Neural Effects of Ethanol in the Blood

BLOOD ALCOHOL CONCENTRATION (%)	NEURAL EFFECTS
0.05	Relaxed feeling; lowered alertness
0.10	Slowed reactions; decrement in motor coordination
0.12	Impairment of judgment and mental faculties
0.15*	Slurred speech; blurred vision
0.20	Severe ataxia; mental confusion
0.30	Stupor
0.40	Unconsciousness
0.50	Deep coma
0.60	Death (respiratory failure)

*Legal intoxication in all states of the Union.

both substances. The result is that the blood level of each drug remains higher than usual, leading to an overwhelming sedation and depression of the breathing center in the medulla oblongata.

Cirrhosis and Liver Damage

The impairment of liver function is a predominant complication of habitual ethanol consumption, and the chronic drinker is faced sooner or later with some degree of liver disease. Even a large, single dose of ethanol promotes a significant accumulation of triglycerides in the liver, and persistent drinking soon leads to a fatty liver (Figure 14-6). Up to a point the fat accumulation is reversible when drinking ceases. On the other hand, fatty changes can be a preliminary step toward a filling in with fibrous connective tissue. At this point the cells are not as effective in carrying out the usual hepatic functions.

When fibrosis begins to spread throughout the liver, various parenchymal cells show irreversible changes in their ultrastructure. Mitochondrial swelling is observed, leading to large decaying hyaline structures, known as *Mallory bodies*. When necrotic degeneration appears, the term *cirrhosis* is used to distinguish this form of pathology (Figure 14-7).

It has been shown that the damage to the liver is caused mainly by alcoholic metabolites such as acetaldehyde and hydrogen. Acetaldehyde damages the mitochondria, and the excess hydrogen appears to be involved in the increased accumulation of fat.

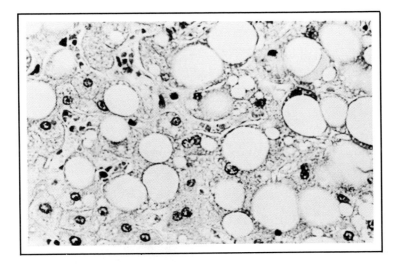

FIGURE 14-6   Fat accumulation in liver. The large, clear-looking inclusions are vacuoles that contained lipid globules which were dissolved during histologic preparation. Photomicrograph 500 X. (From S. A. Price and L. M. Wilson, *Pathophysiology—Clinical concepts of disease processes.* Copyright © 1978 by McGraw-Hill, Inc. Used with permission of McGraw-Hill Book Co.)

Even though fatty livers are often a consequence of drinking, they do not always progress to cirrhosis. Despite the fact that over three-fourths of all alcoholics have abnormal liver function, only 10% develop cirrhosis. But this is still 8 to 10 times the frequency found in the general population. Obviously other variables play a part in the susceptibility to cirrhosis. Viral infections and malnutrition are foremost among contributing factors. A high protein diet with a liberal intake of vitamins has been shown to prevent the development of a fatty liver (Figure 14-8).

Alcoholism

When the consumer of alcohol can no longer control drinking, and the habit begins to interfere with his or her occupational and social behavior, then the individual is said to suffer from *alcoholism*. The disease slowly develops from a background of biochemical and psychologic factors, and is seen among all classes of society. Industrial employees in large cities have the highest incidence, 1 in 13. More and more teenagers and people of college age are joining the ranks of alcoholism. The number of women drinkers has been growing at

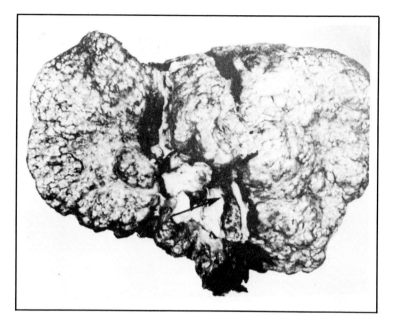

FIGURE 14-7   Cirrhotic liver. The gross features of liver cirrhosis, inferior aspect. Note the hardened, shrunken appearance and surface distortion. At the arrow a portal vein is thrombosed. (From W. Boyd and H. Sheldon, *An introduction to the study of disease.*)

twice the rate for men, bringing the number of female alcoholics to well above one-third of the total. Especially frightening are the facts that women drinkers reach the alcoholic stage much faster than men, and women alcoholics have twice the incidence of cirrhosis of the liver.

Alcoholism has been studied intensively. It has been shown that most addicts pass through a series of predictable phases. The prealcoholic phase begins with controlled social and/or family drinking. About one of ten of these drinkers develops a later drinking problem, and about one in four begins to appreciate that drinking provides an occasional escape from tension. In the next stage the escape afforded by alcohol is sought more frequently, and the drinker finds that more alcohol is required to achieve the previously desired effect. Progressively more preoccupation with alcohol in leisure moments follows, leading to temporary blackouts, or alcoholic amnesia. Such chronic bouts of intoxication begin to promote feelings of guilt, leading to secretiveness and solitary drinking. By this time addiction has become well established.

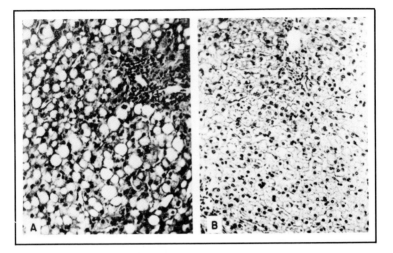

FIGURE 14-8   Nutritional effect on fatty liver. A. Fat infiltration is noted in the liver of a drinker with nutritional deficiencies. B. Liver of the same patient who continued to drink but was supplied with a diet high in protein and vitamins. Note the absence of lipid-containing vacuoles.

Psychologically, alcoholics are insecure and deeply dissatisfied with themselves. They are often immersed in a sense of boredom and despair. Of course, habitual use of ethanol only deepens the depression. In the terminal stages of alcoholism, the loss of brain cells (*Wernicke disease*) leads to a complete mental disorientation known as *Korsakoff psychosis*.

Once addicted, the drinker who stops consumption experiences a more severe withdrawal syndrome (*delirium tremens*) than that associated with narcotic drugs. The uncontrollable tremor, convulsions, and hallucinations exemplify torture at its worst.

CAFFEINE AND SALICYLATES

The two drugs consumed in the greatest quantities by the largest number of Americans are caffeine, a stimulant of the central nervous system, and acetylsalicylic acid (aspirin), that is used primarily as an analgesic. Fortunately, neither is very toxic at usual concentrations. However, both drugs possess physiologic effects that are undesirable in certain types of individuals. Furthermore, the use of caffeine is addictive.

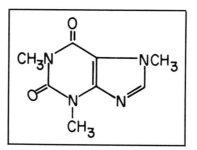

FIGURE 14-9   **Molecular structure of caffeine.** All xanthines are double-ringed structures with methyl groups, but caffeine is the only one that is trimethylated.

Seventy percent of Americans over 10 years of age drink coffee daily, and about 25% drink tea. In addition, over 45% regularly drink colas, and about 4% drink cocoa. All of these beverages contain caffeine. As for aspirin usage, estimates of daily consumption approach 45 million tablets.

Caffeine

Caffeine, along with the related alkaloids, theophylline and theobromine, is a methylated xanthine (Figure 14-9). Caffeine, theophylline, and theobromine are all nerve stimulants, but caffeine is by far the most potent. The amount of caffeine present in commonly used beverages is shown in Table 14-4. The onset of the effects from caffeine begins within 30 minutes of intake, and these actions reach a peak in about an hour. The halflife of the drug in the body is only 3 to 5 hours, due partly to its diuretic action.

At caffeine doses of 200 mg (2 cups of coffee), the cerebral cortex is activated, and the EEG shows an arousal pattern. At the same time the output of epinephrine and norepinephrine from the adrenals is increased, accompanied by an elevation in blood pressure. Initially the heart rate is decreased, but it increases at about an hour after intake. There is also an increase in breathing rate.

A recent finding has shown that caffeine stimulates the output of renin from the kidney. This action in addition to the mobilization of catecholamines makes it clear that caffeine intake may be inadvisable for persons disposed to hypertensive cardiovascular problems. In some persons the drug may also promote increases in serum lipids and glucose, probably through catecholamine mediation. However, in individuals disposed to hypoglycemia, a rapid ele-

TABLE 14-4

Caffeine Content of Common Beverages

BEVERAGE	AVERAGE CAFFEINE CONTENT (mg PER oz)
Regular coffee	25
Instant coffee	16
Decaffeinated coffee	9
Tea	9
Cocoa	1
Coca-Cola	4
Pepsi-Cola	2.5

vation in blood glucose prompts an insulin response, which may then lower the blood glucose to uncomfortable levels about 2 to 3 hours following intake of caffeine. Thus the drug can aggravate reactive hypoglycemia, and when there is sugar in the coffee, or when the drink is a cola beverage, then the extent of the hypoglycemic reaction is compounded.

In some individuals the gastric mucosa is quite sensitive to caffeine. Periodic digestive distress has been reported in about one-third of all habitual coffee drinkers. In addition, there are caffeine withdrawal symptoms, indicating the addictive nature of the drug. In regular consumers several hours of abstinence result in measurable muscle tension and a subjective sense of anxiety, both of which are relieved by resuming caffeine intake.

Recently, a significant statistical correlation has been shown between habitual coffee intake and pancreatic cancer. Because such an association does not exist for tea, it is doubtful that caffeine is a factor in the coffee–cancer association.

Salicylates

Aspirin has three effects: the primary one is analgesic action. Aspirin can dull somatic pain of moderate intensity. It also has an antipyretic effect and a capacity for reducing inflammation. In addition, aspirin decreases fibrinogenesis by suppressing synthesis of prostacyclin, thereby increasing the clotting time of blood. The mechanisms underlying some of these actions are not completely understood, but the antipyretic and anti-inflammatory effects are believed to be due to inhibiting the synthesis of several forms of prostaglandins.

Excessive use of aspirin disrupts the body's acid-base balance, and can induce gastric hemorrhage in many individuals, especially

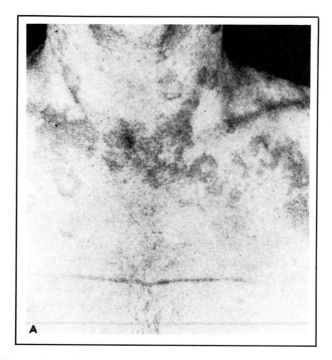

FIGURE 14-10   Allergic reaction to aspirin. Observe the acute urticaria on the neck and upper chest. (From J. M. Sheldon, R. G. Lovell, and K. P. Mathews, *A manual of clinical allergy,* 2d ed. Philadelphia: W. B. Saunders Co., 1967.)

if they are disposed to gastrointestinal ulcers. Another problem more widespread than is generally known is the development of allergic sensitivity to salicylates (Figure 14-10).

ADVERSE EFFECTS OF PRESCRIBED PHARMACEUTICALS

Two-thirds of the United States populace regularly use prescription drugs, of which there are at least several for practically every human ill. Most of the same people, as well as many others, also use over-the-counter drugs that do not require prescriptions. For the most part, there is greater danger in using prescription items, which of course is why their use must be authorized by physicians. In 1980 4.5 billion prescriptions were written—double the volume of ten

TABLE 14-5
Onset of Effect and Duration of Action of Barbiturates

GENERIC NAME	BRAND NAME	ONSET OF EFFECT (HRS)	DURATION OF ACTION (HRS)
Pentobarbital	Nembutal	0.25	2– 3
Secobarbital	Seconal	0.25	2– 3
Amobarbital	Amytal	0.50	5– 6
Barbital	Veronal	1.00	6–10
Phenobarbital	Luminal	1.00	6–10

years before. Furthermore, market analysts predict drug sales will double again during the 1980s.

Prescribed medications have relieved much suffering and permitted many individuals to live normal lives. On the other hand, the fact remains that practically all prescription drugs produce various degrees of chemical stress on the body, particularly when administered for extended periods, and when taken by especially susceptible individuals, such as children and the elderly. Most medicinal drugs are alien to the natural body chemistry; thus, therapeutic advantage must be seriously weighed against so-called side effects, most of which are toxic or allergic in nature. Unfortunately there is no way to predict beforehand what the administration of a given drug will do to any one individual. In many instances the chemical mechanisms underlying drug effects are not clearly understood.

It must be pointed out that pharmaceutical preparations, as effective as they may be, rarely *cure* anything. For example, in antibiotic treatment of pneumonia, the curing is done by the body's own defense mechanisms, though the drug may suppress bacterial multiplication enough to offer defense activity a better chance of succeeding.

To describe the adverse effects of the hundreds of known prescription items is much beyond the scope of this chapter. *The Physicians' Desk Reference* and *The Essential Guide to Prescription Drugs* (listed in For Further Reading section) have complete accounts. Attention here is restricted to a few groups of commonly prescribed drugs, the consumption of which has been known to become abusive.

Hypnotic Depressants

The major hypnotic sedatives are the barbiturates, which are potent depressants of the central nervous system. They are often grouped according to their duration of action (Table 14-5).

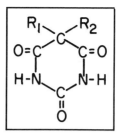

FIGURE 14-11   The reduced pyrimidine ring of barbiturates. R_1 and R_2 each vary according to the particular barbiturate in question.

The molecular structure of barbiturates is based on a reduced pyrimidine ring (Figure 14-11), and their chemical effect is thought to be directed at the neural synapse. Multisynaptic pathways, such as those of the RAS, are among the first to be affected. However, a depression of neural activity spreads to all regions of the brain and cord.

Barbiturates are prescribed to alleviate anxiety, insomnia, and epileptic seizures. As with alcohol their use can lead to addiction. Withdrawal of the drug produces anxiety, muscle-twitching, and even convulsions.

Common adverse effects of barbiturate usage include mental confusion, ataxia, stupor, and mental depression. Almost all consumers experience a residual hangover effect. As a result barbiturate use at night is sometimes coupled with the taking of stimulants, such as amphetamines, by day. Barbiturates are the single most used class of drugs for suicide. Some 5000 deaths and 25,000 trips to hospital emergency wards each year are attributed to sleeping pills.

Stimulants and Antidepressants

The most widely prescribed stimulants of the central nervous system are the amphetamines. These drugs markedly stimulate the RAS, even in the absence of sensory input. The RAS then transmits the excitation to all regions of the brain. Corticular activation results in alertness, arousal, euphoria, and hyperresponsiveness to stimuli. In the hypothalamus the drug stimulates the satiety center, which suppresses appetite. The overall neural stimulation from amphetamines elevates the BMR and produces a notable increase in heart rate and blood pressure. In addition, there may be insomnia, tremor, headache, and dryness of the mouth.

Amphetamines are strongly adrenergic, which accounts for most of their effects. The drugs cause norepinephrine to leak spon-

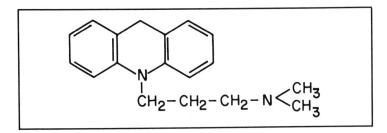

FIGURE 14-12   Chemistry of a tricyclic antidepressant. This is imipramine (Tofranil). Note the three rings.

taneously from presynaptic sites in brain neurons. In addition, they prompt an increase in the volume of released norepinephrine as well as block the presynaptic reuptake of this transmitter.

Amphetamines are prescribed for narcolepsy, hyperkinesis, and weight control, although recently restrictions have been imposed on their use as an appetite depressant. Consumption of amphetamines is especially dangerous to persons disposed to cardiovascular and hypertensive pathology, and there is evidence of drug dependency resulting from use of these stimulants.

The antidepressant drugs of choice for treating endogenous mental depression are the tricyclic compounds, so called because of their three-ring structure (Figure 14-12). The two most commonly prescribed are imipramine (Tofranil) and amitriptyline (Elavil). Tricyclics enhance adrenergic action in the brain by preventing presynaptic reuptake of released norepinephrine. It is believed that chronic, endogenous depression is associated with an underbalance of norepinephrine action in the limbic system of the brain.

Anticholinergic action of the tricyclics tends to produce dryness of the mouth, diminished urination, and constipation. Also, the drugs may suppress libido and promote blood glucose fluctuations. Other adverse reactions to tricyclic antidepressants include palpitations, irregular rhythm of the heart, jaundice, Parkinson-like symptoms, and depression of the bone marrow.

Major and Minor Tranquilizers

Modern drugs used for relieving anxiety, panic, agitation, and general mental unrest have come to be known as *tranquilizers*. The so-called major tranquilizers are the phenothiazines. Major refers to the degree of effect; thus, phenothiazines are commonly administered to calm the acute anxiety and excitability in mental patients with psy-

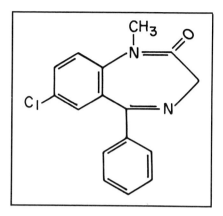

FIGURE 14-13   Molecular structure of diazepam (Valium). This drug is prescribed more than any other in the United States.

chotic tendencies. The three most commonly prescribed phenothiazines are chlorpromazine (Thorazine), prochlorperazine (Compazine), and thioridazine (Mellaril).

The phenothiazines suppress action of all the transmitting mediators in the brain. Thus they are considered antiadrenergic, antidopaminergic, anticholinergic, antiserotonergic, and antihistaminic. Chlorpromazine blocks neural receptor sites for norepinephrine and especially dopamine. In addition, it depresses action of hypothalamic centers and the RAS, thereby diminishing the arousal of the cerebral cortex. Phenothiazines are not as addictive as barbiturates, but they tend to promote what are known as *extrapyramidal* effects. Such effects are characteristic of Parkinson syndrome, and they are due to the blocking of dopamine from receptor sites.

There are two groups of minor tranquilizers, both of which diminish the mind and body aspects of anxiety and emotional tension. Meprobamate (Equanil and Miltown) appeared first (1955). After 1960 came the benzodiazepines, represented first by chlordiazepoxide (Librium), then diazepam (Valium), and more recently lorazepam (Atavan). Librium and Valium are consumed in greater quantities by more people than any other prescribed drug. In 1976 more than 30 million Americans took over 3 billion capsules of diazepam (Figure 14-13).

The site of action of both meprobamate and the benzodiazepines is the limbic system of the brain. This system mediates the emotional expressions, and it serves as an intermediary between the hypothalamus and the cerebral cortex. Apparently the tranquilizers suppress informational exchange between these two levels of emotional reaction. In breaking the circle of action-reaction, there is a decrease in the experience of any emotion as well as in the associated body changes. The minor tranquilizers are superior to barbiturates in that they do not depress cortical functioning nearly as much; hence the individual can reasonably perform and think without undue drowsiness. The thought processes become more calm and are devoid of emotional overtones.

At one time the minor tranquilizers were considered safe and nonaddictive. However, many cases of addiction are now on record—not only of psychologic dependence, but real chemical addiction with serious withdrawal symptoms. Moreover, consumption of these drugs over long periods can promote mental confusion, jaundice, depression, anemia, and allergic sensitivity.

Antibiotics

Chapter 1 alludes to the fact that before the last half century, infectious disease had been a major cause of death. The advent of effective antibacterial medications began to change this, especially after World War II, when antibiotic drugs made their appearance. However, in frequent instances antibiotics are needlessly prescribed. This is especially true in respect to acute upper respiratory distress, much of which may be due to viruses, or even allergy.

One important concern with all antibiotics is that continued use paves the way for the development of resistant strains of pathogenic bacteria. Another point is that antibiotic consumption drastically alters the body's bacterial flora, eliminating beneficial forms, and disturbing normal microbial balance. The consequent loss of the usual competition among microbes leads to risks of overwhelming superinfections from resistant organisms.

The "cillins" such as penicillin and ampicillin are not very toxic, but they can be strongly allergenic in susceptible individuals. Originally penicillin was the drug of choice for combating infections from a variety of gram-positive bacteria. Unfortunately many pathogens have become resistant to penicillin; this is especially true of strains of *Staphylococcus.* Broad-spectrum antibiotics such as the tetracyclines are usually effective against both gram-positive and gram-negative bacteria. However, these types of antibiotics can be toxic to various degrees. Use of tetracyclines can lead to superinfections of yeast organisms, and cause permanent discoloration and malformation of children's teeth. In some cases, long-term consumption of tetracyclines has resulted in bone marrow depression and impairment of liver and kidney function. Perhaps the most dangerous antibiotic is chloramphenicol (Chloromycetin). In a number of isolated instances, use of this drug has been followed by fatal aplastic anemia.

Drugs for Hypertension

Most persons afflicted with hypertension seem to be able to decrease their blood pressure with a tandem of drugs. The tandem consists of a diuretic to alleviate retention of sodium and fluid, in conjunction with an antiadrenergic agent to decrease vasoconstriction. The diuretic is usually a thiazide such as chlorothiazide (Diuril). Such drugs promote the excretion of potassium as well as sodium, and without adequate potassium replacement the resulting hypokalemia can lead to muscle weakness and heart irregularities. In addition, the thiazides tend to cause an elevation in blood sugar and uric acid, which makes their use risky in individuals disposed to adult diabetes and gout, two conditions which unfortunately are often associated with hypertension. Other adverse effects of thiazides that have been reported include jaundice, bone marrow depression, allergic reactions, and a seriously reduced libido associated with impotence in male patients.

An antiadrenergic agent that has been employed in hypertension therapy is reserpine (Serpasil), which also has been prescribed as a tranquilizer. This drug blocks the uptake of norepinephrine into the synaptic vesicles of sympathetic nerves, resulting in a relaxation of the smooth muscle of the blood vessels. Common side effects of reserpine are lethargy, apathy, nasal stuffiness, acid indigestion, and diarrhea. Other documented developments in patients taking reserpine include mental depression, Parkinson-like disorders, activation of gastrointestinal ulcers, and impaired sexual potency. The drug is contraindicated in persons susceptible to depression and peptic ulcer.

Another antiadrenergic agent that is being prescribed increasingly for hypertension is propranolol (Inderal), which acts on the vasomotor center in the brain as well as on the beta receptors localized in blood vessel walls. Propranolol also can cause emotional depression, and it often produces lethargy, fatigue, and various degrees of bronchoconstriction. Its use is contraindicated in those with an asthmatic disposition.

Hypoglycemic Agents

Sulfonylureas, which are chemical derivatives of sulfonamides, an early group of antibacterial drugs, are known to stimulate insulin response in individuals whose beta cells are functional. Tolbutamide (Orinase) and chlorpropamide (Diabinese) are two sulfonylureas that are often prescribed for stable, adult-onset diabetes.

In 1970 a comprehensive, long-term study by the University Group Diabetes Program (UGDP) clearly indicated that adult-onset diabetics who had consumed oral hypoglycemic agents for over 5 years had almost three times the incidence of fatal cardiovascular disease than did those who depended upon dietary control alone. The publication of these data touched off a storm of controversy pertaining to choice of therapy for adult-onset diabetes, and the matter has yet to be completely resolved. However, many specialists contend that over 80% of all so-called diabetics of the adult-onset type can achieve desirable control of blood glucose levels with appropriate weight loss, proper diet, and exercise.

There is no evidence that sulfonylurea therapy corrects the hyperlipidemia or prevents the atherosclerosis associated with diabetes. Nor does it necessarily prevent other diabetic complications such as retinopathy, neuropathy, and nephrosis. On the other hand, extended use of sulfonylureas can suppress thyroid function, which in itself retards carbohydrate metabolism and promotes hyperlipidemia. In addition, long-term use of these drugs may entail risks of hepatitis with jaundice, hemolytic anemia, and the aforementioned development of heart disease. Moreover, chlorpropamide is an antidiuretic and has been used therapeutically in this way, but antidiuresis in turn aggravates hypertension, a condition often associated with adult-onset diabetes.

Steroids

The adrenal-type steroids, cortisone and prednisone, are prescribed therapeutically for a number of conditions, among them are rheumatoid arthritis (and other autoimmune disorders), prevention of transplanted organ rejection, asthma (and other allergic conditions), and various instances in which tissue inflammation arises. Extended use of these hormone preparations is dangerous. Adrenal steroids precipitate glucose intolerance in those so predisposed. Moreover, these hormones suppress immune competence, which greatly enhances the susceptibility to infectious disease and tumorigenesis. Continued use of cortisone or prednisone also can induce mental changes, and eventually Cushing syndrome may develop (see Chapter 4).

More widely prescribed steroids are of the ovarian-type: the estrogens and progesterone that are incorporated into the contraceptive pill. Despite much controversy it is becoming apparent that long-term use of steroid contraceptives is not advisable, at least in women with certain predispositions, and in those past 30 to 35 years of age. Of special concern is the risk of developing *thrombophlebitis.* In addition, regular consumption of progesterone in some women leads to weight gain, blood sugar elevations, and increases in blood pressure. There also are data linking use of oral contraceptives with liver tumors. Several studies have implicated the pill in the development of heart disease. It appears that this particular risk is substantially compounded in smokers and in those past 35 years of age.

Estrogens are also prescribed to relieve symptoms of menopause, or similar problems in younger women who have had ovariectomies. These hormones also increase bladder tone in older women. However, prolonged use of estrogen preparations has been shown to be associated with the development of uterine cancer.

PHYSIOLOGIC IMPLICATIONS OF ILLEGAL DRUGS

Much attention has been drawn to illegal drugs because of the increased usage and addiction since 1960. Most of these substances can be grouped as narcotic depressants, stimulants, and hallucinogens. Only the major drugs of each group are discussed here.

Opiate Narcotics

The substance opium, produced by the poppy, *Papaver somniferum,* has been known and consumed as an analgesic for centuries. The principal opium derivatives are listed in Table 14-6. All but heroin are administered medically, although laws regulating and restricting usage are becoming more strict. The basic molecular structure of opium derivatives is shown in Figure 14-14.

The primary therapeutic value of narcotics is in reducing the suffering from pain and providing relief from chronic diarrhea. Much of opiate action is directed to the limbic system of the brain and certain sensory centers of the thalamus and cerebral cortex. Patients taking these drugs are still aware of pain, but apparently it is

TABLE 14-6

Principal Opium Derivatives

DRUG	ONSET OF EFFECT (INJECTION)	DURATION OF ACTION	EQUIANALGESIC DOSES (MG)
Morphine	45 min	5 hrs	10
Codeine	45 min	3 hrs	120
Heroin	15 min	5 hrs	3
Methadone (synthetic)	30 min	6 hrs	9
Meperidine (Demerol) (synthetic)	10 min	3 hrs	90

Source: New York State Narcotic Addiction Control Commission.

no longer aversive. It is the emotional response to pain that is abolished.

Narcotics also depress the respiratory centers. This is potentially their most dangerous side effect. In addition, narcotics decrease peristalsis and glandular secretions in the gastrointestinal tract. The sedation from the drugs is believed to be associated with serotonergic enhancement. In the use of some narcotics, various degrees of euphoria often accompany the analgesia, indicating that adrenergic processes also may be involved.

Continued use of all narcotics promotes strong addiction, and herein lies the essential problem with them that has led to strict legal control. Heroin is three times as potent analgesically as morphine, and it arouses feelings of euphoria that are much more heightened and intense. Because of this, heroin is much more addictive than other narcotics. There are over 250,000 heroin addicts in this country. Methadone, which exhibits cross-tolerance with other narcotics, is frequently used to ease heroin withdrawal symptoms.

A synthetic narcotic, propoxyphene hydrochloride (Darvon), is a prescription drug that is increasingly being obtained by illegal means. It is used primarily as an analgesic, and has become the third most widely prescribed drug in the United States. However, after abuse of Darvon usage was shown to be linked to a thousand or more deaths each year, the FDA has placed the drug in a more restricted category.

A new and apparently nonaddictive painkilling pill that is more effective than morphine injections has just been approved by the Food and Drug Administration. The drug is called *Zomepirac*, and it seems to prevent pain by a mechanism similar to that of salicylates, by blocking the production of prostaglandins.

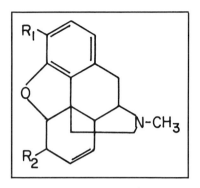

FIGURE 14-14   Chemical structure of opiate narcotics. R_1 and R_2 are variables, depending upon the drug in question. In morphine each R is represented by an O-H group.

Neural Stimulants

The two major stimulants in illegal use are amphetamine and cocaine. Concentrated dosages of cocaine are used medically as a local narcotic anesthetic. Amphetamine has already been described as a prescription drug. Injecting and sniffing cocaine has become fashionable throughout some affluent segments of society, particularly among individuals who are impressionable and bored. Cocaine activates the cerebral cortex and stimulates norepinephrine action, resulting in feelings of exhilaration.

Hallucinogens

A hallucinogen is a drug that can induce the visual and/or auditory mental distortions that we call hallucinations. Most such substances produce these effects by drastically altering the brain action of the neurotransmitter serotonin. There are other hallucinogens, however, that interfere with norepinephrine. An example of the latter is *mescaline*, which is prepared from the peyote cactus of Mexico. The most notorious serotonin blocker is *d-lysergic acid diethylamide* (LSD), which is a test-tube concoction. LSD, an odorless, colorless, and tasteless substance, is an extremely potent hallucinogen. Much of its effect stems from action on the limbic system and RAS of the brain. The normal monitoring of neural flow from sensory input becomes severely altered by LSD. Usage of the drug produces intense dreamlike or nightmarish experiences characterized by complete loss of emotional control, paranoid delusions, and psychedelic hallucinations. The effects are similar to effects in schizophrenic episodes. The psychosis from a dose of LSD can be prolonged over several weeks,

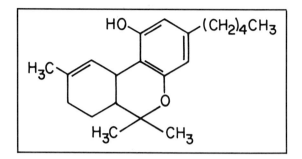

FIGURE 14-15 Molecular configuration of tetrahydrocannabinol. The site of action of the drug is obscure, though one might guess that thalamic centers are affected.

and even after remission, flashbacks may occur much later, in which feelings of paranoia, unreality, and estrangement are reexperienced. LSD also can be responsible for genetic damage.

Marijuana

There are those who consider marijuana to be a hallucinogenic drug. Others do not; a relaxant and euphoriant perhaps, but not a hallucinogen at usual doses. This singular example of diversified opinion typifies the overall public and scientific view of this drug—it is highly controversial.

The active ingredient in marijuana is sometimes termed the *THC isomer* of tetrahydrocannabinol (Figure 14-15), and it is most concentrated in the resin of the flowering tops and leaves of the plant, *Cannabis sativa* (Figure 14-16). Smoking is the typical mode of use in the United States. In initial experiments there appeared to be few marked physiologic changes with usual dosages of cannabis. However, as more data accumulated, a number of adverse effects began to be noted, which has prompted some researchers to revise their view that marijuana is merely a mild intoxicant that is relatively harmless. It has been suggested that marijuana research is at a point similar to tobacco research of two or three decades ago. On the other hand, THC has been put to clinical use. There are indications that glaucoma patients and those suffering the effects of cancer chemotherapy are benefited by the drug.

A recent finding of considerable alarm indicates that marijuana smoke possibly contains 50% more carcinogens than a comparable amount of tobacco smoke. In addition, it has been shown that marijuana smoke reduces the body's ability to rid the lungs of bacteria and other noxious materials. Indeed, experiments with ani-

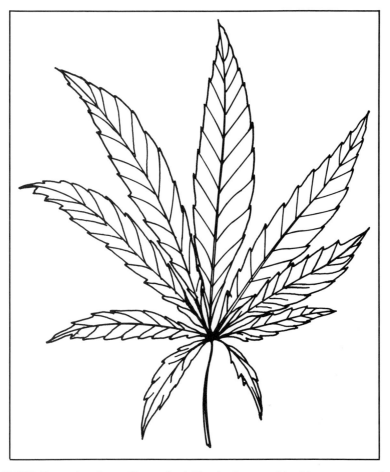

FIGURE 14-16   A marijuana leaf. Tetrahydrocannabinol is concentrated in the sticky resin. The leaf is palmately compound with 5 to 11 leaflets. Leaves have a characteristic odor and are covered with fine hairs.

mals indicate that two to three years of exposure to marijuana smoke severely inflames the respiratory passages, leading to abnormalities far greater than those associated with tobacco smoke.

It has been known for some time that ingredients in marijuana smoke are capable of stimulating sympathetic nerve impulses, causing quickened heart rates and irregular heart rhythm. Well documented also are data clearly showing that tetrahydrocannabinol (THC) reduces sperm production and sexual drive in male monkeys.

Investigations are under way to confirm preliminary studies that indicated that both the immune system and chromosomes are damaged by chronic intake of THC. In view of many of these potential effects, there is particular concern about the recent evidence revealing that marijuana being smuggled into the United States today contains as much as 2% to 6% THC compared to the 0.002% to 0.01% of THC found in plants used in the 1960s.

Consumers of marijuana use it to obtain mental manifestations, although these seem to vary considerably in degree and quality. A primary mental effect, agreed upon by practically all investigators, is that the user experiences an overestimation of the passage of time, which is associated with an impairment of short-term memory. Some investigations have shown that there appears to be a certain amount of learning involved in being able to experience any mental effects at all, indicating that the power of suggestion and possibly other psychologic variables are strategic in determining both the quantity and quality of the subjective experience. Just how the drug produces the mental effects is not clear.

Substantial doses of potent forms of cannabis can produce a toxic psychosis characterized by confusion, disorientation, delusions, and visual hallucinations. Even in instances where average doses are the rule, some investigators have described a nonpsychotic amotivational syndrome that is common among habitual marijuana consumers. An unwillingness to carry out complex long-term plans, an inability to concentrate for long periods, and a poor appreciation for cause and effect relationships are among the mental qualities typifying this syndrome. A recent scare among users of cannabis developed when it was discovered that due to a United States-sponsored defoliation program in Mexico, a substantial amount of marijuana from that country contained paraquat, an herbicide which can cause permanent lung damage, and for which there is no known antidote.

Whether or not marijuana is addictive has become a debatable point. Psychologic dependence does occur. However, chemically based reinforcement is not nearly as apparent as it is with alcohol, barbiturates, opiates, nicotine, and amphetamines. There is an enormous use of marijuana in this country, and over 10% of consumers smoke it daily. Effects of the most commonly used psychoactive drugs, legal and illegal, are summarized in Table 14-7.

SUMMARY

Many serious impairments of health are directly due to the habitual use of tobacco, ethyl alcohol, and other countless varieties of drugs.

Continual inhalation of the nicotine and carbon monoxide in

TABLE 14-7

Common Psychoactive Drugs

TYPE DRUG	MENTAL EFFECT	DANGER FROM ABUSE
Barbiturates	Depressant-sedative-hypnotic	Addiction—respiratory failure
Meprobamate	Diminishes emotional tension	Addiction—depression
Benzodiazepines	Reduce tension associated with anxiety	Addiction—confusion
Phenothiazines	Antipsychotic—diminish agitation and excitability	Parkinson symptoms
Tricyclic antidepressants	Elevate mood, curb agitation	Palpitation—heart irregularities
Ethyl alcohol	Relaxation, release of inhibitions	Addiction—damage to liver and brain
Opiates	Subdue sense of pain—euphoria	Strongly addictive—convulsions
Cocaine	Excitation, exhilaration	Convulsions, mental impairment
Amphetamines	Hyperactivity, euphoria	Hallucinations, hypertension, heart damage
Caffeine	Increases alertness	Hypertension, heart irregularities
Nicotine	Elevates mood, psychologically relaxing	Hypertension, cardiovascular damage
LSD	Hallucinations, expands and distorts sensorium	Chronic psychotic episodes
Marijuana	Mild euphoria	Mental disorientation, sensory distortion

tobacco smoke can lead to premature coronary heart and artery disease, whereas long-term inhalation of nitrogen oxides and aldehydes has much to do with the development of emphysema and chronic bronchitis. The particulates of cigarette smoke convey polynuclear hydrocarbons into the lungs, initiating malignant changes there.

Ethanol toxicity is expressed as a depressive effect throughout the central nervous system. Higher centers of the brain are affected first, resulting in an impairment of judgment and discrimination. Habitual consumption of alcohol promotes a fatty infiltration of liver cells, which can lead to liver damage and cirrhosis.

In some individuals caffeine significantly elevates blood pressure and exacerbates reactive hypoglycemia, whereas excessive use of salicylates (aspirin) can produce gastric hemorrhage and provoke allergic reactions.

Barbiturates are neural depressants that may produce confusion, ataxia, and stupor, and they are especially dangerous in combination with alcohol. Amphetamines are neural stimulants that can stress the cardiovascular system. Phenothiazines are strong tranquilizers used to calm psychotics, whereas meprobamate and the benzodiazepines are minor tranquilizers, used for reducing chronic anxiety.

Thiazide diuretics are frequently prescribed together with an antiadrenergic agent in order to control high blood pressure. Continued use of thiazides entails risks of impotence in males, whereas antiadrenergic agents promote lethargy and emotional depression.

Morphine, heroin, and other opiate narcotics effectively dull the emotional sensitivity to pain and produce varying degrees of euphoria. Compared to the others, heroin is three times as potent and much more addictive.

The most dangerous of the hallucinogens is LSD, which interferes with serotonin action at synapses in the limbic system and reticular activating system of the brain.

In long-term use of marijuana there may be risks of lung cancer development, bronchial pathology, sterility, and genetic damage. The drug also promotes an overestimation of time passage and impairment of short-term memory.

Chapter Glossary

analgesic   an agent that alleviates pain

aplastic anemia   a critical anemia resulting from severe depression of erythropoiesis in the bone marrow

bone marrow depression   reduced activity affecting production and maturation of erythrocytes and granulocytes

ciliary action   beating motion of microscopic, hairlike structures lining the respiratory tract. The action clears particles and noxious materials from the tract.

dopamine   an important neurotransmitter in specific areas of the brain

euphoria   an exaggerated sense of well-being

halflife   an index of how long it takes for a substance to remain unchanged in the body; a halflife of 3 hours means that in that time half the substance has been transformed or eliminated

narcolepsy   a condition marked by a frequent, uncontrollable desire for sleep

neuropathy   functional disturbances in the peripheral nervous system; a complication of diabetes mellitus

Parkinson like   neurologic symptoms similar to those of Parkinson disease

presynaptic   refers to the axon terminals of a nerve fiber which secrete neurotransmitters into the synapse

psychedelic   distorted, intensified sensory perceptions, especially visual hallucinations

retinopathy   noninflammatory pathology of the retina; a complication of diabetes mellitus

serotonergic   nerve fibers that secrete serotonin

superinfections   rapid, uncontrolled growth of infective microbes

synergistic   referring to cooperative action from two or more agents such that the total effect exceeds the sum of the various individual effects

thrombophlebitis   formation of blood clots in veins, brought about by inflammatory changes in the veins

For Further Reading

Aranow, W. S.; Goldsmith, J. R.; Kern, J. C.; et al. 1974. Effect of smoking cigarettes on cardiovascular dynamics. *Arch Environ Health* 28:330.

Begleiter, H., ed. 1980. Biological effects of alcohol. In *Advances in experimental medicine and biology. Vol. 126. New York: Plenum Press.*

Goroni, L. E., and Hayes, J. E. 1978. *Drugs and nursing implications.* 3d ed. New York: Appleton-Century-Crofts.

Gross, M. M., ed. 1977. Alcohol intoxication and withdrawal: Biological aspects of ethanol. In *Advances in experimental medicine and biology.* Vol. 85A. New York: Plenum Press.

Huff, B. B., ed. 1981. *The physicians' desk reference.* 35th ed. Oradell, N.J.: Medical Economics Co.

Israel, Y., and Mardones, J. 1971. *Biological basis of alcoholism.* New York: Wiley-Interscience.

Jones, K. L.; Shainberg, L. W.; and Byer, C. O. 1973. *Drugs and alcohol.* 2d ed. New York: Harper & Row Pubs.

Lieber, C. S. 1976. The metabolism of alcohol. *Sci Am* 23:25.

Long, J. W. 1977. *The essential guide to prescription drugs.* New York: Harper & Row Pubs.

Majchrowicz, E., ed. 1975. Biochemical pharmacology of ethanol. In *Advances in experimental medicine and biology.* Vol. 56. New York: Plenum Press.

Maugh, T. H., II. 1977. Drug-free therapy for diabetics. *The Sciences* 17:16.

Meyler, L., and Herxheimer, A., eds. 1975. *Side effects of drugs.* Vol. 8. New York: Exerpta Medica.

Nahas, G. G., and Paton, W. D. M., eds. 1980. *Satellite symposium on marijuana: Marijuana biological effects: Analysis, metabolism, cellular responses, reproduction and brain.* Elmsford, N.Y.: Pergamon Press.

Niewoehner, D. E.; Kleinerman, J.; and Rice, D. B. 1974. Pathologic changes in the peripheral airways of young cigarette smokers. *N Engl J Med* 291:755.

Ray, O. S. 1978. *Drugs, society, and human behavior.* 2d ed. St. Louis: C. V. Mosby Co.

Romano, C., and Goldstein, A. 1980. Stereospecific nicotine receptors on rat brain membranes. *Science* 210:647.

Schuckit, M. A. 1979. *Drug and alcohol abuse: A clinical guide to diagnosis and treatment.* New York: Plenum Press.

Seiden, L. S., and Dykstra, L. A. 1977. *Psychopharmacology: A biochemical and behavioral approach.* New York: Van Nostrand Reinhold Co.

Soldatos, C. R.; Kales, J. D.; Scharf, M. B.; et al. 1980. Cigarette smoking associated with sleep difficulty. *Science* 207:551.

Tinklenberg, J. R., ed. 1975. *Marijuana and health hazards.* New York: Academic Press.

U. S. Department of Health, Education, and Welfare, PHS. 1975. *The health consequences of smoking.* Washington, D. C.: Government Printing Office.

White, B. C.; Lincoln, C. A.; Pearce, N. W.; et al. 1980. Anxiety and muscle tension as consequences of caffeine withdrawal. *Science* 209:1547.

PART FIVE

STRESS AND DISEASE FROM BIOLOGIC AND CULTURAL STRESSORS

Much physiologic stress and consequent illness is related to our interactions with living organisms, foremost of which are infective microbes and other human beings who make up our cultural society. As biologic entities, we encounter specific forms of stress and disease coincident with particular periods of life.

Stress and Disease from Infection and Immune Response

|| **Objectives:** Upon completing this chapter you should:

1. Understand something of the nature of injury initiated by pathogenic microbes, and be familiar with some of the more significant bacterial, viral, and fungal infections.
2. Know the essential principles involved in immune reactions.
3. Recognize the important relationship of immune response mechanisms to disease processes.
4. Be acquainted with the cause, diagnosis, and therapy of atopic disease.
5. Be informed about slow viral infections and the phenomenon of autoimmunity, and perceive how these conditions relate to specific forms of degenerative pathology.

Despite the availability of antibiotic therapy, infectious disease and associated host reponses continue to be among the most damaging of stressors and producers of desease. This is especially true of viral infections, for which antibiotics are not generally effective. For that matter, bacterial disease itself is still responsible for a surprising amount of morbidity and mortality. Reference to Table 2-5 indicates that pneumonia is the fifth leading cause of death in the United States. Moreover, the number of bacterial venereal infections surpasses yet the incidence of pneumonia. Fortunately venereal disease is not usually fatal.

Of more potential pathologic significance than the mere presence of infective microbes are the variables pertaining to the immune response of the host. Irregularities in immune response to any foreign material (not just living microbes) have much to do with certain forms of disease. Therefore a discussion of immune reactions occupies a considerable part of this chapter.

Not only do infections incite immune responses, but the stress that is associated with the overall disturbance can activate the pituitary-adrenal system, resulting in increased secretions of ACTH and STH (growth hormone). With infections more insulin is required, and the effect of fever on metabolism makes a greater demand on thyroid output.

TOXICITY AND TISSUE DAMAGE FROM INFECTIVE AGENTS

Just how stressing, or how pathogenic, parasitic microbes can be depends upon numerous variables, some of which are: the microbe's ability to invade the system, the microbe's ability to grow and replicate in host tissue, the potential toxigenicity of the parasite, and the general defensibility and immune reaction of the host. Generalizations about these matters cannot be very meaningful without specifying whether the parasite is bacterial, fungal, or viral. Hence each of these infection types is discussed separately.

Bacterial Infections

The mechanisms by which bacteria produce disease are complex and not completely understood. Bacteria generally are extracellular parasites, growing and multiplying in tissue fluid, blood, and lymph. The tissue damage associated with their presence results from a combined effect of their toxins together with the host reaction to the disturbances they produce. The host reaction is characteristically inflammatory in nature, and it is confined primarily to microcirculation and associated perivascular tissues.

The initial derangement of the host biochemistry is attributed largely to the bacterial toxins, which are incidental to the microbes' metabolic activities, and are classified in three groups. Extracellular *exotoxins* are specific proteins which may be potent enzyme inhibitors, whereas *endotoxins* are found within the bacterial cell wall and are usually not released until the bacterium is dead. A third group of bacterial toxins is comprised of a heterogeneous assortment of enzymatic-type secretions such as *hemolysins,* which diffuse freely among host cells. Some of these substances can produce cellular destruction by breaking down cell membranes and organelles.

The majority of exotoxins are derived from gram-positive organisms, while most endotoxins are associated with gram-negative bacilli. As a rule, exotoxins are much more toxic than endotoxins, yet they are more specific and therefore antigenic, which makes them more susceptible to neutralization with antibody.

Inflammation is the basic host response to the altered chemistry induced by pathogenic bacteria. Inflammatory tissue damage is described in Chapter 2. The inflammatory response itself is somewhat nonspecific and can be elicited by stressors other than infective microbes, UV radiation for example. The overall function of the response is to bring plasma proteins and phagocytes to the disturbed area so that any foreign elements can be immobilized, removed, and tissue repair initiated. The primary mediators promoting the vascular changes characterizing inflammation are histamine and the kinins, which in turn may be associated in certain ways with the mobilization of specific types of prostaglandins. Histamine is released from mast cells, basophils, and platelets. It is a potent vasodilator and can affect nonvascular smooth muscle as well. The

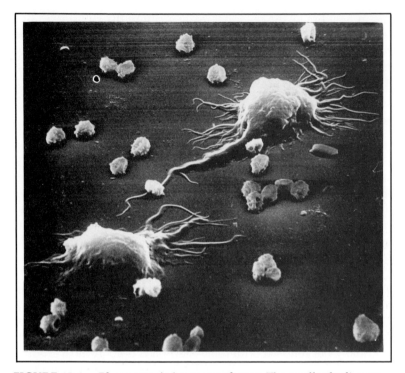

FIGURE 15-1   Phagocytosis by macrophages. The smaller bodies are spores of *Aspergillus*, a commonly inhaled fungus. Two lung macrophages are depicted engulfing the spores. ×4200. (From G. L. Waldbott, *Health effects of environmental pollutants.* (Courtesy Dr. B. Holma and Dr. M. Lundborg, Karolinska Institute of Environmental Health, Stockholm, Sweden.)

kinins are small polypeptides represented primarily by bradykinin. Their vascular effects are similar to those of histamine. In addition, kinins exert marked effects on afferent neuron terminals, which accounts for much of the discomfort and pain associated with inflammation.

Following the initial vasodilation and increased capillary permeability of inflammation, there is a progressive exudation of leucocytes into the disturbed site. Huge numbers of neutrophils appear within 35 minutes. Much later monocytes follow, and once in the tissue they are transformed into macrophages which phagocytize foreign matter (Figure 15-1). Hydrolytic enzymes from macrophagic lysosomes degrade the microbial material.

Inflammatory reactions can be systemic as well as local. Bacterial toxins, particularly exotoxins, may circulate in the bloodstream. Among various bacterial secretions are the exogenous pyrogens, some of which stimulate the release of endogenous pyrogens from neutrophils. As explained in Chapter 7, the pyrogens, through the mediation of certain prostaglandins, elevate body temperature (fever) by resetting the hypothalamic thermostat. Systemic inflammation from bacterial infection is often associated with a generalized leucocytosis.

The transient showering of pathogenic bacteria into the bloodstream is termed *bacteremia.* This effect is usually asymptomatic, although there can be mild sensations of flushing and chills. The microbes are usually cleared by host defense mechanisms. On the other hand, *septicemia* denotes persistent or recurrent bacteremia due to the inability of host defenses to effectively localize the infection. The major sequential steps occurring in a typical localized bacterial infection are elaborated in Figure 15-2.

Bacterial growth locates commonly in the mucous membranes of the sinus cavities, pharynx, middle ear, and in the urinary tract. Infections in these areas are sometimes difficult to eradicate, some of them becoming chronic. The infection usually comprises a mixture of microbes, which may include viruses. The major pathologic forms of bacteria infecting respiratory locations are the gram-positive cocci *(Staphylococcus, Streptococcus,* and *Pneumococcus).* Streptococci are shown in Figure 15-3. Beta-hemolytic Streptococcus is especially virulent. It is the causative agent of septic sore throat, scarlet fever, and erysipelas. Furthermore, it is especially dreaded because immune reactions to it in some individuals result in rheumatic fever with its risk of permanent damage to heart valves and renal glomeruli.

As a result of the widespread use of antibiotics, there has been a changing pattern in the incidence of pathologic microflora. Both streptococci and pneumococci have less clinical importance than they did formerly, but there are resistant staphylococci that remain problematic, and certain gram-negative bacteria such as *Pseudomonas* and *Aerobacter-Klebsiella* have become much more prevalent. A particularly stubborn staphylococcus infection is impetigo (see Color Plate 5). It is a superficial skin infection that is especially contagious among children.

Likewise, there has been a shift in the predominance of organisms producing venereal disease. Almost unheard of only ten years ago, an infection called *nongonococcal urethritis* (NGU) has become our most common venereally transmitted disease. It is estimated that the infection afflicts over 2.5 million Americans in every segment of society. No gonococcus is present in NGU. The causative

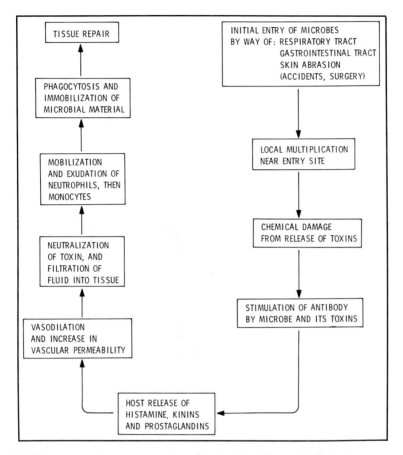

FIGURE 15-2   Course sequence of a localized bacterial infection.
When pathogen multiplication is more prolific than usual and/or antibody
responses become inadequate, the above sequence is altered and
prolonged. A delay in later steps risks spread of the infection to other sites
of the body.

organism in most cases is *Chlamydia,* a ricksettsial-type bacterium
that is sometimes designated erroneously as a large virus. Penicillin
is not effective in treating NGU. Antibiotics of broader spectrum,
such as tetracycline, are required.

Mycotic Infections

In regions where warm, moist seasons occur, there appears to be an
increasing incidence of infections from fungi. One reason for this is
that the administration of antibiotics tends to eliminate bacterial

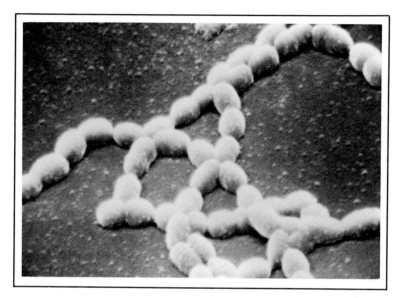

FIGURE 15-3   Electron micrograph of pathogenic Streptococcus mutans. Cells as seen under the scanning electron microscope, ×6000. Note chainlike appearance of the cocci. Strains such as beta-hemolytic strep can be especially virulent. (Courtesy Naval Dental Research Institute, Great Lakes, Ill.)

competitors, thus permitting unrestrained growth of yeastlike and moldlike microorganisms, most of which are not highly pathogenic. The so-called superficial mycoses of the skin and mucous membranes are by far the most common. Skin infections caused by dermatophytes such as *Microsporum* (ringworm) and *Tinea* are not usually serious, although moniliasis of the mucous membranes by *Candida albicans* can assume the proportions of an overwhelming superinfection. Less common but more serious are the deep-seated fungal infections that localize in the viscera. One of the better known examples is histoplasmosis caused by *Histoplasma capsulatum*. The spores of this fungus, which are spread by bird droppings, can be inhaled, leading to a chronic infection of the lungs in susceptible individuals.

Viral Infections

Viruses are submicroscopic, half-crystalline arrays of protein and nucleic acids (DNA or RNA). Outside of living cells they are merely inert chemicals. However, in order to replicate they become *obligate intracellular parasites.* Therefore, unlike bacteria, they are not as openly exposed to host defense mechanisms, and it is difficult to halt their action without harming the host's body cells. In the typical cycle of cellular infection, the virus particles first attach to the cell membrane, then penetrate the cytoplasm and in some instances the nucleus as well. At this point both the viral genome and other viral constituents are replicated, taking over the nutrients and energy provision of the host cell in order to do so. When the maturation of the replicate particles is complete, the new viruses are released from the cell, whence they are carried by the blood and lymph to other cells, or are removed from the body.

Each type of virus has a propensity to invade a specific type of body cell, and the nature of the invaded cell is an important variable in determining the course of the resulting disease. Cytopathic effects of viruses also depend upon many other varying conditions within the host. Foremost among these variables are body disturbances from other stressors. When relatively large amounts of foreign viral material are replicated intracellularly, there is risk of a complete disorganization in cellular metabolism, culminating in cytoplasmic vacuolation. In many instances cell death occurs; in other cases the damage is reversible and repairable. The matter is especially critical for nerve cells in that they have no regenerative capability.

Clinical virology is one of the most challenging areas of modern research. Viral diseases are extraordinary in their diversity. They range from the relatively benign adenovirus infections responsible for the common cold, to *rabies*, one of the deadliest diseases known. Viral infections are not nearly as easy to identify or treat as bacterial infections. Investigative attempts to isolate a virus and grow it in living material, such as fertile hens' eggs, are not always successful. Detecting blood levels of antibodies to known viruses by serologic tests is probably the most practical diagnostic procedure. Unfortunately most viral infections are not controllable with antibiotics. In some acute viral diseases gamma globulin injections are given. Gamma globulin is the blood plasma fraction containing antibodies. If the gamma globulin is from an individual recovering from an illness caused by the same virus, such injections can be especially effective.

Injections of *interferon*, a substance naturally released from viral-infected cells that tends to convey resistance to noninfected cells, has proven to be of some success in combating viral infections in animal experiments. More significantly, the injections appear to offer some protection against tumorigenesis. The interferon molecule itself does not have antiviral activity. Its binding to the plasma membrane of an infected cell stimulates synthesis of antiviral proteins within the cell. Apparently these proteins interfere with synthesis of macromolecules the virus requires for its replication.

Recently, much attention has been given to interferon as an anticancer agent. Previous reports from Europe were encouraging, but more recent studies in this country have been less impressive. There appear to be varying responses among cancer patients being treated with interferon. It is now thought that there may be different forms of interferon.

A few drugs have been effective in trial treatment of such viral infections as herpes, influenza, and hepatitis. However, most of them are not being generally prescribed because of their dangerous side effects. Recently, the National Institute of Allergy and Infectious Disease (NIAID) has recommended that the drug *amantadine hydrochloride* (Symmetrel) be used for both prevention and therapy of all types of influenza A. Clinical trials with amantadine have demonstrated effective antiviral activity.

In many instances all that can be done for viral infections is to support the organism's natural immunity and inclination toward homeostasis with adequate rest, nutrition, and freedom from other stressors, thus allowing the disease to take its course. Much effort is being concentrated to prevent outbreaks of viral disease in the first place by developing vaccines that stimulate natural immunity. A list of some of the more notable virus diseases is provided in Table 15-1.

Most viral infections are acute. They tend to develop rather quickly, reach a climax, then succumb to host defenses (or overwhelm them). However, there are some infections that tend to establish an intermittent or chronic pattern, especially in predisposed hosts. These so-called slow virus infections play such a significant role in a number of chronic, degenerative ailments that the subject is enlarged upon in a subsequent section of the chapter. Indeed, practically every chronic degenerative disease of unknown origin has been linked to a viral cause.

It is beyond the scope of this section to describe the individual stress effects and specific pathology of the many viral infections. However, a few such infections have become progressively problematic in recent years. One is *viral hepatitis,* which occurs in two forms. Infectious hepatitis is spread through personal contact as well as through contamination of food and drink, whereas serum hepatitis is transmitted chiefly through contaminated hypodermic needles. Infectious hepatitis has a shorter incubation period; otherwise the two forms are quite similar in many respects. The initial

TABLE 15-1
Diseases Caused by Viral Infections*

GROUP CHARACTERIZATION	DISEASE
Usually childhood occurrence	Chicken pox
	German measles (Rubella)
	Mumps
	Reye syndrome
Respiratory	Common cold
	Influenza
Systemic	Infectious hepatitis
	Serum hepatitis
	Mononucleosis
Neurologic	Encephalitis
	Meningitis
	Poliomyelitis
	Rabies
	Shingles
Other localized conditions	Herpes infections
	Gastroenteritis

* Exclusive of slow virus involvement.

symptoms of hepatitis are nausea, headache, and fatigue. This is followed by jaundice, gastrointestinal disturbances, and fever. Recovery is slow. The production of key hepatic enzymes such as glutamic oxalacetic transaminase (SGOT) and glutamic pyruvate transaminase (SGPT) may not be normal for many weeks following an infection. Prolonged jaundice may signal permanent liver damage.

Infectious mononucleosis is a debilitating viral disease common among young adults. Headache, chills, fever, and weakness mark the onset, which is shortly followed by a noticeable swelling of the lymph glands. Blood examinations reveal an increased percentage of monocytes and the presence of a heterophil antibody. Epstein-Barr virus is believed to be the causative organism. In over half the cases of mononucleosis, there is enlargement of both the spleen and liver. Liver inflammation is associated with jaundice, and liver damage is a complication that can prove to be serious. Susceptibility to infectious mononucleosis is often stress-related.

Perhaps the most widespread of the more serious viral diseases is *influenza*, which is primarily a respiratory infection that is often accompanied by symptoms of generalized illness and debilitating weakness. Influenza is highly epidemic, with an incubation time as short as 24 to 48 hours. Body temperature may rise quickly to 40 C. In influenza there can be extensive damage to the mucous membrane cells of the nose, throat, and pulmonary passages. The more generalized symptoms, such as headache, muscular aches, and lassitude, are believed to arise from accumulation of large amounts of cellular debris to which the body develops sensitivity reactions. In true influenza, gastrointestinal disturbances are not common. (So-called stomach flu is a gastroenteritis caused by a different form of virus.) The nucleic acids of influenza virus are constantly mutating, which means that the emerging strains are elusive in respect to establishing host immunity. Thus new vaccines are always the order of the day. Individuals most likely to incubate any strain of influenza virus are the aged, the infirm, and those under stresses of various kinds. Bacterial diseases, such as pneumonia, may develop in those already weakened from influenza.

Perhaps the most dreaded disease associated with viral infection is *Reye syndrome*, first reported in 1963. This acute ailment occurs primarily in children, sometimes in a localized epidemic pattern, and is fatal in over 40% of the cases. Since 1977, over 350 deaths have been attributed to this disorder.

Reye syndrome develops in the wake of such viral infections as influenza and chicken pox, and there is some suspicion that giving aspirin during the infection heightens the susceptibility to the syndrome. The disease is characterized by uncontrollable vomiting, delirium, convulsions, and coma. The basic pathologic findings are a fat-filled, damaged liver, and encephalopathy. As the liver becomes affected, it no longer removes impurities from the blood, and the accumulated impurities produce a toxic effect on the brain, causing it to swell. It is the increased pressure within the skull that leads to brain damage or death. Reye syndrome is further discussed in Chapter 18.

IMMUNE RESPONSE

Our immune systems are complex homeostatic devices designed to provide the necessary counteraction to a variety of foreign, noxious materials within our bodies. These devices are sometimes referred to collectively as the *reticuloendothelial system* (RES), which includes tissue in the liver, spleen, lymph nodes, bone marrow, thymus gland, and lungs. Although the RES is reputed to confer resistance to microbial invaders, it has more diverse functions than this. For example, the system is involved in eliminating damaged or worn-out cells. The RES also destroys altered or abnormal cells that may

TABLE 15-2

Four Major Classes of Immunoglobulins

CHARACTERISTIC	CLASS			
	IgG	IgM	IgA	IgE
Molecular weight	150,000	900,000	150,000	200,000
Mean serum concentration (mg/dl)	1,200	150	300	0.025
Complement fixation	+	+	−	−
Effects histamine release	+	+	−	++++
Elevated level in atopic disorder	−	−	−	+

Source: Compiled from various sources.

arise. Even though the immune system is essential for survival, it nevertheless is capable of producing stress, suffering, and disease. When immune mechanisms misfire, overreact, or are deficient, they themselves become disease-producing. For this reason a brief, simplified account of the nature of immune response is helpful as a prelude to subsequent sections of the chapter. Immunology has become an actively investigated subject of far-reaching significance. The understanding of certain chronic diseases and the potential control of cancer rest upon advances in this field.

Immune responses are specific, and they are mediated either by circulating antibodies produced by B lymphocytes, or directly by T lymphocytes. T lymphocytes undergo development in the thymus gland, whence they are released to various lymphoid tissues where they remain under the influence of a thymic hormone. The B cells and their antibodies are usually more effective against bacteria, whereas the T lymphocytes more often respond to viruses, fungi, and foreign tissue. It is the cell-mediated immunity from T cells that suppresses tumor growth and rejects organ transplants. Both antibodies and T lymphocytes respond to specific *antigens*, resulting in *antigen-antibody complexes* and sensitized T cells. There are four or five different kinds of antibodies (Table 15-2). IgG and IgM are the primary antibodies protecting us from infectious microbes, whereas IgE is involved in allergic reactions. Severe deficiencies in antibody production are known as *agammaglobulinemia*. Such conditions are uncommon and usually are due to inherited defects.

Antigen-antibody complexes are capable of activating a nonspecific system of plasma proteins known as *complement*. Activated complement facilitates phagocytosis and triggers the release of mediators associated with inflammation. Both bacterial surfaces and their toxins can be antigenic, leading to the antibody-antigen complexes that activate complement and result in the neutralization of toxins or the immobilization of bacterial cells. The neutralization of virus is effected by preventing viral attachment to the membranes of host cells. The T cells become sensitized to the appropriate antigen whenever it combines with receptor sites on their surfaces. When these lymphocytes encounter the same antigen again, they release a battery of cytotoxic chemicals that immobilizes the antigenic matter along with some of the cells with which this matter is associated.

A major question in immunology asks how the immune system distinguishes between *foreign* antigenic material and its own body proteins. It appears that antigens present during embryonic and early neonatal life are recognized as *self*. Such antigens are thereby protected from immune attack throughout later life. Apparently materials that enter the body or arise from endogenous antigenic alterations after this critical time of development are considered foreign, and therefore provoke immune reactions. However, as we shall see later on, the body does not always maintain the ability to discriminate between self and nonself.

ALLERGIC STRESS: ATOPY

When lymphocytes (B or T) become sensitized from the presence of antigen to the degree that subsequent exposures to the antigen elicit damaging immune reactivity, we say that the individual has become *allergic* or *hypersensitive* to the offending substance. Allergic reactions are often distinguished as immediate or delayed. In the former case the antigen reacts with antibody, either in the circulation or fixed to certain tissues. A release of potent chemical mediators follows within several minutes. On the other hand, delayed hypersensitivity is cell-mediated. In this case the antigen reacts directly with sensitized T lymphocytes in a slower fashion. Maximum intensity may not be reached for over 24 to 36 hours. The clinical allergic response that we commonly associate with the word *allergy* is known as *atopic* allergy. (Autoimmunity, a special form of chronic allergic reaction, is discussed later.)

Atopy

About 15% to 20% of the population has a genetic constitution that endows lymphocytes with an especially phenomenal memory storage for recognizing and reacting to many substances that ordinarily

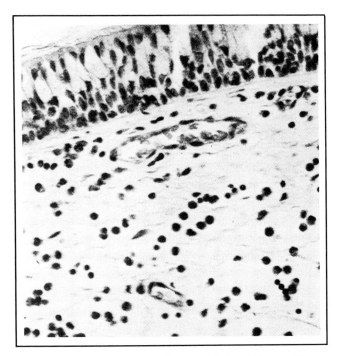

FIGURE 15-4   Nasal mucosa in allergic rhinitis. Edema of the surface epithelium and increased activity of nasal mucin-producing cells. The dark inclusions scattered throughout the submucosa are eosinophils. Their presence here and in nasal secretions is indicative of allergic sensitivity. (From Sheldon, Lovell, and Mathews, *A manual of clinical allergy.*)

are innocuous to most individuals. Such persons easily become sensitized. In atopic individuals pollen grains, mold spores, dusts, animal dander, feathers, microbes, foods, bee venom, and an almost infinite array of chemical substances can become antigenic. Such materials are then capable of unleashing progressively stronger immune reactions with repeated exposures. Most atopic reactions are of the immediate type, and although the antigens typically are proteins, simpler compounds (*haptens*) can become antigenic by coupling with larger molecular weight materials such as proteins or polypeptides. Hence practically any chemical compound is potentially allergenic (see Color Plate 6).

In allergic individuals antigenic material stimulates the synthesis of IgE. This immunoglobulin circulates from plasma cells to mast cells and basophils to which it binds. When an antigen combines with the mast cell-IgE complex, histamine and other vasoactive mediators are released. It is the mediator action that produces the inflammatory stress. Inflammatory damage is often localized due to restricted distribution of antigen. In allergic rhinitis, for example, the symptoms are confined largely to the nose and sinus cavities (Figure 15-4). Other well-known shock organs are bronchial airways, gastrointestinal tract, skin, and nervous system. Indeed, those of us who are predisposed to atopy are well aware that there is no symptom unknown to an allergic sufferer (Table 15-3).

Some allergic reactions become systemic when large amounts of mediators are released and enter the circulation. A consequence of systemic allergy is generalized hypotension, which can lead to various degrees of shock. Severe shock of this nature is known as *anaphylaxis*. Although histamine is the predominant mediator in allergic reactions, bradykinin, serotonin, acetylcholine, and one known as *slow-reacting substance* (SRS) also have been shown to be involved. The release of acetylcholine in allergic reactions is consistent with the idea that there tends to be parasympathetic predominance in hypersensitive states. Such well-known allergic effects as hypotension, bronchoconstriction, hypersecretion, and gastrointestinal motility are alleviated by sympathomimetic and anticholinergic drugs. Apparently histamine and acetylcholine are somewhat synergistic in action.

A classic example of the immediate type of hypersensitive reaction is inflammatory rhinitis, better known as *hay fever*, which is initiated by exposure to seasonal plant pollens. This type of allergy is easy to identify by skin-testing, and it also responds effectively to desensitizing injections. By comparison, sensitivity to molds and dusts is more perennial and less easy to control. It has been shown that the allergenic component of house dust is a microscopic mite (Figure 15-5). Molds and fungi can be ingested as well as inhaled. Several foods and beverages that are likely to contain fungus spores are listed in Table 15-4.

The presence of chronic infections can sensitize the immune system. Antigens from bacteria, viruses, and fungi are common sensitizers in delayed hypersensitivity. Sensitivity to bacteria in the respiratory tract can significantly aggravate bronchial asthma.

An effort to identify offending allergens can be made by injecting an extract of a suspected substance intracutaneously and waiting several minutes to determine if there is localized inflammation from histamine release (Figure 15-6). However, the demonstration of antibody by skin-testing cannot be taken as proof that its corresponding antigen is initiating the suffering. Nor does an elevation in IgE always imply that histamine is being released. Actually experiencing symptoms offers the best evidence of histamine release.

TABLE 15-3

Some Signs or Symptoms of Allergic Stress

Sneezing

Throat-clearing

Nasal congestion

Itching

Burning sensations

Coughing

Hypersecretions (nasal, tear ducts, salivary glands, gastrointestinal)

Bronchoconstriction

Dyspnea

Vertigo

Tinnitus

Edema

Nervousness, irritability

Depression

Palpitations

Fever

Chills

Gastrointestinal spasms

Tremor

Visual disturbance

Insomnia

Eczema

Hives (urticaria)

Mental disorientation

Diarrhea

Constipation

Rheumatic pain and discomfort

Fatigue

Cystitis

Erythema

Nausea

Once an offending allergen has been identified, there are three therapeutic measures. The most effective is avoidance; however, avoidance is frequently not possible. Symptomatic relief can be

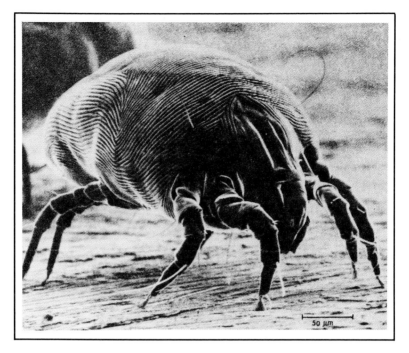

FIGURE 15-5   House dust mite. The microscopic protonymph of *Dermatophagoides farinae* is believed to be the major allergic constituent of house dust. ×300. (From G. W. Wharton, Mites and commercial extracts of house dust. *Science* 167:1382, 1970. Copyright © 1970 by The American Association for the Advancement of Science.)

obtained from the use of antihistamines, sympathomimetics, cortisone, ACTH, and anticholinergics. Some of these treatments, notably use of steroids and ACTH, can be dangerous, especially when used frequently (see Chapter 14). None of them should be taken habitually. A third therapeutic measure is in the form of desensitization, or more correctly *hyposensitization*, whereby minute amounts of the offending antigen are injected periodically. According to theory, a minute amount of antigen given frequently tends to favor responses from IgG (blocking antibody) over IgE. With IgG there is much less release of vasoactive mediators, hence diminished symptoms. However, desensitization does not always help, especially if started later in life.

Research of the past several years has revealed that autonomic nervous regulation and the secretion of certain hormones and other mediators are highly significant variables in determining the output of histamine. For example, an increase of *cyclic adenosine monophosphate* (cAMP) in mast cells inhibits IgE-mediated histamine release,

TABLE 15-4
Foods and Beverages Usually Containing Fungus Spores (Yeasts and Molds)

Mushrooms (mushroom soup)

Cheese (most kinds)

Vinegars

Soy sauce

Mayonnaise

Salad dressing

All fermented beverages (beer, wine, gin, whiskey)

All malted products

Frozen and canned fruit juice

Dried fruits (prunes, raisins, dates)

Pickles

Any baked goods made from enriched flour

Sour cream

Sauerkraut

Milk fortified with vitamins

Catsup

Mince pie

Olives

Tomato sauce

Source: Courtesy of Hollister-Stier Laboratories, N. 3525 Regal Street, Spokane, Wash. 99220.

and of course it is well established that catecholamine action increases synthesis of cAMP by stimulating the activity of the enzyme adenylate cyclase. Xanthines, such as caffeine, also increase cAMP by blocking the phosphodiesterase activity that normally suppresses production of cAMP. In addition, prostaglandin E is an adenylate cyclase stimulator, and therefore a histamine inhibitor. In Chapter 7 reference is made to the fact that asthmatics under stress do not appear to mobilize catecholamines as readily as normal individuals. Could this be the case generally with individuals disposed to allergic problems?

AUTOIMMUNITY AND THE PATHOLOGY OF IMMUNE RESPONSE TO VIRUS

In a preceding section of the chapter it was pointed out that viral infections in some persons are characterized by a slow course, and

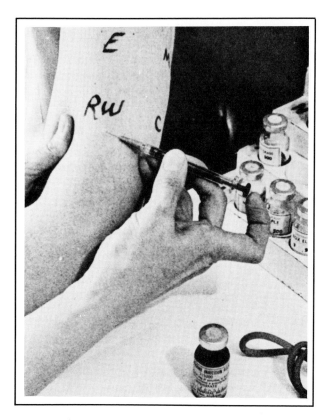

FIGURE 15-6   Skin-testing. A quantity of 0.02 ml of test extract containing a suspected allergen is injected intracutaneously. When an interval of time has elapsed, the site of injection is examined for the presence of allergic inflammation (wheal formation). (From Sheldon, Lovell, and Mathews, *A manual of clinical allergy.*)

that such patterns of chronic infection appear to be related in some way to degenerative tissue damage. In these cases the host fails to adequately clear the virus, and ultimately the immune reaction evolves pathologic changes.

When the viral particles replicate very slowly, the viral nucleic acid may become associated with the host cell's own DNA molecules, replicating along with them and being transmitted to daughter cells in cell division. Such viruses may remain in host cells for many years and alter the host's antigenic properties so that the immune system may no longer recognize these cells as self, thereby risking the development of autoimmune disorders.

The slow virus process is not to be confused with latent infections in which inactive virus persists and can be reactivated to produce acute disease. An example of latent infection is chicken pox virus, which, after the initial outbreak, may remain inactive in the body for many years, only to reappear as the acute, painful inflammation along nerve roots, known as *shingles*. The reactivated virus is called Herpes zoster, and the reactivation appears to be precipitated by stresses such as emotional tension, seasonal weather change, malnutrition, drug intake, or sun exposure. *Herpes simplex*, the virus that produces fever blisters and cold sores, and Epstein-Barr virus which produces mononucleosis, also can be latent and easily reactivated by stress. Apparently stress disturbs the immune equilibrium that is necessary in checking viral replication.

In the true slow virus infections it has been shown that the virus is responsible for the formation of viral antigens on the infected cell's surface. Much of the time viruses are actually within host cells; thus they are relatively protected from host immunity. However, the surface viral antigens can be recognized by sensitized lymphocytes. The host cells possessing such antigens are then subject to attack from these lymphocytes or from mediators released from complement components that the lymphocytes have activated through the formation of antigen-antibody complexes. The immune reactions to infected host cells are displayed in simplified diagrammatic form in Figure 15-7.

Following cell damage from involvement with slow virus, the antigen-antibody complexes are free to circulate in the bloodstream. When they become trapped in the delicate glomerular capillaries of the kidney, they can initiate inflammatory changes that progressively impair glomerular filtration and lead to chronic glomerulonephritis, a form of immune-complex disease. Antigen-antibody complexes resulting from persistent virus activate the components of complement, which then generate the release of mediators and tissue-injuring enzymes that produce chronic inflammatory damage. Most of these pathologic manifestations can be alleviated by steroids and ACTH, potent drugs that typically suppress immune response.

Pathology resulting from immune reactions to microbes is not restricted to viral infections. The bacterial antigens of beta-hemolytic Streptococcus are evidently similar to the protein components of some human cell membranes, since it is known that immune responses stimulated by strep infections can become directed to human tissues (rheumatic fever). Likewise, the lung damage in tuberculosis is caused by the cell-mediated immunity of the host to the bacilli.

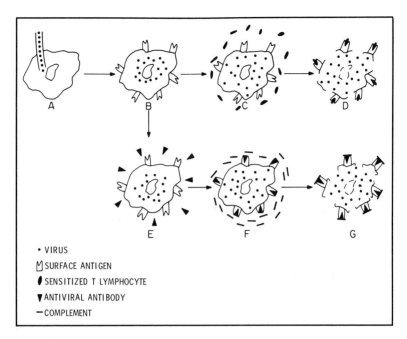

• VIRUS

Ⓜ SURFACE ANTIGEN

❢ SENSITIZED T LYMPHOCYTE

▼ ANTIVIRAL ANTIBODY

− COMPLEMENT

FIGURE 15-7   Immune reaction to slow virus. A. Virus invades a cell, which then establishes viral antigens along B., cell surface, C. These antigens are recognized by sensitized lymphocytes, or attract antibodies, E., which activate complement, F. The reaction of both T lymphocytes and the antibody-complement system results in disorganization of the host cell, D. and G.

Autoimmunity and Autoimmune Diseases

Autoimmunity, or *autoallergy,* is the term used to denote the immunologic reaction of antibody and/or sensitized lymphocytes of an organism with the normal cellular components of that same organism. When such immune reactions are persistent and severe enough to damage tissue, the consequent pathology is termed *autoimmune disease.* It would appear that some of our most incapacitating and debilitating chronic ailments are autoimmune in nature. In many autoimmune diseases it is believed that viruses initiate the process. An important variable in determining susceptibility to autoimmune processes is the particular combination of antigenic markers that appear on the surfaces of the sensitized lymphocytes. Before we examine the details of two or three of the more important diseases in which the body slowly self-destructs through immune action, let us identify and classify those ailments thought to be autoimmune.

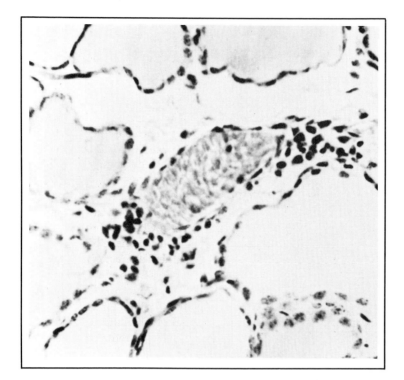

FIGURE 15-8   Experimental autoimmune thyroiditis. In this tissue section of guinea pig thyroid there is an infiltrate of lymphocytes and macrophages around a venule (shown in the very center). Such infiltrations characterize delayed hypersensitivity reactions. (From J. R. Anderson, W. W. Buchanan, and R. B. Goudie, *Autoimmunity—Clinical and experimental,* 1967. Courtesy of Charles C Thomas, Publisher, Springfield, Ill.)

Autoimmune maladies are sometimes distinguished as either organ-specific, or generalized. Examples of autoimmune diseases that are organ-specific include chronic forms of thyroiditis, gastritis (including pernicious anemia), idiopathic Addison disease (adrenal cortex), myasthenia gravis (skeletal muscle), and multiple sclerosis (MS) (central nervous system). Also included in some accounts of autoimmune pathology are ulcerative colitis (colon), the severe juvenile form of diabetes mellitus (pancreas), and certain skin disorders. In all of these diseases the affected tissue may show chronic inflammatory changes with aggregations of infiltrating lymphocytes and plasma cells (Figure 15-8). Autoantibodies can be demonstrated in the serum. However, the mere detection of antibody does not establish a cause and effect relationship to autoimmune pathology. In fact, there may be no close correlation between the autoantibody titer and the severity and rate of progress of the lesions. In some forms of autoimmune pathology, delayed hypersensitivity that is cell-mediated may be more pertinent than autoantibody titers. The generalized autoimmunities are often referred to as the *connective tissue diseases* (collagen diseases) in view of the fact that the disease process usually involves a progressive degradation of collagen in connective tissues throughout the body (see Color Plate 7).

The connective tissue diseases include rheumatoid arthritis, lupus erythematosus (LE), scleroderma, rheumatic fever, ankylosing spondylitis, and polyarteritis nodosa. Systemic lupus erythematosus (SLE) is usually cited as the classic prototype of an autoimmune disease in this group. SLE was mentioned in Chapter 6 in regard to sun exposure. Lupus may be acute or insidious in onset, but it eventually becomes a chronic, relapsing, febrile illness characterized by damage to the skin, kidney, joints, heart, and other sites as well. There is no questioning the fact that the pathology is due to a heightened immune response to self-antigens. Apparently genetic, viral, hormonal, and environmental factors are important contributors. In SLE the autoantibodies are directed at cellular DNA. A reduced suppressor T cell function is suspected.

There appears to be a certain relatedness among all autoimmune diseases in that individuals with thyroiditis, for example, often show autoantibodies specific for other tissues such as the gastric mucosa and the adrenal cortex. The age of onset varies considerably among individuals as well as among the various maladies. However, in general there seems to be a predilection for the second, third, and fourth decades of life. The incidence of autoimmune pathology is significantly higher in women. This is particularly true in respect to lupus, myasthenia, ulcerative colitis, and the rheumatoid ailments. A complete listing and classification of diseases thought to have an autoimmune basis is presented in Table 15-5.

There is reason to believe that autoimmune involvement underlies additional pathologies besides those diseases usually acknowledged as autoimmune. For example, autoantibodies to beta-adrenergic receptors have been demonstrated in some patients with bronchial asthma and allergic rhinitis—conditions believed to be related to an imbalance in autonomic control of airway diameter due to diminished beta-adrenergic sensitivity in bronchial smooth muscle, mucous glands, and mucosal blood vessels. It is speculated that the beta-adrenergic receptors in these patients are dulled by autoantibody action.

TABLE 15-5
Diseases Believed to Have Autoimmune Involvement

CLASSIFICATION	DISEASE	TISSUE OR ORGAN AFFECTED
Organ-specific	Thyroiditis (Hashimoto disease)	Thyroid gland
	Gastritis (pernicious anemia)	Gastric mucosa
	Idiopathic Addison disease	Adrenal cortex
	Myasthenia gravis	Skeletal muscle
	Multiple sclerosis	Central nervous system
	Ulcerative colitis	Mucosa of sigmoid colon
	Juvenile diabetes mellitus	Beta cells of pancreas
	Hemolytic anemia	Red blood cells
Collagen diseases*	Rheumatoid arthritis	Synovia of joints
	Lupus erythematosus	Skin, kidney, other viscera
	Scleroderma	Skin
	Rheumatic fever	Joints, heart, kidney
	Ankylosing spondylitis	Articulations of spine
	Polyarteritis nodosa	Connective tissue of blood vessels

*Even though the pathology may be most noticeable at certain sites, these ailments involve the connective tissues throughout the body.

Rheumatoid Arthritis

There are several forms of arthritis, the most common of which is *osteoarthritis*, a condition that seldom appears in those under 40 years of age. Thus this form of arthritis is largely a degenerative ailment of old age. The degeneration often occurs in joints that are used a great deal and exposed to temperature change; therefore the body site most commonly affected is the hand. Injury, weight-bearing, physical stress from habitual use, and normal wear and tear over long periods of time are among factors contributing to osteoarthritis. Autoimmunity does not appear to be a major factor in this form of joint disease. Two other forms of arthritis, *gout* and *ankylosing spondylitis*, occur much less frequently. Gout is a metabolic disorder, occurring primarily in men, in which excessive uric acid from faulty purine metabolism tends to form urate crystals in the joints. The development of ankylosing spondylitis (arthritis of the spine) is considered to have an autoimmune involvement.

By far the most serious form of arthritis, and one that is increasing in incidence, is rheumatoid arthritis (RA). Over 8 million Americans are chronic sufferers of RA. Though the disease strikes

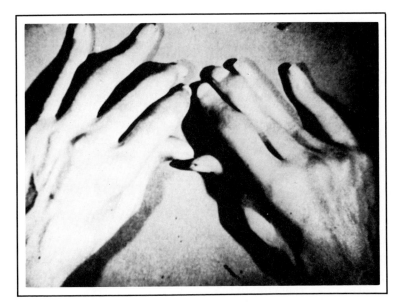

FIGURE 15-9   Rheumatoid hand. A case of rheumatoid arthritis of the joints of both hands. The change shown on the left fourth digit is known as *Boutonniere deformity.* Note the muscle-wasting between thumb and forefinger. (From S. A. Price and L. M. Wilson, *Pathophysiology—Clinical concepts of disease processes.* Copyright © 1978 by McGraw-Hill, Inc. Used with permission of McGraw-Hill Book Company.)

persons of all ages, women between the ages of 18 and 40 are most susceptible (Figure 15-9).

Unlike osteoarthritis, rheumatoid arthritis is relatively modern. The principal hypothesis in explaining the cause of RA is that chronic infection initiates autoimmune reactions. However, attempts to isolate virus or bacteria are not always successful. Some investigators assume that the synovial membrane of the joints is the focus for both the infective process and the immune response. Others believe that immune complexes move into the joints from other parts of the body through the bloodstream, as happens with immune complex glomerulonephritis.

Another theory of RA etiology is that traumatic injury to a joint exposes previously protected tissue protein to the immune system, thereby inviting autoimmune reactions. There does appear to be some autoimmune involvement in rheumatoid arthritis. Histological sections of synovial tissue reveal a progressive accumulation of inflammatory cells and collagen degradation. There is evidence also of activated complement. Some investigators consider the B cell

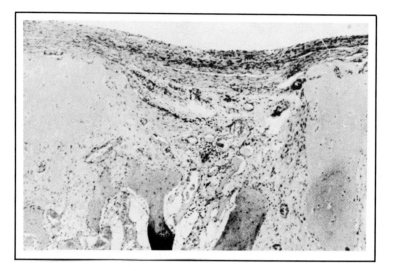

FIGURE 15-10   Cartilage erosion in rheumatoid arthritis. This section is of a knee joint. The clear area at top is the joint cavity. Through the middle of the section, cartilage is being replaced by granulation tissue. (From Anderson, Buchanan, and Goudie, *Autoimmunity—Clinical and experimental*, 1967. Courtesy of Charles C Thomas, Publisher, Springfield, Ill.)

system to play the significant role in the pathogenesis of RA. Evidently some auto-IgG is produced locally in synovial tissues. As the pathology of RA progresses, there is erosion and replacement of articular cartilage by granulation tissue as well as involvement of the underlying bone. The granulation tissue, which grows over the articular cartilage, is referred to as *pannus* (Figure 15-10).

There are specialists who consider juvenile rheumatoid arthritis as a separate form of pathology, and they strongly suspect rubella virus as the etiological agent. Children with the disease show a prolonged IgM response to the virus. There is much stronger evidence for the role of slow virus and autoimmunity in juvenile RA than in the adult form.

Rheumatoid arthritis is not just a disease of the joints. Connective tissue all over the body can be affected. Tissue destruction can become so severe that the patient is incapacitated. Unused muscles surrounding painful and swollen joints waste away, and the patient may eventually be confined to a wheelchair or hospital bed. Steroids, such as cortisone, dramatically relieve the inflammation and pain of rheumatoid arthritis, but when the treatment is withdrawn, the suffering and crippling immediately return. Unfortunately it is dangerous to take cortisone and ACTH on a regular basis (see Chapter 14).

Multiple Sclerosis

One of the most common neurologic diseases in North America and Europe is *multiple sclerosis* (MS). The disorder affects approximately 500,000 people in the United States alone. The basis for the pathology of MS is the deterioration of myelin, the lipid substance that insulates nerve fibers. Diseased myelin is replaced by scar tissue that interrupts and distorts nerve impulses. The result is tremors, loss of coordination, loss of balance, numbness, and paralysis. Sooner or later locomotion is severely restricted, leading to wheelchair confinement. The onset of MS is usually between the ages of 20 and 40, followed by progressive disability for which there is no cure.

Recent discoveries indicate that MS is produced by slow virus that precipitates an autoimmune attack on the myelin of nerve fibers. The viral infection, which in all likelihood is measles (rubella), is acquired sometime during childhood. Much higher titers of antibody to rubella antigen are present in both the serum and cerebrospinal fluid of patients with MS than are ever found in normal controls. Apparently those with MS have an abnormal immune response to measles virus. In some manner there is a defect in cell-mediated immunity that apparently is influenced by the genetic makeup of the individual, a point pursued further in the next subsection. The defect in the cell-mediated response to measles antigen results in a failure to completely eliminate the virus from the host.

Autoimmune conditions in general are characterized by faulty cellular immunity and the production of unusual antibodies. In addition, there often are unusually large quantities of normally occurring antibodies, particularly IgM. All these phenomena could be related to decreased numbers of functional T lymphocytes. There appears to be some correlation of susceptibility to autoimmune disease with susceptibility to certain forms of cancer. Defects in cell-mediated immunity (inherited or acquired) is the suspected common denominator. As such, autoimmunity is looked upon as an immune deficiency.

It is becoming clear that the development of autoimmune disease appears to require an infection (usually viral) coupled with an inherited predisposition to mobilize a relatively incompetent type of cell-mediated response which permits the virus to remain long enough to progressively damage host cells so that previously unex-posed protein then becomes exposed to the host's immune system. This system then fails to recognize the newly exposed protein as self, thereby inciting autoimmune attack. Generalized stress may contribute to autoimmune development. The onset of several of the autoimmune ailments has been known to follow some sort of psy-chologic trauma, or other stressing experience such as illness.

HLA and Disease

One of the most exciting developments in clinical biology is the re-cent discovery that individual differences among surface antigens of our lymphocytes significantly relate to susceptibility to certain dis-eases. Leucocyte antigens are now being typed and classified. The system of classification is referred to as human leucocyte antigens (HLA), and it is far more complex than the classification of the anti-gens of red blood cells. There are two large major groupings of leu-cocyte antigens, the As and the Bs, but the possible combinations in each division run into the millions. As is the case with red blood cells, the determination of leucocyte antigens is gene-controlled. In humans the sixth chromosome carries these genes.

Lately significant statistical associations between certain anti-genic combinations and specific diseases have begun to come to light. The first convincing associations were those described for cel-iac disease and ragweed allergy. By far the most noteworthy associa-tion is of *antigen B27* with ankylosing spondylitis. The correlation is of such a high percentage that the disease can practically be pre-dicted on this basis. Most other disease associations are not nearly so strong, yet many of them are statistically significant. Among other HLA-disease associations are juvenile-onset diabetes mellitus, MS, autoimmune thyroiditis, SLE, and idiopathic Addison disease. (Adult-onset diabetes is not associated with any HLA antigens.) The relative risks of disease development for various HLA antigens are charted in Table 15-6. It is noted that most of the diseases listed in the table are thought to be autoimmune, which implies that virus is probably involved.

In juvenile-onset diabetes there is strong suspicion of the mumps virus, which has a known predilection for glandular cells. It would appear that the combination of virus infection with the ap-propriate type of lymphocytes imposes a risk of beta cell damage from the infection and the immune response to it. In vitro studies have demonstrated that human beta cells can be infected and de-

TABLE 15-6
Risks of Disease Development for Various HLA Antigens

DISEASE	PERTINENT HLA ANTIGEN(S)	RISK RELATIVE TO OTHER CLASSIFICATIONS
Ankylosing spondylitis	B27	87.8 times
Juvenile rheumatoid arthritis	B27	4.7 times
Multiple sclerosis	A3, B7	5.3 times
Myasthenia gravis	B8	4.4 times
Psoriasis vulgaris	B13, B$_w$17	8.8 times
Juvenile diabetes mellitus	B8, B18	3.8 times
Idiopathic Addison disease	B8	3.9 times
Systemic lupus erythematosus	B8	2.0 times

Source: Courtesy of Community Blood Center, Dayton, Ohio.

stroyed by both mumps virus and certain forms of Coxsackie virus. Moreover, Coxsackie B4 virus has been isolated from the damaged beta cells of children who have died following the comatose complication of juvenile-onset diabetes.

Recently it was demonstrated that injections of rabbit antiserum to rat lymphocytes reversed hyperglycemia in spontaneously diabetic rats and prevented diabetes in susceptible nondiabetic controls. Such data strengthen the hypothesis that cell-mediated autoimmunity plays a role in the pathogenesis of juvenile, insulin-dependent diabetes mellitus.

GENERALIZED STRESS AND ALTERED IMMUNITY

Much of this chapter deals with how immune reactions can be stressful to the body. Other stressors as well can significantly affect immune responses. It was pointed out in Chapter 4 that glucocorticoids and ACTH suppress action of the immune system, and the adverse effect of noise exposure on immune competence was cited in Chapter 8. Active investigation today concerns the mechanisms by which the autonomic nervous system can alter normal patterns of immunity.

It is acknowledged from both animal experiments and clinical studies that generalized stress can distort immune reactivity by such means as interfering with the production and maturation of B and T lymphocytes, suppressing the synthesis of immunoglobin, restricting macrophage transformations, and reducing interferon production. It seems that T lymphocyte activity is more readily inhibited in this way than the B lymphocyte system. By generalized stress we mean stresses that are mediated primarily through the hypothalamic-pituitary-adrenal axis, resulting in elevated levels of cortisol; in other words, the Selye form of stress. Although exposure to many stressors stimulates the secretions of ACTH and cortisol, the major ones in this regard are temperature change, noise, fatigue, physical restraint, emotional tension, and some forms of injury or illness.

Recall once more that the stress Selye imposed upon his rats resulted in shrinkage of the thymus gland and the lymph nodes. Since that time innumerable reports have substantiated that susceptibility to infections, particularly viruses, is substantially heightened in stressed animals. The stressors most commonly employed are of a psychosocial nature. For example, when mice are exposed to the presence of predators, they exhibit a depression in acquired immunity to the parasite *Hymenolepis nana* (a tapeworm), and their circulating plasma reveals higher than usual concentrations of corticosterone. Daily exposure of mice to such stressors as avoidance-learning and confinement has produced increased susceptibility to viruses among which are Herpes simplex, polio, Coxsackie B, and polyoma. The degree of immunosuppression was highly correlated with increases in plasma corticosterone, which was two to ten times higher than normal. Continuation of the regime over many weeks resulted in a slow involution of thymus and spleen associated with adrenal hypertrophy and pronounced lymphocytopenia. Interestingly, vitamin A tends to show a protective effect against thymic involution.

Is the elevated adrenal output always responsible for the suppressed immunity, or is the nervous system more directly instrumental in some way? Lesions in certain regions of the hypothalamus (ventromedial nuclei) can result in protection against anaphylaxis, an overpowering immune reaction. However, the mechanism involved is not understood, although a restricted release of histamine has been suspected. Other studies have shown that the central nervous system itself can modify effects from histamine. Whether cortisol-mediated or otherwise, generalized forms of stress must be considered as significant factors in our susceptibility to infections, autoimmunity, and cancer.

SUMMARY

Stress and disease from bacterial infections are produced by their toxins together with host reactions to the disturbance.

Gram-positive cocci are responsible for most clinically significant infections of the respiratory tract, beta-hemolytic Streptococcus being especially dangerous because of the heart and kidney damage that can result from the body's immune reaction to it.

Viruses are obligatory intracellular parasites whose replication is difficult to control without harming host cells.

In pathologic significance virus diseases range from the common cold to fatal diseases like rabies and Reye syndrome. Viral hepatitis and mononucleosis are noteworthy because of risks of permanent liver damage and because of their increasing incidence.

A predisposition for lymphocytes to become easily sensitized to many substances that are innocuous to most individuals is recognized as atopic allergy. In the immediate allergic reaction, the antigen reacts with antibody (IgE), and histamine release shortly follows. In delayed hypersensitivity the reaction is much slower and is cell-mediated by T lymphocytes.

In some viral infections the immunity of a particular host fails to clear the virus, leading to subdued, chronic infection (slow virus) that persistently stirs immune reactivity that assumes an autoimmune nature. Viral antigens on the surface of infected cells progressively sensitize lymphocytes, and the resulting antigen-antibody complexes mobilize a continuous autoimmune attack on chronically infected cells.

Rheumatoid arthritis (RA), multiple sclerosis (MS), lupus erythematosus (LE), myasthenia gravis, idiopathic Addison disease, and forms of thyroiditis, glomerulonephritis, gastritis, and juvenile diabetes are among ailments suspected of having an autoimmune basis.

In addition to a viral stimulus, autoimmune diseases seem to require a certain combination of inherited surface antigens (HLA) on the host lymphocytes. There is a remarkable association of specific antigen classifications with risks of developing certain diseases.

Chapter Glossary

anaphylaxis   a hypotensive shock reaction produced by sensitization to foreign protein

antigen-antibody complex the combination of immunoglobulin with cell-bound antigen

articular pertaining to a joint

celiac pertaining to abdominal viscera

Coxsackie name given to a heterogeneous group of enteroviruses

gastroenteritis inflammation of the gastrointestinal tract

gram-negative refers to bacteria that do not retain a blue stain

gram-positive refers to bacteria that retain a blue stain

hapten simple nonantigenic substance that acts as an antigenic determinant by coupling with a large molecule

idiopathic disease of unknown, self-originated cause

involution the shrinkage and functional decline of an organ or tissue

mast cells connective tissue cells that release histamine

polyoma a virus producing tumors in mice and hamsters

sympathomimetic produces effects of sympathetic nerve impulses

thyroiditis inflammation of thyroid tissue

For Further Reading

Anderson, J. R.; Buchanan, W. W.; and Goudie, R. B. 1967. *Autoimmunity— clinical and experimental.* Springfield, Ill.: Charles C Thomas Pub.

Barrett, J. T. 1978. *Textbook of immunology.* 3d ed. St. Louis: C. V. Mosby Co.

Beers, R. F., Jr., and Basset, E. G., ed. 1976. *The role of immunological factors in infectious, allergic, and autoimmune processes.* Miles International Symposium Series No. 8. New York: Raven Press.

Braun, W. E. 1979. *HLA and disease: A comprehensive review.* Boca Raton, Fla.: CRC Press, Inc.

Burke, D. C. 1977. The status of interferon. *Sci Am* 236:42.

Finland, M.; Marget, W.; and Bartmann, K., eds. 1971. *Bacterial infections.* Bayer Symposium III. New York: Springer-Verlag.

Gordon, B. L., II. 1974. *Essentials of immunology.* 2d ed. Philadelphia: F. A. Davis Co.

Holborow, E. J., and Reeves, W. G., eds. 1977. *Immunology in medicine.* New York: Academic Press.

Holland, J. J. 1974. Slow, inapparent and recurrent viruses. *Sci Am* 230:32.

Like, A. A.; Rossini, A. A.; Guberski, D. L; et al. and Appel, M. C. 1979. Spontaneous diabetes mellitus: reversal and prevention in the BB/W rat with antiserum to rat lymphocytes. *Science* 206:1421.

Litwin, S. D.; Christian, C. L.; and Siskind, G. W., eds. 1976. *Clinical evaluation of immune function in man.* New York: Grune & Stratton.

Locke, D. 1978. *Virus diseases.* New York: Crown Publishers.

Maugh, T. H., II. 1977. Multiple sclerosis: genetic link, virus suspected. *Science* 195:667.

Middleton, E., ed. 1978. *Allergy: Principles and practice.* Vols. 1 and 2. St. Louis: C. V. Mosby Co.

Mudd, S., ed. 1970. *Infectious agents and host reactions.* Philadelphia: W. B. Saunders Co.

Notkins, A. L., and Koprowski, H. 1973. How the immune response to a virus can cause disease. *Sci Am,* 228:22.

———. 1974. Viral infections: Mechanisms of immunologic defense and injury. *Hosp Practice,* 9:65–75.

Panayi, G. S. 1977. *Rheumatoid arthritis and related conditions.* Annual Research Reviews. Montreal: Eden Press, Inc.

Sheldon, J. M.; Lovell, R. G.; and Mathews, K. P. 1967. *A manual of clinical allergy.* 2d ed. Philadelphia: W. B. Saunders Co.

Snyderman, R.; Pearlman, O. S.; and Patriarca, G. 1972. *Mediators of the allergic state: Recent investigations I.* New York: Mss Information Corp.

Stein, M.; Schiavi, R. C.; and Camerino, M. 1976. Influence of brain and behavior on the immune system. *Science* 191: 435.

Stewart, W. E., ed. 1977. *Interferons and their actions.* Boca Raton, Fla.: CRC Press.

Svejgaard, A.; Hauge, M.; Jersild, C.; et al., eds. 1979. *The HLA system. An introductory survey.* 2d ed. New York: S. Karger.

Vander, A. J. 1976. In Introduction to *Human physiology and the environment in health and disease.* San Francisco: W. H. Freeman and Co. Part 5, articles 20, 21, 22.

Vander, A. J.; Sherman, J. H.; and Luciano, D. S. 1980. *Human physiology: The mechanisms of body function.* 3d ed. New York: McGraw-Hill Book Co. Chapt. 17.

Venter, J. C.; Fraser, C. M.; and Harrison, L. C. 1980. Autoantibodies to beta-adrenergic receptors: A possible cause of adrenergic hyporesponsiveness in allergic rhinitis and asthma. *Science* 207:1361.

Zeman, W.; Lennette, E. H.; and Brunson, J. G., eds. 1974. *Slow virus diseases.* Baltimore: Williams and Wilkins Co.

Psychosocial Stress and Functional Nervous Disorder

|| **Objectives:** Upon completing this chapter you should:

1. Perceive the importance of the modern environment in creating unrelenting emotional tensions.
2. Be acquainted with the neural basis of emotional stress reactions.
3. Understand the development of emotional insecurity and how it becomes conditioned.
4. Recognize the role of positive reinforcement in reducing stress.
5. Be informed about biofeedback and muscle relaxation as means of combating stress.
6. Have an insight into the nature of functional nervous disorders.

To most people the word *stress* implies psychologic tension; but to the physiologist a psychologic stimulus is just another stressor, albeit a very significant one. Human consciousness, an expression of the 9 billion neurons of the cerebral cortex, is constantly being bombarded by social stimuli, and all personal interactions promote unique conditioned neural patterns that inevitably have some emotional or motivational aspect. Meaningful stimuli direct impulses from the cerebral cortex through the limbic system to the hypothalamus, from which the autonomic and hormonal systems mediate the physiologic manifestations of emotion. In turn, body changes promoted by ANS impulses and hormonal actions return impulses to the hypothalamus, which then relays discharges through the reticular activating system to the cerebral cortex, thereby maintaining a powerful positive reinforcement.

We are mental beings, and it is probably true that much of the physiologic stress residing in the bodies of many of us is mentally provoked. More than any other organism, we can perceive and anticipate other stressors. Thus, when we enter an environment *knowing* that it is excessively noisy, hot, crowded, and polluted, our dread entails an added stress that is perhaps even more stressing than that provoked by the other stressors. Therefore it must be acknowledged that there is always a significant psychologic stress component associated with many physical and chemical stresses. It is difficult to determine how much of the resulting chemical imbalance in the body can be attributed purely to physical stress alone as opposed to that prompted by mental arousal.

Because we are knowing animals, we spend much of our time in mental unrest. Indeed, psychologic stress is sometimes defined as the *perception* of impending threat to physical or psychologic well-being along with *sensing* that the individual's responses are inadequate to cope with it.

The role played by the mind in stressing the body and promoting disease has undergone a history of varied interpretations. During World War II, psychosomatic medicine came of age and began to flourish, only to be subdued later by the avalanche of discoveries in genetics and molecular biology, which drew attention away from the concept that disease may have much to do with adaptive failure of the whole organism. More recently, however, there has been a return of attention to the health significance of psychologic tensions emanating from inability to cope with modern-day demands. As R. S. Lazarus has stated: "It has become increasingly apparent that [mental] stress is important as a factor in illness in general and in chronic illness in particular. Most present day illnesses cannot be explained in terms of a single cause. Research suggests that a significant portion of the population seeking medical care is suffering from a stress-based illness."[1]

It would appear that many of us do face difficulty in adapting to the rapid pace of the nuclear-jet age. Nervous tension is unavoidable, and negative emotions are easily aroused. Establishing emotional security was a simpler matter in yesterday's world. Today, proper medical care must recognize the emotional requirements of each patient.

The subject of psychologic stress is more often the domain of the psychologist rather than the physiologist. Of the major schools of thought in clinical psychology, *behaviorism* appears to have taken a commanding lead.[2] Freudian psychoanalytic theory, by comparison, seems to be diminishing in importance. Even though Freudianism and gestalt theory may claim a certain degree of validity, their principles are not easily testable and they do not lend themselves to the observation and measurement of real stimulus-response relationships. It may be true that followers of the behavioristic school tend to oversimplify the complexities and powers of the mind; yet behaviorism is the most objective approach to a field that is far from an exact science. Perhaps the most penetrating, scientific approach to mental phenomena and behavior rests with the biochemists. It is their efforts that are beginning to provide intriguing insight into the workings of the mind and emotions.

1R. S. Lazarus, "Proceedings of the National Heart and Lung Institute Working Conference on Health Behavior," DHEW (NIH, 77-868), Washington, D.C., 1977.

2An approach to psychology based upon the study of overt responses to specific psychologic stimuli. Such responses may be variously conditioned and reinforced. This approach is opposed to introspective, less objective methodology.

Psychosocial stressors are stimuli originating from interpersonal interactions and social arrangements whose initial effects are mediated through the senses and the higher neural processes. This input to the brain is evaluated in reference to past feelings and then is selectively relayed through the hypothalamus to the autonomic nervous system, pituitary, adrenal glands, and skeletal muscles. Therefore the background material of Chapter 4 is especially pertinent to discussions here and in the following chapter. Also, it must remain clear that the physiologic stress produced by psychosocial stimuli is essentially chemical in nature: body chemistry is altered. These chemical effects are explored at greater length in Chapter 17.

Psychosocial stress is considered to be a widespread problem in today's society as attested by the incidence of suicide, mental illness, crime, divorce, depression, smoking, and consumption of alcohol and drugs. Psychosocial stress tends to occur in the form of debilitating emotions, particularly negative ones. Legacies of past hurts, neglected childhood needs, parental overindulgence, and overcoercion often set the stage for later stress because an individual is not prepared realistically for life.

METHODS OF ASSESSING PSYCHOSOCIAL STRESS

Attempts to investigate emotional stress objectively have been beset with numerous problems. One of these lies in identifying and measuring the particular body reactions that are being produced by psychic stimulation. Even more difficult is the correct identification and measurement of the psychosocial stimuli themselves. We cannot weigh guilt or calculate an effective dose of fear. For that matter, we cannot be sure whether a certain reaction in the body is due to a psychologic stimulus or perhaps to some other physical or chemical stressor. Furthermore, when human subjects are exposed experimentally to specific psychologic stressors, how can we be sure that some of the controls are not being psychologically stressed by some other mental factor peculiar to them but unknown to the investigator? Still another problem in assessing the effects of psychologic stimuli is that psychologic reactions are uniquely individual. They are readily modifiable in subtle ways by numerous variables and therefore are not easy to predict. Each mind has been programmed differently.

Distress that may appear to be psychologic in origin is often due to changes in the body chemistry. In such cases some internal

TABLE 16-1
Frequently Employed Measurements of Response to Psychosocial Stimuli

TYPE OF ASSESSMENT	PARAMETER MEASURED
Autonomic activity	Heart rate
	Systolic blood pressure
	Galvanic skin resistance
	Saliva volume
Level of hormones (blood or urine)	Total catecholamines
	Epinephrine
	Norepinephrine
	Vanillylmandelic acid (urine)
	17-hydroxycorticosteroids
	Cortisol
	ACTH
Brain activity	EEGs (surface and depth)
	MHPG (urine)

chemical stress is responsible for the mental condition rather than the other way around. Fluctuations in blood glucose can appreciably affect brain metabolism, particularly when the glucose swings to low levels. The release of chemical mediators in allergic sensitivity is known to be capable of producing considerable irritability and depression. Indeed, allergy to foods and other ingested chemicals is purported to elicit transient episodes of mental illness in some persons. Likewise, hormonal imbalances, both temporary and extended, can promote emotional disturbance. It is well known that hypothyroidism can be associated with depressive reactions, whereas shifts in blood levels of ovarian hormones are capable of inciting agitation and nervous tension.

Despite all these difficulties, a substantial battery of physiologic and biochemical measurements has emerged and are employed in efforts to assess the body's reaction to psychosocial stressors. Such methods apply exclusively to the objective aspects of emotion that are typically physiologic and are mediated primarily by the autonomic nervous system (ANS) and the endocrine system.

The major means of assessing responses to psychosocial stressors are listed in Table 16-1. Several of these such as heart rate, systolic blood pressure, saliva volume, and galvanic skin resistance (GSR) are designed to reflect sympathoadrenomedullary activity. A higher electrical resistance (impedance) at the skin surface indicates less apocrine gland output, hence more sympathetic activity (Figure 16-1). Determinations of plasma glucose, free fatty acids, and cholesterol are tests that indirectly reveal changes in both sympathetic and

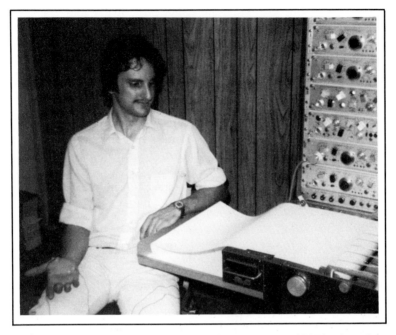

FIGURE 16-1   Monitoring galvanic skin resistance (GSR). The subject has electrodes attached to the palm of the hand that are sensitive to electrical resistance along the skin surface there. Leads from the electrodes carry current to the amplifying console (upper right), which regulates the deflection of a pen writing on moving chart paper. (Courtesy Dr. S. D. Nau, Psychology Department, University of Dayton, Dayton, Ohio.)

glucocorticoid activity, whereas increased sedimentation rates of red blood cells and decreased white blood cell counts (leucopenia) suggest immune alterations that involve only the ACTH-glucocorticoid system.

More direct evaluations of psychosocial stress include measurements of the stress hormones themselves. There actually are no set norms for these hormones. All of us experience fluctuations in their levels. However, significant increases or decreases can be determined. Measurement of urinary catecholamines or their metabolite, *vanillylmandelic acid* (VMA), has been employed for some time in research on psychologic stress. Furthermore, individual levels of epinephrine and norepinephrine can be determined from blood as well as urine. The measurement of *17-hydroxycorticosteroids* (17-OHCS) from urine samples has also become a well-established practice in assessing response to stress. These steroids include cortisol, cortisone, and most of their metabolites. In addition, adrenocorticotropin (ACTH) and cortisol can be individually identified and measured from both blood and urine.

Quite recently methods for detecting mental stress have been developed that are directed at the brain itself. Surface electroencephalogram (EEG) power spectrum analyses, and depth electrode EEG recordings are now being utilized. Direct measurements of brain neurotransmitter metabolism that can detect regional differences in brain neurophysiology are new improvements in the methodology for investigating biochemical responses to psychologic stressors. For example, it has been shown that the measurement of 3-methoxy-4-hydroxyphenylglycol (MHPG) from urine samples provides a valid index of norepinephrine metabolism in the brain.

MODERN PSYCHOSOCIAL ENVIRONMENT

The body's physiologic mechanisms for reacting to emotional stimuli were slowly developed eons ago during a time when psychosocial environments were vastly different from those of today's advanced civilizations. Such mechanisms are marvelously adapted for the overt activities of fight or flight, as postulated by W. B. Cannon. However, because of social or behavioral restraints, we no longer resolve anger or fright in this manner. The contemporary human organism frequently mobilizes physiologic preparedness for what once was life-saving exertion only to do little or nothing in the way of muscular activity. Thus there is much physiologic preparation for action that is never realized. Since these physiologic preparations are not well suited for doing nothing, they may deter homeostasis rather than help to restore it.

When responses that remain primarily psychologic in nature replace muscular action, then physiologic mobilization remains largely unresolved and thereby becomes maladaptive. Frequent occurrences may even become damaging. The functional disengagement of the musculoskeletal system from other target organs sustains emotional tension by maintaining a prolonged state of hormonal readiness. This point may help us appreciate why vigorous exercise helps to rid the body of tension. Persistent emotional tension can stress such systems as those responsible for cardiovascular and immune regulations.

The advent of industrialization and the mass migrations from country to city have been major factors in altering both the quality and quantity of psychosocial stimuli. These developments introduce

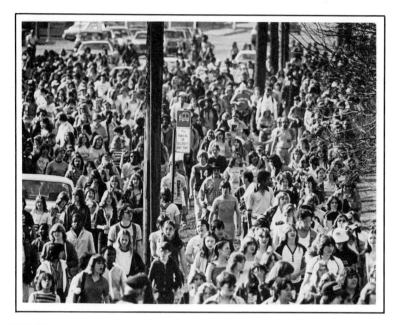

FIGURE 16-2   Urban crowds. City people today spend much of their time and carry out many of their activities in crowded conditions. This is especially true of young people. In December 1979, 11 people died (trampled and suffocated) in a huge throng attempting to enter a coliseum to see a rock concert in Cincinnati, Ohio.

a whole new class of stimuli to which the human organism must adapt. Today's world is much more hurried and competitive. Changes occur with extreme rapidity, and the social order has become more emotionally and intellectually demanding. The mere increase in numbers of individuals underlies much of the problem. The primitive sense of territoriality and the need for privacy are severely thwarted by the intense crowding that characterizes the modern urban environment. Indeed, there are psychologists who feel that much of today's psychosocial stress is simply a consequence of the perpetual frustration attending attempts to function in situations in which other human beings are constantly in the way or are carrying out opposing actions (Figure 16-2).

It has been said that cities are stimulating. For some of us they are probably too much so: the urban environment can overload the nervous system with excessive stimuli. Crowding, noise, and compulsiveness in competing socially and professionally may provoke a habitual mental state of urgency and rush. For many people this demands too much psychologic energy, and they find it increasingly difficult to cope with the multiple and often conflicting stimuli. It has been observed that some inner-city dwellers expend more psychic energy in attempting to avoid stress than they do in their efforts to cope with it. The result is a withdrawal from normal social behavior. Drugs may be implicated in this turning off process.

There are several environmental situations that typically provide us with most of our psychosocial stress. These include jobs, homes (families), recreation and entertainment, illnesses and need for clinical services, and the ever-present threats of crime in the streets and nuclear war.

Occupational Stress

There was a time when the principal factor of concern in occupational stress was work overload. This is not so much the case anymore. It is true that some professionals and executives drive themselves excessively, and there are those who overdo in striving for advancement. However, many employees these days do less work on the job than did previous generations. Hours are shorter and rest breaks longer and more frequent. Therefore, occupationally related stress today is more likely to derive from other matters such as concern with pay scales and promotion, or the fear of losing employment.

Labor union squabbles and interpersonal frictions with superiors and peers are other well-known sources of occupational tension. Various reports indicate, however, that today's principal occupational stressor is simply boredom with routine. It is estimated that over one-third of us are not particularly interested or happy in our work.

Tension in the Home

Within the past 25 years more psychologic turmoil has been generated by changes in home and family life than has been witnessed in occupational situations. Family stability has noticeably diminished. Establishing a high living standard and the desire for material things have become the major priority. Managing a home with small children in addition to employment outside the home provides a significant stress for some of the mothers attempting it. On the other hand, the limited role of housewife has come to be looked upon as menial, boring, depressing, and financially nonproductive by many women. The entire matter inevitably creates conflict. Many young adults are attempting to sidestep domestic strife by avoiding marriage altogether. Despite their achieved freedom, tensions and guilt do not necessarily vanish. Neither does boredom or disillusionment.

Most of the stimuli that signal the initial sensing of insecurity or security originate during our early years in the midst of the family constellation. The conditioning that transpires there determines how we later respond and to which stimuli.

Illness and the Clinical Environment

Perhaps the greatest source of anxiety and depression in many persons is illness, at least in severe and/or chronic cases. This is especially true when the patient must leave the familiar surroundings of home and enter the hospital or nursing home. Many persons have a morbid dread of the clinical environment, even a physician's office. The sights and smells in such places often have become conditioned stimuli that are aversive; and the anticipation of what is going to be done to them and the feeling of loss of personal control over their fate promote much anxiety in most patients. Both the dread of physical suffering and the resignation to it amount to a substantial load of mental stress in anyone. Awareness of such realities often escapes the minds of those who are well, yet health care personnel have come to realize that anticipating and administering to the emotional needs of clinical patients warrants a high priority for improving their overall health and well-being. Indeed, in many illnesses there is a strong emotional component in the etiology. This is especially valid in conditions such as alcoholism and drug abuse.

Not only is the ill, confined patient subjected to much mental stress, but persons around him or her likewise may be anxious or overworked in their efforts to care for such patients. Unusual psychologic and physical demands are frequently made upon close relatives, nurses, and other attendants. In some instances attempting to cope with the emotional and physical needs of patients may be more taxing than the patients' own efforts to cope with their illnesses. This is especially true in cases in which patients have become passively resigned in regard to their clinical condition. When such resignation occurs, the patient may not appear to be under mental stress; nevertheless, a mental attitude of hopelessness is a very damaging emotion that makes the prognosis of the illness much less favorable.

National and International Tensions

As this book goes to press, we are forced to focus much concern on escalating international tensions, threats, and military preparedness.

The anticipation of nuclear holocaust is ever present. In addition, there are inflation/recession spirals, energy shortages, and significant increases in violent crime. That such conditions as these pose an unrelenting source of anxiety and fear for all of us goes without saying.

NEURAL BASIS OF EMOTION

We equate psychologic stress with emotional activation, and all of us have experienced feelings of fear, anger, happiness, and sadness. Such feelings in turn can prompt characteristic forms of behavior, though overt expression does not necessarily have to follow. In association with these feelings our bodies show characteristic changes in certain functions. There may be heart palpitations, trembling limbs, flushing skin, changes in breathing, goose bumps, changes in blood pressure, and spasms of gastrointestinal smooth muscle. Moreover, we are sensitively aware of these bodily sensations. The word *emotion* is used to encompass all of the above manifestations, which are mediated by a complex interplay of neural pathways, some of which cannot be identified in detail. Even though we commonly conceive of emotion as something distinct and transient, it is really always present to a greater or lesser degree. All perception and awareness has an emotional component that colors our impressions. Our knowing is inevitably associated in some way with such mood overtones as satisfaction, pleasure, apprehension, resentment, surprise, or disappointment.

In Chapter 4 it is emphasized that the hypothalamus is intimately involved in the regulation of the bodily changes associated with emotion. Many of these effects are directly attributable to the actions of the ANS and the pituitary-adrenal system. In addition, there are descending pathways through the brain stem and cord that induce widespread tension of the skeletal muscles. How does a psychosocial stressor activate the hypothalamus? What are the sources of the afferent input? What is the relationship between subjective emotional feelings and the objective physiologic changes in the body that are measurable?

The current physiologic view of emotion holds that its principal centers of integration reside in various portions of the limbic system of the brain (Figure 16-3). It is here that experiences filed away in various cerebral centers are selectively appraised in terms of feeling whenever stimuli arouse the system. It is believed that the perception of external events mediated by the cerebral cortex is re-

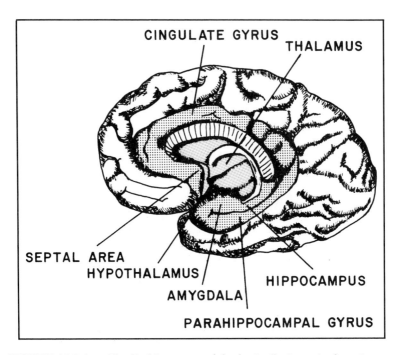

FIGURE 16-3 A.   The limbic system of the brain. Brain sagittal section depicting the structures collectively termed the limbic system (shaded areas).

ferred first to the reticular activating system (RAS) (Figure 14-5), which stimulates various degrees of arousal of the entire brain, but particularly the limbic circuits. These exercise a reference to previous sensory impressions through their connections from sensory nuclei in the thalamus to various cortical association areas. Recall of former sense impressions requires a circuit that can switch into the appropriate neural area whenever afferent input is appraised as worth investigating.

Subjective emotional feeling is initiated when ascending thalamic input reaches the cerebral cortex. However, at the same time that upward discharges from limbic components begin to activate cortical areas, other portions of the limbic circuitry are discharging descending impulses to selective hypothalamic nuclei, which then initiate the characteristic physiologic effects of emotion in the body (Figure 16-4). These peripheral effects throughout the body rapidly spark relays back to various portions of the limbic system where they are interpreted as sensations and whence they further excite both the cerebral cortex and the hypothalamus, thus intensifying

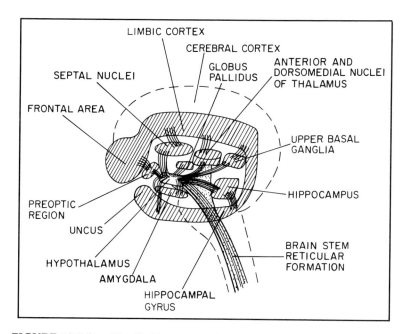

LIMBIC CORTEX

CEREBRAL CORTEX

GLOBUS PALLIDUS

ANTERIOR AND DORSOMEDIAL NUCLEI OF THALAMUS

SEPTAL NUCLEI

FRONTAL AREA

UPPER BASAL GANGLIA

HIPPOCAMPUS

PREOPTIC REGION

UNCUS

BRAIN STEM RETICULAR FORMATION

HYPOTHALAMUS

AMYGDALA

HIPPOCAMPAL GYRUS

FIGURE 16-3 B. The limbic system of the brain. Diagrammatic concept of the limbic system isolated and shown in greater detail, with the major neural pathways (fiber bundles) connecting the various individual structures. Note the convergence of bundles on the hypothalamus.

and prolonging both the subjective feelings and the body sensations. Enhancing the excitation of the body pathways enhances the excitation of cerebral centers and vice versa. Thus, emotional arousal tends to gain momentum in typical positive feedback fashion, as described in Chapter 3. Eventual fatigue or relaxation of skeletal muscle helps to break the cycle, hence the value of muscular exertion in subduing emotional states. A simplified model of these neural interactions is diagrammed in Figure 16-5.

Perhaps a hypothetical example of a pronounced type of emotional arousal can lend some reality to the model. Suppose that an individual has developed a strong fear reaction (phobia) to speaking before a large audience (stage fright). Such a situation is an excellent example of marked psychologic conflict, because the individual consciously wishes to perform and do well, yet continues to be tormented by strange nervous reactions when attempting to do so. In a true phobia the individual is often willing to do almost anything to avoid the stressing situation, ranging from making up all kinds of excuses to simply not making an appearance. For our purposes here

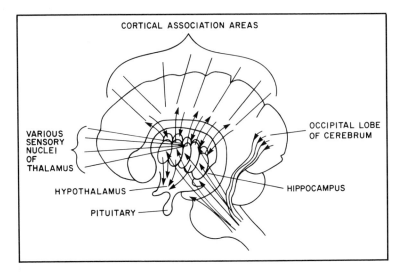

FIGURE 16-4   Functional interactions believed to occur among thalamic centers, the cerebral cortex, and the hypothalamus. Thalamic sensory nuclei serve as a selective clearinghouse in determining which mental stimuli are emotionally meaningful. Mental arousal may be initiated by visual impressions mediated by the occipital cerebrum, thereby stimulating RAS pathways that ascend from the brain stem into the thalamus and other limbic regions. Note the two-way paths between thalamus and cerebrum.

we need not know how the emotional reaction originated except to say that disturbing sensations of some sort must have attended this particular type of experience at one time or another.

In a phobia the sufferer realizes that the fear is irrational, but this is of no help in overcoming it because essentially the fear is not of external things. Rather it refers to the morbid dread of the alarming, menacing sensations that surge through the body, forcing conscious attention away from the surroundings and directing it inwardly to the unpleasant feelings.

Sooner or later the stage fright sufferer will become concerned with the audience detecting his or her terrorized state. This reinforces the feelings even more. Eventually the thought processes themselves begin to lose stability. When internal panic sufficiently overrides rationality, the victim may feel compelled to escape by the nearest exit.

In the reaction described above, stimuli that are responsible for the identification of the dreaded situation also stimulate the RAS, which especially arouses various limbic centers. These in turn un-

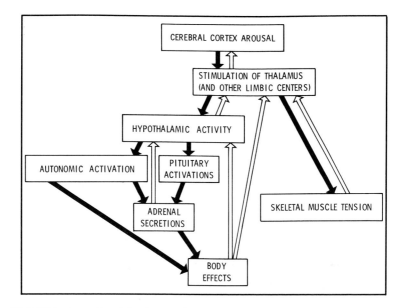

FIGURE 16-5   Model of neural interactions underlying the cyclic buildup of emotional arousal. Observe how the visceral and skeletal muscle effects of arousal intensify emotion through feedback (light arrows) to the mediating centers of the brain.

lock the strong sensations associated with the same type of past experience, prompting the hypothalamus to unleash powerful autonomic and somatic impulses throughout the body. The feedback to the limbic system from the body's peripheral activation influences the cerebral cortex in such a way that subjective feelings of fright and panic are intensified.

So-called will power is not very helpful in attempting to overcome a phobic reaction. The more the victim vows to be unafraid, the worse the reaction is likely to become. In this instance the conscious mind does not control the limbic system and hypothalamus. Once a phobic reaction has become established in the nervous system and is easily unleashed by the appropriate stimuli, the quickest and surest attack on the problem is to break up the positive feedback cycle at some point, possibly by employing muscle relaxants, or medications that diminish RAS activation of limbic circuits. This is essentially what the drugs meprobamate and diazepam do. In alleviating phobic reactions, a more stable function of the nervous system must first be restored before psychologic measures can be of much help.

It is apparent from the foregoing descriptions that emotion is

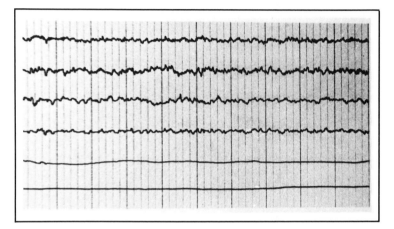

FIGURE 16-6   An electroencephalogram (EEG) depicting emotional arousal. This record shows a fast (beta) activity, low voltage pattern in which the spikes appear to be run together. Each of the four patterns (from top downward) represents activity in a different cerebral location. (Courtesy Psychology Department, University of Dayton, Dayton, Ohio.)

not a fixed entity that has a specific location in the body, but is a unique amalgam of our perception of external events together with our perception of internal body sensations. Emotional experiences are essentially physical phenomena that exist in our bodies largely as proprioceptive sensations. The phenomena are products of complex interactions involving the cerebral cortex, which is the center of conscious awareness; the limbic system, which performs as a clearinghouse; and the hypothalamus, which regulates the body through the ANS and the pituitary.

Differentiation of Emotions

Physiologically speaking, how is fear different from anger? Are different neural pathways involved in each? Are the chemical mediators different? For that matter, does emotion come in distinct forms, or are these just subjective impressions? It has been known for a long time that the mucous membranes of the nose and stomach redden and swell during anger, but become pale and shrink with fear.

Yet in all emotions the EEG record shows a similar type of low voltage, fast activity pattern that characterizes general arousal (Figure 16-6). Furthermore, as far as we can tell, the cortical-limbic system interactions appear to be generally the same regardless of

TABLE 16-2

Autonomic Activities Having Differences in Reaction Depending Upon Anger or Fear

AUTONOMIC PARAMETER	ANGER	FEAR
Rate of respiration	Relatively unchanged	Increased
Heart rate	Relatively unchanged	Increased
Skin conductance (GSR)	Unchanged or transiently increased	Sustained increase
Diastolic blood pressure	Increased	Unchanged
Skeletal muscle tension	Sustained increase	Unchanged or intermittent increase
Gastrointestinal secretion	Reduced	Increased
Peripheral vasomotion	Sustained constriction	Intermittent constriction or unchanged

whether the subjective feeling is one of fear or anger. However, of 14 measures of autonomic activity, 7 show significant differences between the reactions of fear and anger. These are listed in Table 16-2. Apparently each of the two emotions is associated with the predominance of a different chemical mediator. Whereas the response pattern in anger depends upon the combined action of norepinephrine and epinephrine, epinephrine alone is associated with fear reactions. In fact, states of aggressive excitability characterized by action appear to be associated with excessive norepinephrine levels. In states of anxious waiting and expectation that are passively devoid of action, epinephrine levels are elevated.

SORTING OUT STIMULI

What kinds of psychosocial events stimulate the RAS and incite the kind of cortical-limbic system interaction that we recognize as emotional activation? One certainly would consider that such situations as threatened loss of status, identity, health, or income are high priority sorts of stimuli. Yet a separation of psychosocial stimuli into those that are noxious and those that are not is totally unrealistic if not impossible. *A psychosocial event is stressful only when it is perceived as such.* What one individual may take in stride, another finds emotionally exhausting. What is at most a slight delay for one person may mean excruciating frustration for the next individual. The difference between them resides in the way the higher centers of the brain interpret the particular set of environmental circumstances.

Emotional responses are highly personal and individualized. Even the same individual may respond quite differently to the same stimulus at different times. What is the basis for these variations in responsiveness? One important factor is the physiologic state of the individual at the time. It is inferred in a previous section of this chapter that blood glucose levels, allergic states, infections, fatigue, drugs, and hormonal changes are of great importance in respect to both the quality and quantity of mental reactability. The previous psychologic history of the individual is also of the utmost significance in determining which stimuli are capable of unlocking the neural pathways that operate the emotions. To appreciate this point, the concepts of emotional insecurity and conditioned stimuli are introduced below, with a brief consideration of their interrelationship.

Emotional Insecurity and Conditioned Stimuli

Humans are considered to have two instinctive fears at birth; meaning that from the beginning there are two stimuli capable of inciting nervous responses of the type we call fear reactions. One of these fear reactions involves sensing a lack of support for the body (falling), and the other is produced by a sudden loud sound. The type of sensations that stimuli such as these can provoke are elicited to a greater or lesser degree by new stimuli arising again and again throughout life. Such sensations might be termed feelings of emotional insecurity. Very soon following birth additional stimuli begin to provoke the same type of sensation. The new stimuli are called *conditioned stimuli.* In conditioned reactions old responses answer to new stimuli. For example, in Pavlov's dogs (Figure 16-7), salivation (an old response) began to occur at the ringing of a bell (new stimulus) after the bell had been rung each time food was presented and sensed by smell and sight (the original stimuli). Of particular interest among these experiments was a case in which the dog's salivation was conditioned to the sight of a circle, whereas the sight of an ellipse produced no conditioned response. The ellipse was then progressively made more like a circle. When the ratio of the axes of the ellipse was reduced to 9 to 8 (Figure 16-8), the usual neural responses became disrupted, and the dog howled, trembled, and struggled to escape. Of special interest is the fact that afterward, even perfectly obvious ellipses and circles gave the dog trouble. Remarkably, there were no painful stimuli such as electric shocks employed in the experiment; yet simple conflicting stimuli had

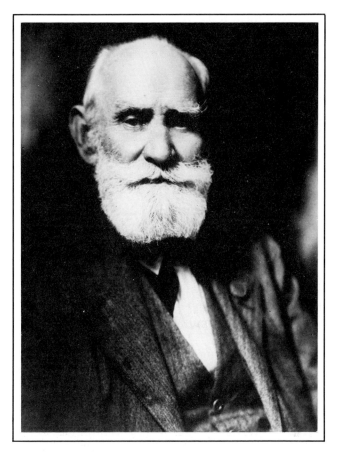

FIGURE 16-7   Ivan Pavlov (1849-1936). Pavlov, a Russian physiologist, conducted extensive experiments with dogs in which he clearly demonstrated the important principle of conditioned response. His classical experiments helped to initiate sound insight into the neural basis of human behavior. (Brown Bros. Photos, Sterling, Pa.)

produced a nervous breakdown—without need to resort to deeper psychologic explanations such as guilt and Oedipus complexes.

Practically all mental responses in humans are elicited by conditioned stimuli. As we proceed through life from early infancy, the provocation of sensations of insecurity becomes transferred to more and more stimuli. Regardless of how vague these sensations may be, they essentially are an expression of fear, which is our most common and basic form of emotion. Indeed, some psychologists consider anger to be a special projection of fear, in that it is generated from threats to security.

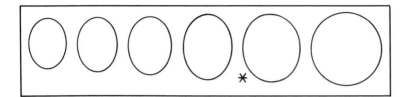

FIGURE 16-8 **An ellipse progressively made circular.** The figure far left is an ellipse and the figure far right a circle. As the figures proceed from left to right, they become less elliptical and more circular. In the figure with the asterisk, the axes have become reduced to 9:8.

Regardless of how fundamental fear is to our being, individual reactions to it vary considerably. It is even possible to develop a fear of fear. How one has learned to respond to fearful events is frequently more important than how afraid one is. It is in such matters as this that conditioning is so all-important. Moreover, chemical changes in the body are generated just as easily by a conditioned stimulus as they are with the original stimulus. Rats clearly show the same stress changes in brain norepinephrine metabolism in response to harmless stimuli previously paired with inescapable shock.

There also are feelings of security as well as feelings of insecurity. The first and foremost stimuli in our lives that promote security feelings are our mothers, the loss of whose presence and touch arouses sensations of insecurity. Feelings of security can be described as pleasant, satisfying, and relaxing. Much of our lives is spent seeking those stimuli that induce feelings of security while attempting to avoid events that provoke sensations of insecurity. Throughout life both types of stimuli are conditioned and reconditioned to the point that they become disguised and are no longer recognized for what they are. Thus the impatient competitor with an exaggerated sense of time urgency and easily aroused hostilities in striving for status and position may merely be responding to a need to obtain long-lost feelings of security that somehow disappeared and were replaced by feelings of rejection. Such an individual seeks attention (acceptance) and therefore must prove worthiness. So it is with the obsessive perfectionist who unconsciously feels that anyone or anything that has flaws thereby risks rejection. This person's behavior is likely to reveal a desperate search for the security that one feels acceptance provides, and in this individual's mind the more perfect one is, the more acceptable. Stress then ensues when the individual cannot meet the demands which he or she has placed upon himself or herself.

Another common source of psychologic conflict concerns comparing what is perceived with what is expected. When we cannot accept features of the real world in terms of our previously established beliefs and attitudes, the provoked discrepancy inevitably generates anxiety.

The particular social situation in which one finds oneself can be an additional variable in determining which psychologic stimuli are effective in stressing the body. An individual usually reacts differently when in a group from when alone. Therefore, in considering which stimuli are important in psychologic stress, we must include the particular social context along with the nature of the threat itself, the individual's habitual strategy of coping, and one's physiologic state at the time.

The individual's habitual strategy in attempting to cope is an especially important variable. The operation of neural pathways in critical situations tends to be based upon ingrained neural involvements that may have been beneficial in previous emotional situations, even though in the present situation such a response may be poorly adapted, leading to an inability to cope.

POSITIVE REINFORCEMENT

For some time psychologists have been observing and analyzing what is called *reinforcement behavior* in laboratory animals (Figure 16-9). *Positive reinforcement* occurs when the stimulus provokes a rewarding or desirable effect, prompting the animal to attempt renewing the stimulus. *Negative reinforcement*, on the other hand, involves aversive stimuli that provoke punishment, and therefore the animal avoids repeating them. A considerable body of evidence has accumulated indicating that positive reinforcement, or positive feedback[3] as it is sometimes termed, can effectively diminish the body's load of physiologic stress induced by psychosocial stimuli. It has been found that the more positive or relevant the feedback that results from coping attempts, the less the body's neural and hormonal output in response to the stress situation. Indeed, stressed rats obtaining positive reinforcement showing that their coping efforts are successful show little or no gastric ulceration. On the other hand, rats exposed to the same stressor but whose nervous systems receive

3The connotation of the term here is not quite the same as a previous use introduced in Chapter 3, and referred to earlier in this chapter.

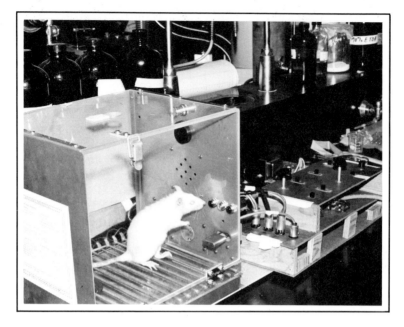

FIGURE 16-9   The study of operant reinforcement behavior. As
shown here, the animal usually employed in these studies is the rat, which
is subjected to a test chamber (Skinner box) where it can be presented with
numerous stimuli. By learning to press the lever to its right, it can obtain a
food pellet. (From the laboratory of the author.)

no relevant feedback from their less successful attempts to adapt
show severe ulceration. Furthermore, it has been repeatedly demonstrated in rats that positive reinforcement greatly inhibits output of
hydrocortisone.

The exact pathways mediating positively reinforcing stimuli
are unknown, but apparently they involve the amygdala of the
limbic system, and probably utilize the short ventral pathway from
the amygdala to the anterior zone of the hypothalamus (Figure
16-10). There is a theory that the hypothalamus is organized into
two reciprocally inhibitory zones in respect to its control of the ANS
and the pituitary in stress. According to this idea, the anterolateral
zone inhibits the response to stress, whereas the posteromedial zone
facilitates these responses (see Figure 16-10). Reciprocal inhibition
could explain the restriction of hydrocortisone output by positively
reinforcing stimuli.

Recently it has been substantiated that the brain catecholamines, norepinephrine and dopamine, are significant in medi-

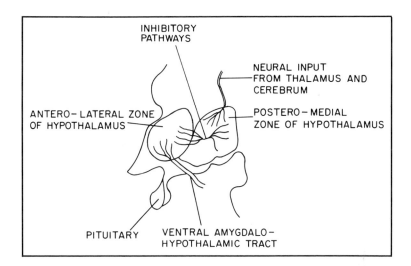

FIGURE 16-10   Concept of how positive reinforcement inhibits hypothalamic-pituitary output in stress. Successful coping is thought to activate the ventral pathway from the amygdala to the postulated anterolateral zone of the hypothalamus, which is believed to subdue pituitary output of stress hormones by inhibiting the posteromedial centers believed to facilitate neurohormonal response to stress. According to this concept negative reinforcement activates the posteromedial zone of the hypothalamus.

ating positive reinforcement, whereas serotonin probably mediates the aversive negative effects. Along these lines it is becoming clear that habitual negative reinforcement is associated with progressive patterns of helpless behavior. Animals developing this type of behavior become deficient in brain norepinephrine and are especially vulnerable to psychologic stress. Such animals remind one of a depressed human who no longer tries.

BIOFEEDBACK AND TRANSCENDENTAL MEDITATION

It had always been assumed that visceral functions controlled by the autonomic nervous system, such as heartbeat and intestinal contraction, could not be influenced by learning. Apparently this is not the case. Both animals and humans can learn visceral responses in the same way that they learn skeletal responses. In fact, rats have been trained to make changes specific to a single structure. They actually can dilate the blood vessels in one ear more than those in the other ear. Following animal experimentation with autonomic conditioning, it wasn't long before human studies were undertaken. It became evident that human subjects could be trained to modify their blood pressure, although the extent of the learning in human subjects has been less than that achieved with animals. The idea of conditioned visceral responses may explain why each of us has a tendency to respond to psychologic stress with our own particular visceral reaction, whether it be headache, queasy stomach, palpitation, or faintness. The fact that it is usually the same psychosomatic symptom suggests that specific autonomic pathways have become conditioned.

The principle of exercising some degree of control over visceral responses through operant, instrumental conditioning procedures is known as *biofeedback*. The theory underlying the principle implies that control over these responding systems is ordinarily impossible because we are not normally aware of what such systems are doing. By providing externalized, augmented information about what is going on in the body, operant control may be achieved. In biofeedback procedures a selected physiologic activity is monitored by an instrument that senses, by electrodes or transducers, signals of information about the particular body function (Figure 16-11).

Biofeedback operations are conducted for both theoretical and therapeutic reasons. Although more attention has centered around functions of therapeutic interest such as blood pressure regulation, application of biofeedback to skeletal muscle tension is especially pertinent to our interest in psychosocial stress. As previously implied, threatening stimuli activate physiologic preparation for action. Without body movement, considerable muscular tension is maintained. This stimulates proprioceptors in the muscle that feed back impulses to various brain centers, thereby enhancing the overall stress reaction throughout the body, including additional tensing of the muscles. Not only do the muscle fibers themselves adapt to higher levels of tension, but there is also a recognized effect in the cerebral cortex that works to maintain and heighten muscle tension. More importantly this effect prevents recognizing the tension. The process of mentally rehashing a disturbing incident over and over has been shown to sustain and increase muscle tension. Indeed, subconscious memories can keep muscles tense during sleep—and dreaming may further increase the tension.

In view of the importance of muscular tension in emotional stress, the electromyograph (EMG) is being employed in biofeedback research, and it is assumed that the muscle-cerebral control sys-

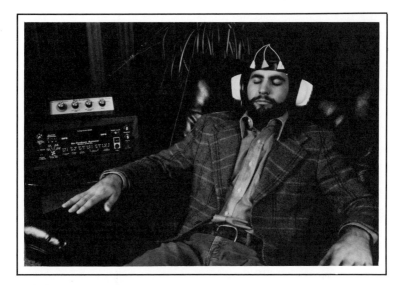

FIGURE 16-11   Biofeedback operation in a human subject.
Physiologic activity is monitored by the instrumentation at the subject's right. The subject is attempting to get the cycle started by self-inducing a relaxed state. (Courtesy Bio-Feedback Systems, Inc., Boulder, Colo.)

tem can be beneficially influenced by positive biofeedback. The initial procedure used with EMG biofeedback in order to get the cycle started employs autosuggestion: "My arm is heavy," or "I am becoming relaxed," are often used phrases. The relaxation from clinical trials of EMG biofeedback supplemented by other therapeutic techniques has been effective in alleviating several physical and emotional conditions (Table 16-3). However, when EMG feedback is used alone, the results are equivocal. For the most part this is the case with biofeedback in general. It has shown positive effects in some instances but not in others. Like many innovations in biomedical science, the therapeutic value of biofeedback procedure is controversial, and its use thus far has been restricted mostly to medical research centers, although more clinical specialists are beginning to design biofeedback programs, and departments of behavioral medicine are beginning to appear in selected clinical medical centers.

The practice of *transcendental meditation* (TM) was popularized almost concurrently with the development of biofeedback. TM was originated by practitioners of meditation systems in the Orient associated with yoga and Zen Buddhism. It has been claimed that the TM procedure, which calls for two 15-minute meditations a day, produces profound physiologic changes conducive to relaxation and

TABLE 16-3

Physical and Emotional Conditions Improving with EMG Biofeedback and Other Muscle-Relaxing Procedures

PHYSICAL CONDITIONS	EMOTIONAL CONDITIONS
Tension headache	Anxiety
Asthmatic bronchoconstriction	Phobias
Menstrual distress	Insomnia
Essential hypertension	Alcoholism and drug abuse
Gastrointestinal ulcers	Depression associated with anxiety
Spastic colitis	
Pain from muscle spasms	
Cerebral palsy	
Migraine headache	
Stiff neck	

Source: Modified from B. B. Brown, *Stress and the art of biofeedback*, Harper & Row Pubs., 1977.

tranquility. In some of the earlier experiments without controls it was reported that several meditating subjects decreased their oxygen consumption by 20% and developed a predominance of alpha waves in their EEG patterns.[4] Other reported changes included diminished respiratory rate and volume, decrease in blood lactate, slowing of the heartbeat, increase in electrical skin resistance, and slight increase in acidity of arterial blood. The subjects undergoing TM were described as being in a "wakeful, hypometabolic" state.

In later TM experiments in which the controls merely rested, there were no significant differences found between the two groups in respect to plasma levels of epinephrine, norepinephrine, and lactate. These investigators concluded that meditation does not induce a metabolic state that is any more unique than that found with complete resting in quiet surroundings.

For individuals who experience no benefit from biofeedback or meditation, other ways of handling stress have been recommended. Regular, strenuous exercise is one such practice. In addition, the habit of seeking quietness and concentrating on positive ideas, such as love, a sense of purpose, and self-acceptance can be effective. And although some psychiatrists may frown upon religious faith as self-deluding, there is no denying the positive effect that such faith has for many persons in coping with life. Probably

4Alpha waves appear as a specific EEG pattern that indicates a relaxed mental state devoid of arousal.

the most desirable human accomplishment of all is the ability to develop a personal, healing inner strength and tranquility that transcends worldly strife.

FUNCTIONAL NERVOUS DISORDER

When an individual is suddenly confronted with a striking conflict between psychologic motives or stimuli, there arises a confusion among signals to the hypothalamus and other brain stem centers. The inability of Pavlov's dogs to distinguish a circle from an ellipse, and the human phobic reaction to speaking before a large audience, were cited earlier as examples of how conflict alters the integrated function of the nervous system. When signals become confused, nerve impulses along the usual, well-established pathways are interrupted and may be switched or rerouted to effectors that produce useless maladaptive responses. Such functional disturbances in sensing and responding to stimuli can vary in degree and duration.

As a consequence of disintegrated neural function, the unfortunate victim feels a loss of control; one's nerves do not perform in the manner one would like. We call this sort of nervous instability a *neurosis*. The practice of psychiatry is full of descriptive classifications of psychoneurotic reaction types. However, the physiologist's concern is focused upon the functional disruption in the nervous system when afferent signals become crossed. More importantly, how does the dysfunction affect the body, and what are the risks of initiating true pathologic development? There are evidences that sooner or later poorly integrated nerve function takes its toll of every organ of the body.

There are thousands of persons who limit their activities and enjoyment of life because they are victims of nervousness. Such individuals regularly undergo physical suffering resulting from their autonomic nerve impulses. In stressful situations these persons experience palpitations, or trembling hands, or they breathe unnaturally; or they may complain of dizziness, a lump in the throat, excessive perspiration, gastrointestinal discomfort, diarrhea, or a backache. A relatively complete grouping of psychophysiologic reactions is displayed in Table 16-4.

Whether a neurotic reaction is classified as phobic, hysteric, depressive, obsessive, compulsive, or anxious, it is based upon some sort of emotional conflict that results in muscular tension and auto-

TABLE 16-4

Psychophysiologic Reactions Frequently Experienced by Neurotics

Tremor

Vertigo

Hyperventilation

Palpitations

Excessive perspiration

Itching

Gastrointestinal hypersecretion

Nausea

Diarrhea

Inability to swallow

Sensations of numbness (hands, feet, face)

Visual disturbance

Fatigue

Headache

Backache

Chest pain

Abdominal pain

Stiff neck

Hot flashes

Chills

Nasal congestion

Dyspnea

Frigidity (women)

Impotence (men)

Premature ejaculation (men)

Vomiting

Hives (urticaria)

Fainting

Excessive muscular tension

Bronchoconstriction

Menstrual distress and irregularity

nomic imbalance. When the ensuing discomfort leads to alterations in behavior, the matter becomes recognized as a nervous disorder, which over periods of time can damage the body through chemical stress.

‖ SUMMARY

Interpersonal and social relationships often give rise to conflicting stimuli that can stress the body chemically through disrupting neural interactions involving the cerebrum, limbic system, hypothalamus, and ANS.

The measurement of hormones such as the catecholamines, ACTH, and cortisol from blood and urine offers a means of assessing the body's response to psychosocial stress.

In responding to psychosocial stimuli our hormonal and muscular systems become mobilized for action, but action that is usually restrained by our modern social order, leading to unresolved muscular tension and chemical imbalances within the body. When these tensions and chemical imbalances persist, they can impair regulation of cardiovascular and immune function.

Emotional reactions are viewed as a duality of body sensations initiated by hypothalamic discharges together with subjective impressions mediated by the cerebral cortex. Portions of the limbic system of the brain integrate interaction between these two components. Feedback from body effects to the limbic system intensifies all aspects of emotion.

Both the quality and quantity of emotional reactivity from psychosocial stimuli depend upon the physiologic state of the individual, the person's particular history of psychologic conditioning, and the social context within which the stimulus is applied.

Positive reinforcement °resulting from effective attempts to cope with threatening stimuli can reduce the body's load of chemical stress by inhibiting secretion of glucocorticoids from the adrenal cortex. Adequate levels of norepinephrine and dopamine in the brain are necessary in mediating positive reinforcement.

Visceral responses may be altered by conditioning, a procedure known as biofeedback. Biofeedback has been successful in controlling blood pressure and heart rate in some individuals.

Conflicting psychologic stimuli can result in a confusion of signals to the hypothalamus, thereby interrupting neural impulses along established pathways and redirecting them to new effector actions that are often inappropriate. Such functional disorders are called neuroses. Neuroses produce many bodily symptoms and can lead to more serious disease.

Chapter Glossary

amygdala   an almond shaped group of neural nuclei making up part of the limbic system

behaviorism a school of experimental psychology devoted to studying overt stimulus–response reactions

electromyograph an instrument measuring electrical changes accompanying tension in skeletal muscle

hypometabolic below average rate of body metabolism

nervous breakdown an ill-defined term indicating a temporary impasse in adjusting to normal living routine

operant (operative) refers to behavior involving operation of instrumentation

proprioceptive neural stimulation originating from receptors in internal tissues

psychoneurosis a nervous disorder of mental origin

psychosomatic a disorder in the body produced by the emotions

reciprocal inhibition when the function of one element of a dual system automatically inhibits the function of the other element

sympathoadrenomedullary sympathetic division of the ANS and its effect on catecholamine secretions from the adrenal medullae

For Further Reading

Anderson, R. A. 1978. *Stress power.* New York: Human Sciences Press.

Archer, J. 1979. *Animals under stress.* Baltimore: University Park Press.

Black, P., ed. 1970. *Physiological correlates of emotion.* New York: Academic Press.

Brown, B. B. 1977. *Stress and the art of biofeedback.* New York: Harper & Row Pubs.

Cassens, G.; Roffman, M.; Kuruc, A.; et al. 1980. Alterations in brain norepinephrine metabolism induced by environmental stimuli previously paired with inescapable shock. *Science* 209:1138.

Chinn, P. L., ed. 1979. Stress and adaptation. In *Advances in nursing science.* Germantown, Md.: Aspen Systems Corp.

Colligan, D. 1975. That helpless feeling: The dangers of stress. *New York Magazine,* July 14, pp. 28–32.

Gellhorn, E., and Loofbourrow, G. N. 1963. *Emotions and emotional disorders: A neurophysiological study.* New York: Harper & Row Pubs.

Goldwag, E. M., ed. 1979. *Inner balance—The power of holistic healing.* Englewood Cliffs, N.J.: Prentice-Hall, Inc.

Gray, J. A. 1971. *The psychology of fear and stress.* New York: McGraw-Hill Book Co.

Greenfield, N. S., and Sternbach, R. A., eds. 1973. *Handbook of psychophysiology.* New York: Holt, Rinehart and Winston.

Grings, W. W., and Dawson, M. E. 1978. *Emotions and bodily responses: A psychophysiological approach.* New York: Academic Press.

Henry, J. P., and Stephens, P. M. 1977. *Stress, health and the social environment: A sociobiological approach to medicine.* New York: Springer-Verlag.

Ittelson, W. H.; Proshansky, H. M.; Rivlin, L. G.; et al. 1974. *An introduction to environmental psychology.* New York: Holt, Rinehart and Winston.

Lazarus, R. S.; Cohen, J. B.; Folkman, S.; et al. 1980. Psychological stress and adaptation: Some unresolved issues. In H. Selye, ed., *Selye's guide to stress research.* Vol. 1. New York: Van Nostrand Reinhold Co.

Levi, L., ed. 1972. *Stress and distress in response to psychosocial stimuli.* International Series of Monographs in Experimental Psychology. Vol. 17. New York: Pergamon Press.

Loraine, J. A., and Bell, E. T. 1971. *Hormone assays and their clinical application.* 3d ed. Baltimore: Williams and Wilkins Co.

McLean, A., ed. 1974. *Occupational stress.* Springfield, Ill.: Charles C Thomas Pubs.

Michaels, R. R.; Huber, M. J.; and McCann, D. S. 1976. Evaluation of transcendental meditation as a method of reducing stress. *Science* 192:1242.

Miller, N. E. 1980. Effects of learning on physical symptoms produced by psychological stress. In H. Selye, ed., *Selye's guide to stress research.* Vol. 1. New York: Van Nostrand Reinhold Co.

Miller, N. E., and Dworkin, B. R. 1977. Effects of learning on visceral functions-biofeedback. *N Engl J Med* 296:1274.

Moyer, K. E. 1971. *The physiology of hostility.* Chicago: Markham Publishing Co.

Newton, G., and Tiesen, A. H., eds. 1974. *Advances in psychobiology.* Vol. II. New York: Wiley-Interscience, John Wiley and Sons.

Olds, J. 1977. *Drives and reinforcements: Behavioral studies of hypothalamic functions.* New York: Raven Press.

Ray, W. J. et al. 1979. *Evaluation of clinical biofeedback.* New York: Plenum Press.

Schwartz, M. 1978. *Physiological psychology.* 2d ed. Englewood Cliffs, N.J.: Prentice-Hall, Inc. Chapts. 7, 11.

Selye, H. 1976 a. *The stress of life.* New York: McGraw-Hill Book Co.

———. 1976 b. *Stress in health and disease.* Boston: Butterworths.

Vander, A. J. 1976. In Introduction to *Human physiology and the environment in health and disease.* San Francisco: W. H. Freeman and Co. Part 4, articles 13, 17, 18.

Vernikos-Danellis, J., and Heybach, J. P. 1980. *Psychophysiologic mechanisms regulating the hypothalamic-pituitary-adrenal response to stress.* In H. Selye, ed., *Selye's guide to stress research.* Vol. 1. New York: Van Nostrand Reinhold Co.

17

Disease from Emotionally Induced Chemical Imbalance

|| **Objectives:** Upon completing this chapter you should:

1. Understand how pathology can result from sympathoadrenal and adrenocortical responses to psychosocial stress.
2. Be acquainted with the mediative action of neurotransmitters in the brain, and perceive how psychologic tensions alter the balance among these mediators.
3. Recognize the interrelationship of brain norepinephrine, mental depression, and coping with stress.
4. Know about the endorphins in the brain, and appreciate their significance in such matters as stress, pain, and metabolic regulation.
5. Know something of the chemical basis of functional forms of mental illness.
6. Fully apprehend the role of mental stress in producing cardiovascular disease.
7. Be able to evaluate the importance of emotions in diseases associated with immunologic dysfunction.
8. Be informed of the role of psychologic stress in causing gastrointestinal disease.

      When and how does psychologic stress become physiologic stress? From a practical standpoint it is of the utmost importance to know if chronic emotional tension harms the body, and if so, by what means. It already has been stated in general terms that emotional states provoke significant chemical changes within the body. Both the intensity and duration of the emotion are important variables. The neural interactions mediating emotional responses to psychosocial stimuli were discussed in Chapter 16. Despite the multitude of neural circuits involved, projections from these interactions are directed to final, common pathways in the hypothalamus, which regulates the ANS and the pituitary-adrenal system. Hence a great deal of the ensuing chemical stress in the body is hormonally induced. Indeed, it has been generally acknowledged that the body's hormonal system can get "bent out of shape" by chronic mental stress. In addition, it has been found that disturbances in the chemical balance of several neurotransmitters in the brain itself can accompany and follow psychologic stress. The resulting chemical imbalances in turn affect mental states and behavior, and they may set the stage for mental illness in susceptible individuals.

      Since much of the physiologic impact of emotional tension

on the body would be expected to be translated through hypothalamic influence on both the medulla and cortex of the adrenal glands, discussion of tension influence on these systems follows.

RESPONSE OF THE SYMPATHOADRENOMEDULLARY AND PITUITARY–ADRENAL SYSTEMS

Sympathoadrenal Response

It is firmly established that stimulation of the sympathetic division of the ANS and the consequent secretion of catecholamines from the adrenal medullae can be executed by a great variety of psychosocial stimuli in humans as well as in animals. This is concluded from numerous investigations where it has been clearly demonstrated that emotional reactions influence the quantity of catecholamines excreted in the urine. The catecholamine response can be surprisingly strong as well as rapid, typifying the fight or flight reaction. Separate measurements of epinephrine and norepinephrine from both blood and urine have shown that fear reactions are associated mostly with elevations of the former, whereas rage is more often characterized by increases in norepinephrine.

The physiologic effects of sympathetic stimulation and catecholamine action are described in Chapter 4. Studies of psychologic stress in which urinary catecholamines become elevated reveal a characteristic battery of physiologic changes (Table 17-1) that include elevations in plasma concentrations of LDL cholesterol, triglycerides, and glucose. In addition, systolic blood pressure, heart rate, and BMR noticeably increase, whereas blood clotting time decreases. Psychosocial stimuli provoking this overall response are of a threatening nature, whereas security types of stimuli are expected to diminish sympathoadrenomedullary activity in the body.

Persons encountering emotionally arousing situations would be expected to have increased levels of epinephrine and norepinephrine in the blood and urine. Aircraft pilots and passengers, parachute jumpers, competitive athletes, newly admitted hospital patients, dental patients, automobile drivers, and fans at sporting events all have shown elevated levels of these hormones. Conditions characterized by anticipation and unpredictability especially provoke catecholamine responses.

TABLE 17-1

Physiologic Changes Associated with Elevation of Catecholamines in Urine

Increased heart rate

Increased blood pressure, particularly the systolic

Increased oxygen consumption (BMR)

Increased body temperature

Decreased blood-clotting time

Higher electrical skin resistance (GSR)

Higher levels of glucose in the blood

An elevation of free fatty acids (FFA) in the blood

An increase in serum triglycerides

Increased LDL cholesterol in the blood

Studies of college students have shown that subjective feelings of anxious anticipation, uncertainty, and helplessness can be associated with a threefold increase in epinephrine secretion. Moreover, the average blood pressure of a group of students rose from 118/78 to 152/112 torr during examination time, and remained at 147/108 torr for several hours afterward. Students undergoing final examinations also have shown marked elevations in plasma glucose, triglycerides, LDL cholesterol, and free fatty acids. Note the bar graph of Figure 17-1. It clearly shows that the stress hormones, epinephrine, norepinephrine, and cortisol, are greatly increased among students in an achievement situation.

Adrenocortical Action

It is well documented for humans and animals that psychologic stimuli incite adrenocortical responses. Indeed, psychologic events resulting in fear, anxiety, and frustration are among the most potent stressors that activate the pituitary-adrenal system. As stated in Chapter 3, the secretion of cortisol by the adrenal cortex is so central to the generalized stress response that the two are considered synonymous. The pituitary-adrenocortical system can be remarkably sensitive to subtle psychologic changes. For example, merely transferring a monkey from one cage to another has been shown to be followed by a significant elevation of ACTH.

Apparently glucocorticoid hormones are effective in maintaining homeostasis during periods of emotional stress after the first catecholamine-triggered responses begin to wear off. As increased

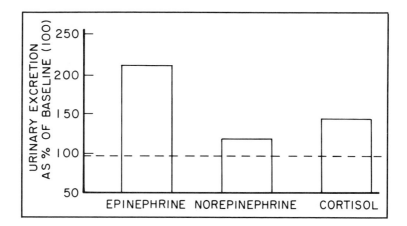

**FIGURE 17-1   Mean urinary excretion of three hormones in
engineering students under stress.** The baseline (100) represents mean
values when the students were not in an achievement situation. (Modified
from data of Collins and Frankenhaeuser, 1978, Stress responses in male
and female engineering students, *Jour of Human Stress* 4:43.)

blood levels of glucose and sodium begin to diminish, secretions of
cortisol and aldosterone intervene and instill antishock measures.
Thus, responses from the adrenal cortex become especially significant when mental strain is sustained.

There are numerous reports indicating that the mounting
tension associated with anticipating an event can significantly increase corticosteroid secretions. Bomber crews awaiting flight, patients awaiting surgery, and those waiting to participate in athletic
competition all show marked increases in plasma levels of both
ACTH and cortisol. Watching movies with themes of sustained,
threatening suspense is associated with increases of 17-hydroxycor-
ticosteroids (17-OHCS) in the urine, whereas watching movies with
secure, benign contents is associated with decreases of these hormones. A number of psychologic events known to activate the pituitary-adrenocortical system are listed in Table 17-2.

Even though persistent anxiety evokes secretions from the
adrenal cortex, this is not the only type of emotion capable of eliciting that response. Overall affective arousal, rather than any one
emotional state, can lead to increased corticoid secretions. For example, chronic depression has been associated with excessive quantities
of 17-OHCS in the urine, even though catecholamine levels remain
normal or even become diminished.

It has already been implied that the pituitary-adrenocortical

TABLE 17-2

Psychologic Events Activating the Adrenal Cortex

Any first experience characterized by novelty or uncertainty

Anticipation of something previously experienced as unpleasant

Situations in which long-standing rules or expectations are suddenly changed

Persistence of an increase in social interaction

Crowding

Awaiting news of any important decision

Awaiting surgery

Aircraft flight

Final exams (students)

Competitive athletics

Anticipation of exposure to cold

Chronic feelings of frustration

A sense of rush or time urgency

Witnessing violence (real or fictitious)

---

system reacts more slowly to psychologic stimuli than does the sympathoadrenomedullary system. This is not surprising in view of the immediate preparation for fight or flight offered by hormones, such as catecholamines, that rapidly promote energy metabolism. On the other hand, slower responding hormones, such as corticosteroids, are important in recovering chemical stability, reconstituting tissues, and maintaining energy stores. In chronic mental stress it is the adrenal cortex that becomes overworked, subjecting the individual to increased risks of immune system impairment, glucose intolerance in those predisposed, and weight loss due to negative nitrogen balance.

Whether psychologic stress is acute or chronic is also of significance in respect to thyroid function. In sudden threats, such as acute anger, thyroid secretion may become excessive along with catecholamine output. However, in unresolved conflicts where anxiety is mild but chronic, and is sometimes associated with inactivity and depression, thyroid output may become diminished.

Much individual variation is apparent in adrenal responses to psychosocial stimuli. In persons disposed to functional instability of the limbic system-hypothalamic circuitry, ACTH appears to be released more liberally. Such individuals are sometimes referred to as stress-prone. There also is great individual variation in adrenal re-

TABLE 17-3

Various Brain Neurotransmitters

Dopamine
Norepinephrine
Epinephrine
Tyramine
Serotonin (5-hydroxytryptamine)
Melatonin
Acetylcholine
Histamine
Gamma-aminobutyric acid (GABA)
Gamma-hydroxybutyrate (GHB)
Aspartate
Glutamate
Beta-endorphin

Source: Modified from J. D. Barchas, A. Akil, and G. R. Elliot, 1978, Behavioral neurochemistry: Neuroregulators and behavioral states, *Science* 200:965.

serve capacity. Persons with a disposition to allergies and parasympathetic response predominance more frequently become exhausted from prolonged periods of psychologic tension.

BRAIN NEUROTRANSMITTERS AND MENTAL ILLNESS

There is compelling evidence that psychologic events alter neurochemical function in the brain, and altered neurochemical function in turn modifies behavior. The chemical mediators involved are known collectively as neurotransmitters or neuromodulators (Table 17-3). The key neurotransmitters implicated in those areas of the brain having to do with emotional reactions and neural regulation of pituitary function are norepinephrine, dopamine, and serotonin (Figure 17-2). Emotional arousal may lead to changes in the proportions of these chemical mediators, especially when the exposure to aversive stimuli is repetitive and prolonged. Such changes were first demonstrated for norepinephrine, the transmitter that is thought to play a major role in mediating positive, assertive responses. Persistent frustration leading to a sense of hopelessness is

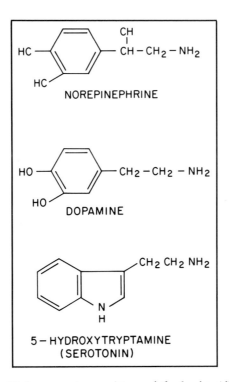

FIGURE 17-2   Major neurotransmitters of the brain. All three substances are biogenic monoamines. Note their molecular structure, and particularly the similarity of norepinephrine to dopamine, which is the precursor of norepinephrine.

believed to result in a relative depletion of brain norepinephrine, resulting in emotional and behavioral depression. According to this idea, the depressive state would tend to be perpetuated in a vicious cycle, since the inability to cope alters the balance of neural norepinephrine, a condition which further accentuates the depression. Dogs given electric shocks from which there is no escaping (and, therefore, no positive reinforcement) soon give up trying and become completely helpless. It was shown that norepinephrine in the limbic areas of their brains had become depleted.

Rats that are able to perform avoidance responses to electric shock have higher levels of brain norepinephrine than do nonshock control animals. On the other hand, yoked rats with no coping response have lower brain norepinephrine than do the controls (Figure 17-3).

Not only can performing a simple, effective coping response increase the level of brain norepinephrine (an effect similar to that

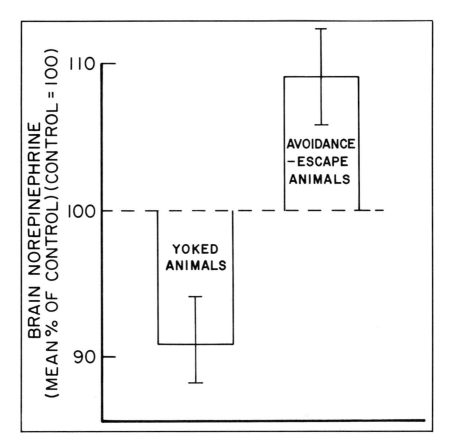

FIGURE 17-3   Comparison of means and standard deviations for brain norepinephrine in rats both able and unable to avoid electric shock. 100 represents the mean line for controls not confronted with shock. Yoked animals are forced to take the shock; they have no way to avoid it. (From N. E. Miller, Effects of learning on physical symptoms produced by psychological stress, in *Selye's guide to stress research*, Vol. 1, 1980. H. Selye, ed. New York: Van Nostrand Reinhold Co.)

produced by antidepressant drugs), but, an inability to do anything about anxiety or pain reduces the level of brain norepinephrine, which in turn can interfere with subsequent abilities to cope. Repeated exposure to stress in animals free to make coping efforts will increase the activity of the enzyme (tyrosine hydroxylase) that synthesizes norepinephrine in the brain, thereby enabling more coping responses that are effective.

Depression ranks as the third most common health problem in the United States. Thousands of persons are beset with chronic episodes of pessimism, irritability, feelings of helplessness, discouragement, and general dissatisfaction with everything and everyone, along with a variety of physical complaints. Indeed, depression has been called a great masquerader because of the many physical symptoms that occupy the victim but are in reality due to the depressed mental system. Such symptoms commonly include muscle pains, lethargy, backache, chest pains, gastrointestinal distress, constipation, headache, fatigue, and insomnia. Recently it has been found that exercise can relieve depression, at least the milder cases. Indeed, the concept of the role of brain norepinephrine in depression may explain the elevated mood and euphoria experienced by joggers. Vigorous exercise generates much sympathetic activity and elevates norepinephrine levels throughout the body.

Animals able to learn effective coping responses also have lower levels of plasma corticosterone. Thus it follows that immunosuppression should be less in any organism that can actively cope with aversive psychologic events. Accordingly, the human who can transmute fears and worries into plans and actions should have less undesirable chemical alteration in the body. The fear-reducing ability of effective coping may be the principle involved in the placebo effect. An example of this effect occurs when one is able to reduce anxiety by taking what is believed to be an antianxiety drug, even though it is actually a sugar pill possessing no neurochemical action.

In addition to acknowledged neurotransmitter substances, another group of brain chemicals has been discovered. These were originally called *endogenous opioids,* but they are now known collectively as *endorphins.*[1] The endorphins belong to a growing family of known brain peptides. Pharmacologically, many of the endorphins are opiatelike. Thus they produce analgesia, inhibit respiration, and modulate mood. They bind to the same cell receptors in the limbic system as opiate drugs, and their effects are reversed by naloxone, a selective opiate antagonist.

Some of the endorphin peptides resemble portions of the ACTH molecule, suggesting links between the endorphins and hormonal systems. Moreover, it has been shown that psychologic stress is associated with increases of several endorphins in the blood. In fact, stress may increase plasma beta-endorphin as much as sixfold.

In ways not yet understood the endorphins appear to have some relationship to noradrenergic and dopaminergic systems in the brain. They are thought to be involved with modulating responses

---

[1]Endogenous opioids are sometimes separated into the small enkephalins, with 5 amino acids, and the larger beta-endorphin, with 31 amino acids. However, shorter fragments of beta-endorphin have been isolated. The name *endorphin* is derived from *endo*genous m*orphine.*

to pain and stress. Indeed, a recently discovered natural opioid appears to act in a manner similar to the benzodiazepines (Librium and Valium), a class of tranquilizers described in Chapter 14. Perhaps this is why some individuals have a lower anxiety response level and therefore can cope more effectively with aversive psychosocial stimuli.

There is speculation that opioids may compete with other brain neurotransmitters for receptor sites on nerve cells. This also appears to be true for certain psychoactive drugs that mimic actions of specific natural opioids. For example, it has been shown that there are high-affinity binding sites in the brain for the benzodiazepines. Furthermore, the binding results in an increase in postsynaptic responses throughout limbic centers to gamma-amino butyric acid (GABA), a major inhibitory neurotransmitter. Thus the inhibition is intensified. It is believed that this constitutes the mechanism of action of benzodiazepines in reducing anxiety.

As for the relationship of endorphins to pain, it has been shown that these peptides have little effect on experimental or acute pain alone, but they appear to diminish the reaction to protracted pain as do opiate drugs. Thus their effect is linked to psychogenic pain syndromes and depression. In some instances the administration of beta-endorphin to depressed patients has produced dramatic, though fleeting, improvement.

Release of beta-endorphin from the rat pituitary seems to accompany, almost molecule for molecule, the release of ACTH. Thus the response of this opioid peptide is induced by stress. It has been shown that both ACTH and beta-endorphin are produced in the same pituitary cell by cleavage from a large precursor known as *pro-opiocortin*. Whereas ACTH stimulates the release of glucocorticoids from the adrenal cortex, beta-endorphin appears to stimulate appetite and cause release of insulin from the pancreas. It has been suggested that the so-called common obesity of middle age may be a consequence of chronic overreaction from these two mediators of the pituitary. The obesity of middle age is viewed by some physiologists as a mild version of Cushing syndrome (see Chapter 4), and the characteristic changes in body conformation are sometimes looked upon as a usual part of aging. In the overall process ACTH maintains a tendency to hyperglycemia and can promote protein wasting of the muscles, particularly in the extremities, whereas beta-endorphin promotes hyperphagia and hyperinsulinism, both of which may lead to obesity of the face (moon face), upper back (buffalo hump), and trunk (pot belly). All of these features, when extreme, characterize Cushing syndrome.

Fractions of beta endorphin are also known to be psychoactive agents with profound general effects on the mood and behavior in animals and humans. For that matter, ACTH itself can have dramatic effects on brain function. It has been shown that injections of ACTH into hypophysectomized animals restore normal learning ability and improve habituation to environmental change and novel stimuli. Recent investigations have revealed that the ACTH molecule, like beta-endorphin, has specialized subparts in the form of small peptides. One of these acts directly on limbic centers to elicit fear responses, whereas another fraction can act as a "security" hormone. This points to the possibility that some of the drive mechanisms of the brain may be events that essentially are controlled by various peptides.

Mental Illness

Even though the term *mental illness* may be applied to a broad spectrum of behavioral abnormalities, the majority of individuals afflicted suffer from one of two types of functional psychosis in which no neural lesions can be demonstrated.[2] The two types of mental illness are known respectively as *affective disorders* and *schizophrenic illness.* It is thought that there is some degree of genetic predisposition underlying a particular biochemical deviation in each form of illness. Both types of disorders are found in varying degrees of severity, and mixed forms may exist. Milder cases of psychosis may be difficult to distinguish from severe, incapacitating forms of neurosis.

The prototype of the affective disorders is *manic-depressive psychosis,* characterized by periods of profound depression or manic excitement. The two moods may alternate in the same individual, who typically overreacts emotionally to ordinary situations. Onsets of manic-depressive episodes may be sudden. They are precipitated by stress and usually occur intermittently from young adulthood through middle age. On the other hand, the onset of *schizophrenia* is more insidious, sometimes beginning in early adolescence. Those afflicted with schizophrenia progressively withdraw from reality, mentally and emotionally, and proceed to live in their own world of feeling and ideas which may have little to do with real, external events. Delusions and hallucinations are often present.

The leading biochemical hypothesis for explaining what hap-

2There are psychoses with an organic basis, such as those associated with cerebral arteriosclerosis, alcoholism and drug abuse, head injuries, or paresis, in which the brain is infiltrated with syphilitic organisms.

pens in the affective disorders states that episodes of depression are produced by an underactivity or deficiency in the brain of the neurotransmitter norepinephrine and possibly serotonin as well. Mention has been made already of the relation of norepinephrine depletion to depression. Mania, on the other hand, is thought to be associated with the functional hyperactivity of these neurotransmitters.

The norepinephrine theory in part is based upon the known effects of various drugs used in the effective treatment of depression and mania. For example, the tricyclic antidepressants, such as imipramine, increase the functional activity of norepinephrine and serotonin by preventing their uptake by the neuron that released them into the synaptic cleft. On the other hand, reserpine, used to treat hypertension, depletes brain norepinephrine and serotonin and creates a depressionlike syndrome.

It has been postulated that lithium carbonate, the most effective treatment for mania, decreases the electrically stimulated release of norepinephrine as well as enhances its reuptake from the synaptic cleft. It is of interest that exposure to aversive psychologic stimuli in experimental animals has been shown to be capable of altering the reuptake mechanisms for norepinephrine. In addition, it has been shown that lithium reduces the number of acetylcholine receptors at neuromuscular junctions, and it is now believed that this regulation may be involved in the drug's control of manic episodes.

Recently the demonstration of euphorogenic action by endogenous opioids has led to the idea that some of the endorphins may be responsible for the mood changes in affective disorders. Investigations of this matter are under way.

At first the neurotransmitter serotonin was theoretically implicated in the etiology of schizophrenia, in view of the action of hallucinogens such as LSD, which is antiserotonergic and produces schizophreniclike symptoms. However, accumulating evidence suggests that an imbalance of other brain catecholamines, such as norepinephrine and dopamine, underlies schizophrenic disturbance. The most current hypothesis postulates that schizophrenic symptoms result from a relative excess of dopaminergic transmission in critical cell groups within the brain. The concept is supported by the fact that all known antipsychotic agents used in schizophrenic treatment block dopaminergic transmission. Moreover, amphetamine, which can induce a psychoticlike paranoia, even in nonschizophrenics, is known to enhance dopaminergic activity. It has been shown that chronic paranoid schizophrenics excrete significantly higher levels of urinary phenylethylamine, an endogenous amine chemically and pharmacologically related to amphetamine.

TABLE 17-4

The Three Dopamine Pathways in the Brain

PATHWAY	ANATOMIC LOCATION	HYPOTHESIZED INVOLVEMENT
Nigrostriatal	Substantia nigra to caudate-putamen	Movement coordination Parkinson disease Extrapyramidal symptoms of antipsychotic drugs
Tuberoinfundibular	Arcuate nucleus to median eminence (hypothalamus)	Modulation of certain endocrine functions
Mesolimbic-mesocortical	Substantia nigra and medial area to limbic nuclei and cortical regions	Emotional tone Action of antipsychotic drugs Amphetamine psychosis Schizophrenia

Source: Modified from P. A. Berger, 1978, Medical treatment of mental illness, *Science* 200: 978.

It is thought that dopamine serves as the neurotransmitter in three brain pathways: the nigrostriatal, the mesolimbic-mesocortical, and the tuberoinfundibular (Table 17-4). Antipsychotic drugs, such as chlorpromazine, block dopamine receptors in all three pathways. Blockade of the nigrostriatal pathway can promote Parkinson-like extrapyramidal reactions, whereas blocking the tuberoinfundibular pathway induces changes in endocrine responses. It is the blocking of the mesolimbic-mesocortical pathway by chlorpromazine that presumably yields the desired antipsychotic activity, thus establishing the idea that dopamine neural activity in this pathway is excessive in schizophrenic patients.

Disturbance in brain endorphin levels also has been viewed as a possible involvement in the development of schizophrenia. Opiate agonists such as cyclozocine and nalorphine induce hallucinations and derealization experiences in healthy volunteers. The provoked psychotic episode can then be immediately reversed by naloxone, a specific opiate antagonist.

Another interesting hypothesis has developed about the roles of norepinephrine and dopamine in producing mental disturbance. Apparently the functions of these two catecholamine systems in the brain are dynamically interrelated. When their normal relationship is upset by manipulating one component, as is believed to occur in stress, then it is up to the other to act in a compensatory fashion to maintain a balanced function. The deleterious effects of decreased dopamine activity, for example, could be counterbalanced by a similar decrease in norepinephrine activity, thereby preserving dopamine-norepinephrine ratios. If dopamine activity increases in response to stress without a concomitant increase in norepinephrine, or if dopamine activity remains the same when norepinephrine activity decreases, then it is believed that the system becomes disposed to schizophreniclike reactions. Recall that in Figure 17-2, an enzyme converts dopamine to norepinephrine. Hence it has been suggested that in schizophrenia an overbalance of dopamine to norepinephrine may be due to a deficiency of the hydroxylase enzyme.

The imbalances in brain neurotransmitters underlying mental disturbances are both initiated and aggravated by stress. It has been shown that the presentation of psychosocial types of stressors to laboratory animals can sensitize the animals to later effects of amphetamine and vice versa. Apparently there are similarities between the behavioral and biochemical effects of stress, and drugs such as amphetamines, which are known to induce psychotic states. Such evidence indicates that stress is an important variable in precipitating some forms of mental illness.

Imbalances involving additional brain neurotransmitters are thought to be instrumental in the development of other forms of neuropathology. For example, *Parkinson disease* is considered to involve a preponderance of brain cholinergic activity over dopaminergic activity.

PSYCHOSOCIAL STRESS AND DISEASE

It has long been recognized that the existence of unresolved mental conflict leading to periods of mounting emotional stress produces alterations in normal bodily functioning. Indeed, the development of a variety of specific disorders has been shown to be closely associated with mental stress, and it is evident that neurally induced chemical alterations within the body can eventually promote disease processes. As stated years ago by Hans Selye: "Modern man has created a civilization which subjects him to more worries, pressures and emotional stress than his body is equipped to cope with. These stresses cause physiological change which can make the body prey to heart and kidney diseases and possibly to other ailments."[3]

3From an address to the New York Academy of Medicine, 2 East 103d Street, New York, N.Y., October 7, 1947.

Foremost among the conditions associated with emotional distress are hypertension, cardiovascular disease, bronchial asthma, gastrointestinal ulcers, colitis, chronic headaches, skin disorders, mental disturbances, and hormonal imbalances contributing to diabetes and hyperthyroidism. There are volumes of statistics correlating acute psychosocial changes, such as divorce, death of a spouse, and loss of employment, with the onset and development of various illnesses, both minor and major. Prospective as well as retrospective investigations reveal statistically significant relationships between shocking mental experience and the occurrence of myocardial infarction, accidents, athletic injuries, leukemia, multiple sclerosis, diabetes, and an entire gamut of minor complaints. Although in some instances the precise relationship to psychosocial events is conjectural, it is accepted nevertheless that disorders such as ulcers, hypertension, asthma, and migraine headaches are seriously exacerbated by emotional upsets.

A study of 204 men who were students at Harvard University in the early 1940s revealed that those judged to be the most poorly adjusted suffered much more heart attacks, cancer, emphysema, hypertension, and gastrointestinal disease in later life than well-adjusted men. Other studies have shown that persons denying themselves outlets for emotional expression are especially susceptible to psychosomatic ailments. Indeed, self-disclosing individuals tend to be healthier mentally and physically. By self-disclosing we mean voluntarily revealing one's problems, beliefs, values, and feelings to another person.

Along the same lines the importance of coming to grips with one's problems cannot be overemphasized. The degree or severity of psychologic stress is related to the individual's ability to recognize, know, and understand the stress itself, as well as how much control the individual *feels* he or she has over the situation. A list of important types of disease in which psychosocial stress is believed to play a contributing role is presented in Table 17-5.

Despite significant statistical correlations it remains difficult to prove that emotional stress alone causes disease. Even though sustained hostile impulses are classically linked to the development of high blood pressure while chronic dependency and anxious help-seeking are identified with increased gastric secretion, asthmatic distress, and other allergic suffering, there are other variables to be considered. Especially important are genetic predisposition, dietary habits, immune irregularities, and various kinds of environmental exposures.

As pointed out in Chapter 16, there is an almost insurmount-

TABLE 17-5

Debilitating Diseases in Which Psychosocial Stress Is Considered a Contributing Factor

Hypertension

Cardiovascular impairment

Bronchial asthma

Gastrointestinal ulcers

Ulcerative colitis

Migraine headache

Myocardial infarction

Multiple sclerosis

Most forms of allergies

Certain skin disorders

Susceptibility to viral infection

Diabetes mellitus

Mental illness

Hyperthyroidism

Cancer (?)

able problem in identifying and quantifying the psychosocial stimuli that alone are responsible for biochemical imbalances capable of initiating pathologic changes. We can measure adrenal output and demonstrate that when it is chronically excessive, it exacerbates cardiac and hypertensive disorders, whereas a decreased adrenal output can be shown to aggravate arthritic and rheumatic illnesses. Yet there are investigators who are reluctant to conclude that psychologic factors alone cause these illnesses. Furthermore, the mere elimination of psychologic stressors in most cases cannot be expected to completely reverse the organic aspects of the disease once it has become firmly established. Rather, the social stressor is looked upon as a factor altering the individual's susceptibility to disease at a particular period of time, thereby serving as an important contributor to the biochemical disruptions which precipitate and hasten the onset of organic change in susceptible individuals. Moreover, the presence of psychosocial stress invites other damaging stressors such as accidents, poor dietary habits, infections, and the dependency on drugs and medications.

In general it may be stated that conditions favoring physical breakdowns leading to disease include an *inherent predisposition, pro-*

TABLE 17-6

The Holmes-Rahe Social Readjustment Rating Scale

RANK*	LIFE EVENT	PROPORTIONAL VALUE*
1	Death of spouse	100
2	Divorce	73
3	Marital separation	65
4	Jail term	63
5	Death of close family member	63
6	Personal injury or illness	53
7	Marriage	50
8	Fired at work	47
9	Marital reconciliation	45
10	Retirement	45
11	Change in health of family member	44
12	Pregnancy	40
13	Sex difficulties	39
14	Gain of new family member	39
15	Business readjustment	39
16	Change in financial state	38
17	Death of close friend	37
18	Change to different line of work	36
19	Change in number of arguments with spouse	35
20	Mortgage over $10,000	31
21	Foreclosure of mortgage or loan	30
22	Change in responsibilities at work	29
23	Son or daughter leaving home	29
24	Trouble with in-laws	29
25	Outstanding personal achievement	28
26	Wife begins or stops work	26
27	Begin or end school	26
28	Change in living conditions	25
29	Revision of personal habits	24
30	Trouble with boss	23
31	Change in work hours or conditions	20
32	Change in residence	20
33	Change in schools	20
34	Change in recreation	19
35	Change in church activities	19
36	Change in social activities	18
37	Mortgage or loan less than $10,000	17
38	Change in sleeping habits	16

Source: T. H. Holmes and R. H. Rahe, 1967, The social readjustment rating scale, *Psychosom Res* 11:213.
*Both the relative order and magnitude have been derived from the coefficients of correlation matching a particular event with a subsequent change in the physical, emotional, and social pattern of living that requires readjustments. Proportional values are based on "death of a spouse" as a maximum correlation of 1.00, or 100%.

TABLE 17-6 *(continued)*
The Holmes-Rahe Social Readjustment Rating Scale

RANK*	LIFE EVENT	PROPORTIONAL VALUE*
39	Change in number of family get-togethers	15
40	Change in eating habits	15
41	Vacation	13
42	Christmas	12
43	Minor violations of the law	11

longed psychologic stress that is perceived as stress, and an obvious inability to cope with the stress. The 43 most common stressful life events that may play a part in precipitating disease processes are shown in the Holmes-Rahe Social Readjustment Rating Scale in Table 17-6.

As the following subsection reveals, there is a strong connection between psychosocial stress and hypertensive cardiovascular disease. Likewise, there are considerable data linking failure of psychologic adaptation to susceptibility to infectious disease, cancer, and autoimmune disorders—though the evidences are not as clear or as direct as is the case for heart and artery ailments.

Cardiovascular Disease

More has been written about mental stress in respect to hypertensive cardiovascular disease than any other stress-disease relationship. There is no question that activated emotions can elevate blood pressure, increase serum levels of LDL cholesterol, enhance blood viscosity, and decrease clotting time. Aside from this there is a rapidly accumulating mass of data indicating that atherogenic changes in the aorta and coronary arteries can occur independently of hypertension and hypercholesterolemia. Electrical stimulation of the lateral hypothalamus of rats for periods of 62 days has produced atherosclerotic lesions despite normal blood pressure and cholesterol levels, *suggesting that responses to psychosocial stimuli alone may play a significant role in ischemic heart disease by way of direct neural mediation.* Other animal experiments have shown that chronic stimulation of autonomic nerves directly supplying the aorta can produce advanced lesions in the form of fibrocalcitic arteriosclerosis.

Animals tied down or restrained so that they cannot avoid painful electric shocks frequently show heart cell necrosis, which can lead to death. Furthermore, subjecting dogs to a psychologically stressful environment has been shown to reduce the threshold of their ventricles for repetitive response, indicating the presence of electrical instability and a predisposition to ventricular fibrillation, a mechanism of sudden death.

There also is evidence of this sort of cardiac pathology in humans. Fifteen young people who died apparently as a consequence of having been kept captive by a deranged sadist and subjected to cruel, intense mental horror from which there was no escape were autopsied. Autopsies revealed hearts with bright red patches of dead cells. Such pockets of dead cells interfere with the heart's normal electrical regulation of the contractile cycle. The resulting abnormal rhythm led to cardiac failure.

Of particular interest are data derived from large numbers of highly specialized aerospace professionals (aged 36 to 52) who experienced sudden mass unemployment at Cape Kennedy between 1966 to 1976. With their consequent loss of identity and income, and faced with accepting much less desirable occupations (or none at all), these individuals were suddenly subjected to feelings of alarm, which progressed to mounting frustration and sustained hopelessness. This was reflected in increased rates of divorce, alcoholism, and drug abuse, which of course amounted to additional stress. Physiologic studies of these individuals revealed elevated blood glucose and increased eosinopenia. In addition, there was a remarkable increase in the frequency of abnormal resting ECG patterns. Cholesterol levels were not unusually high, and blood pressure readings, though fluctuating, were not consistently elevated. Nevertheless, despite the absence of these standard risk factors, and others such as obesity, cigarette-smoking, and diabetes mellitus, there was a very high incidence of acute myocardial infarction in this relatively young group. In cases like this, either coronary artery spasms or disturbances in heart rhythm may make up the mechanisms underlying the heart attacks.

Though investigations of the effects of aversive psychologic stimuli on the development of cardiovascular disease are frequent enough, studies in which positive treatments are employed are sparse by comparison. In one investigation of this sort, two groups of rabbits were kept on a 2% cholesterol diet. The animals of one group were individually petted, held, talked to, and played with on a regular basis. Compared to the control group, which was ignored, these rabbits showed more than a 60% reduction in atherosclerotic lesions of the aorta. Along the same lines, medical data from the Plains Indians, who are reputed to live serene, unstressful lives in their rural setting, reveal a very low incidence of heart attacks despite a high incidence of diabetes and dietary cholesterol.

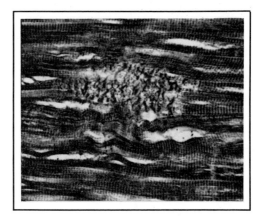

FIGURE 17-4   Catecholamine-induced myocardial necrosis. Observe the severe necrotic damage just above center of the picture. Damage resulted from an infusion of isoproterenol. (From R. S. Eliot, F. C. Clayton, G. M. Pieper, et al., Influence of environmental stress on pathogenesis of sudden cardiac death. *Fed Proc* 36(5):1719, 1977.)

Numerous cardiac specialists have repeatedly emphasized the importance of emotions and behavior in susceptibility to coronary heart disease. Indeed, writers such as Glass, as well as Friedman and Rosenman, have recognized a specific pattern of coronary-prone behavior, known as Type A, in which achievement, striving, time urgency, and hostility dominate the personality. Eugene Braunwald, Chief of Medicine at Harvard's Peter Bent Brigham Hospital, has concluded that aversive psychologic experiences are a foremost factor in triggering heart attacks.[4]

Even though there are indications that vascular pathology can be directly induced by neural stimulation, much of the stress on the cardiovascular system from strong emotion is produced by an overdrive of catecholamine responses. Vasoconstriction is sustained with intense alpha receptor activation. Moreover, excessive catecholamine release is associated with depletion of high-energy phosphate stores in the heart muscle as a result of increased energy demand. Though epinephrine has long been known to stimulate cardiac action, it has not been appreciated until recently that sustained blood levels of the hormone can be toxic to cardiac muscle cells. Infusion of the catecholamine isoproterenol into the heart muscle of dogs exhausts the ATP supply of the subendocardium and induces tissue necrosis (Figure 17-4).

4From an address to the 52nd Annual Scientific Sessions of the American Heart Association, Anaheim, Calif., November 1979.

Psychologic tensions created by various conditions of the modern urban environment can profoundly affect the cardiovascular system through sympathoadrenomedullary mediation. Normal persons driving cars in busy city traffic have developed heart rates of 120 to 130 beats per minute accompanied by significant elevations in plasma norepinephrine and epinephrine. Crowding also can activate the sympathoadrenomedullary system. Controlled experiments with crowding in mice have produced adrenal medullary hyperplasia and hypertrophy as well as hyperglycemia.

There appears to be little doubt concerning the importance of emotional stress as a contributing factor in cardiovascular pathology, especially in those who otherwise have been in good health and have not reached the senescent years.

Cancer

A considerable amount of research data has prompted some clinicians and researchers to tentatively link psychologic stress to tumorigenesis. Also, a number of specialists have noted that a sense of hopelessness along with denial and repression of negative emotions makes for a poor prognosis among cancer patients. Recent evidence that clearly demonstrates hypothalamic influence on immune function has generated considerable speculation about the role of the emotions in cancer susceptibility. It has been stated repeatedly that high levels of corticosteroids suppress the immune surveillance thought to be so important in protecting against the development of malignant neoplasms. And prolonged mental unrest leads to elevated blood levels of ACTH and corticosteroids. Indeed, there is no doubting the fact that hormonal changes induced by prolonged emotional stress can shift the immunologic equipoise to favor tumorigenesis.

In one investigation the function of T lymphocytes was shown to be significantly depressed in 26 people (aged 20 to 65) who were grieving over the loss of a spouse. In another study a single session of inescapable shock in male mice resulted in an early appearance of mastocytoma tumors, exaggeration of tumor size, and decreased survival time in the recipient animals. Escapable shock had no such effects, suggesting that the inability to cope with stress may initiate and aggravate tumorigenesis.

On the other hand, there are those who maintain that there are no extensive data pointing to the importance of psychologic factors in either predisposing people to cancer or in determining how well they will respond to treatment once diagnosis has been made.

At present we must conclude that the relation of the emotions to cardiovascular pathology is much more convincing than is the case with cancer. Nevertheless, the potential role of mental stress in malignant disease should not be dismissed, but warrants further study and elucidation.

Respiratory Disease and Allergy

Allergic diseases bear a unique relationship to the emotional systems of the body. Nasal hypersecretion, hypervascularity, skin reactions (eczema), and mucous membrane swelling can be brought on by feelings of anxiety, depression, and helplessness. It is well known that hay fever reactions to pollen, which are often minimal in settings that are relaxed and secure, become severe whenever there is anxiety and depression. Likewise, the bronchial obstructive syndrome in asthma, due to bronchoconstriction, mucosal swelling, and hypersecretion, becomes reversible to a surprising degree in cases where reassurance and psychologic supportive measures are offered. It is well documented that in certain types of individuals, repressed nervous tension is channelled through parasympathetic pathways, and stimulation of parasympathetic nerves intensifies allergic disorders.

This is not to say that the symptoms of hay fever and asthma do not involve immune responses to allergens. However, immune reactions are profoundly influenced by neuroendocrine mediation, which takes us back to the role of the hypothalamus and limbic system in emotional expressions. Indeed, research with mice has shown repeatedly that susceptibility to viral infections is greatly enhanced by stressing the animals' nervous systems. Likewise, human tears shed from emotion have been shown to contain stress hormones.

At present there is exciting research being done on the association of emotional stress with overall dysfunctions of the immune system. This relationship may well be significant when considering susceptibility to infectious, allergic, autoimmune, and malignant disease.

Gastrointestinal Disease

It is widely recognized that gastrointestinal function is especially vulnerable to psychosocial stress. So-called nervous stomach and irritable bowel are frequent reflections of emotional tension. The increased secretion of gastric acid and pepsin found in anger and anxiety states is usually considered a somewhat normal psycho-

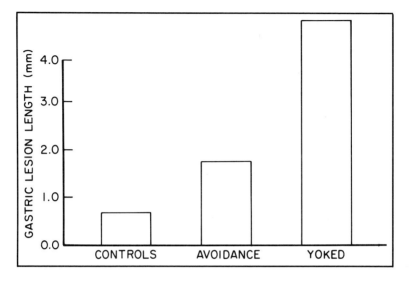

FIGURE 17-5   Comparison of mean length of gastric ulcerations in rats both able and unable to avoid electric shocks. Observe that rats with no opportunity to cope developed lesions that were well over twice the size of the ulcers in those able to avoid the shocks. (From N. E. Miller, in *Selye's guide to stress research,* Vol. 1, 1980.)

physiologic response which may or may not be related to the production of gastrointestinal ulcers. Ulcer development depends upon characteristic changes in the mucosal wall associated with a decrease of protective mucus (Figure 2-8). However, a chronic course of increased secretion of acid and pepsin can set the stage, and once the ulcer is present, any stimulus that increases acid secretion seriously aggravates the lesion.

Extensive studies of psychostimulation in rats have revealed two important facts about gastrointestinal ulceration. One is that the degree of ulceration is invariably correlated with the blood level of the stress hormone corticosterone, an adrenal steroid. Secondly, the animals that could escape or avoid the stimuli (electric shock) developed much less ulceration than did the yoked, helpless animals receiving the same shock patterns (Figure 17-5). Furthermore, those that received a warning signal before shock and thus anticipated it, had more ulceration and higher corticosterone levels regardless of whether they were yoked or not. Of particular note is the role of conflict in producing gastric ulceration. When rats were trained to give themselves a brief electric shock in order to avoid a longer train of shocks, the animals that would so cope found themselves in an

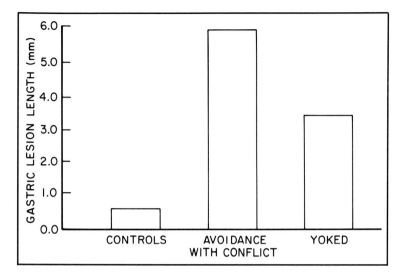

FIGURE 17-6   The significance of conflict in producing gastric ulceration in rats. Mean lesion length was almost twice as great in animals who had to tolerate brief shocking to avoid a longer series of shocks than it was in animals (yoked) who simply could not avoid the usual, brief shocking. The necessity of exposure to aversive stimulation in order to avoid much more such stimulation is conflicting to the animal. (Modified from N. E. Miller, in *Selye's guide to stress research*, Vol. 1, 1980.)

avoidance-avoidance conflict, something like being between the devil and the deep blue sea. Such avoidance conflict resulted in more severe gastric lesions than being yoked (Figure 17-6).

Two other gastrointestinal ailments to which emotional stress strongly contributes by means of autonomic mediation are *spastic colitis* and *ulcerative colitis*. The former condition is characterized by loose, mucus-laden stools, sometimes alternating with bouts of constipation and much gas formation. Ulcerative colitis is much more serious. It is characterized by a progressive development of organic disease in which small ulcerations and petechial hemorrhages occur, resulting in blood loss. The lower colon of patients susceptible to ulcerative colitis responds to emotional activation with increased mobility, hyperemia, congestion, and marked fragility of the mucosa. In this disorder there is an increase in both lysozyme levels and proteolytic enzymes, similar to changes following injections of methacholine chloride, a strong cholinergic agent. Intestinal symptoms are particularly apparent following feelings of anger and resentment, and the personality profile often reveals a person (usually female) who feels injured and degraded. In some cases of ulcerative colitis, autoimmunity has been suspected as a contributing factor.

Vasomotor Lability

There are individuals in whom emotional activation becomes associated with spasm of the smooth muscle of blood vessels, in some cases producing prominent dilation, which may alternate with constriction. Typically there is vasoconstriction during times of tension, but later there is often a prominent letdown associated with marked dilation of some blood vessels. One of the consequences of these changes, and one that can be potentially dangerous, is a sudden lowering of coronary blood flow. An increased viscosity of the blood and decreased clotting time induced by sympathetic activation during the emotion may lag behind the sudden drop in cardiac output and oxygen consumption prompted by the letdown.

Certain individuals experience a collecting of fluid and metabolites in the interstitial area around dilated cranial arteries that have lost their vasomotor tone. The distortion of the vessel wall pressing into the interstitial area produces a throbbing pain, commonly experienced on one side of the head. The best known form of vascular headache is *migraine*—which should not be confused with tension headache. The actual suffering of migraine is usually associated with a relaxation or letdown from tension. Thus, relaxing sedatives may exacerbate the symptoms. Migraine attacks are more likely to occur during evenings, weekends, holidays, and vacations. It is believed that the warning visual distortions that precede migraine attacks, such as seeing bright spots and so on, are associated with arterial constriction, whereas the reversal to vasodilation introduces the painful throbbing. Personality profiles of migraine sufferers reveal individuals who are overly conscientious and meticulous. They often hold deep resentments and are inflexible and tense.

Tension headaches are more common than migraine attacks. They also are related to psychologic stress, but they are produced by sustained contraction of the skeletal muscles of the head and neck as a preparation to engage in physical activity which is never realized.

Still another vasomotor problem provoked by emotional activation is emotional fainting (vasovagal syncope). Upon the sudden ending of an acute emotional crisis, sympathetic tone falls quickly and steeply, but the vagal tone remains high, promoting a loss of central blood supply, coupled with a slowing of the heart. There is allusion to this phenomenon in the discussion of the autonomic nervous system in Chapter 4.

Autoimmune Disease

Emotional stresses, acute and chronic, have been suspected to contribute to the development of autoimmune disorders. The onset of MS often follows emotional trauma, and myasthenia gravis is notably exacerbated by expressions of aggression. The role of the emotions in rheumatoid arthritis has not been resolved. Patients with RA are generally described as overconscientious, compulsive, self-sacrificing, and unable to show hostility. The entire matter of the part played by emotions in immune dysfunction is one of intense interest today.

FURTHER STRESS FROM BEHAVIOR PATTERNS INDUCED BY EMOTIONAL ACTIVATION

When one becomes unsettled emotionally, one tends to be more impatient, more desperate, and more irrational than usual. One's usual behavior is frequently altered, and more often than not the change subjects the person to additional chemical stress. Eating habits may worsen. There may be more smoking, drinking, and dependency on medicines and other drugs. In addition, the susceptibility to accidents may be heightened, sleep lost, and exercise neglected. Not only does psychosocial stress invite further chemical stress on the body from other stressors, but, it in itself tends to become compounded. When the psychophysiologic changes of emotion are initiated, a feedback mechanism is operative that intensifies the existing physiologic changes or even initiates additional ones. For example, emotionally induced muscle tension can become a secondary stimulus that increases emotional arousal, which then further heightens muscle tension. Prolonged muscle tension can reduce blood flow to muscles to the point that metabolites accumulate and pain is produced. The pain then becomes still another input leading to further physiologic and biochemical alterations. This principle of ever-expanding physiologic activation is depicted diagrammatically in Figure 17-7.

It is the mounting tension from the enhancement of positive feedback combined with the likelihood that the resulting behavior will subject the individual to additional chemical stressors that distinguishes psychologic stress as a powerful contributor to eventual body damage. Before we know it, health begins to take a downward course. The involvement of psychosocial stress in pathologic

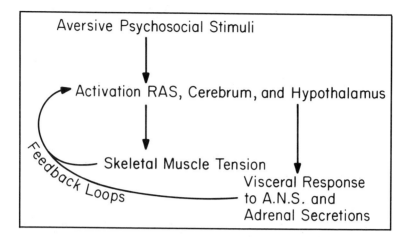

FIGURE 17-7   Sustained emotional activation from body feedback.
Skeletal muscle tension and visceral responses emanating from
psychosocial stimuli further activate emotion-mediating centers of the
brain, thereby prolonging and intensifying emotional states.

changes exemplifies once more that it is not usually a single stressor
that is responsible for the progressive breakdown of homeostatic
mechanisms that leads to disease. *It is multiple stresses reinforcing one
another over periods of time.*

SUMMARY

Unresolved psychologic conflict sustains nervous tensions that may
eventually harm the body and mind through chemical alterations
arising from adrenal responses and neurotransmitter imbalances in
limbic-cortical pathways of the brain.

Sustained activation of the sympathoadrenomedullary system
stresses the cardiovascular system, whereas exaggerated adrenocortical responses lead to dysfunction of the immune system.

Emotional activation alters the proportions of norepinephrine, dopamine, and serotonin in the brain. Depletion of brain norepinephrine in the limbic centers produces mental depression,
whereas excessive norepinephrine action is responsible for manic
moods.

Schizophrenia, characterized by hallucinations and a withdrawal from reality, is thought to be a manifestation of excessive
dopamine relative to norepinephrine in the mesolimbic-mesocortical pathway of the brain.

Brain peptides, called endorphins, are strategically involved along with ACTH in mediating reactions to psychosocial stress. Some endorphins have an antianxiety effect, whereas others diminish sensitivity to pain. One such peptide stimulates appetite and insulin release.

Prolonged emotional tension enhances the susceptibility to cardiovascular disease usually brought about by chronic overdrive of the sympathoadrenomedullary system. However, there is evidence that neural stimulation alone can promote heart disease independently of hypertension and hypercholesterolemia.

Symptoms of hay fever, asthma, and eczema are markedly exacerbated by feelings of anxiety and depression. Likewise, the development of gastrointestinal ulcers and colon disease is strongly associated with emotional states.

Emotional stress can alter immune reactivity through hypothalamic-pituitary-adrenal mechanisms. Therefore, exposure to aversive psychosocial stimuli may contribute to the development of infectious, allergic, autoimmune, and malignant diseases.

Psychosocial stress tends to invite additional chemical stress from malnutrition, drinking, smoking, and drug intake, and it enhances its own action through patterns of positive feedback.

Chapter Glossary

agonist   a positive effector (opposite of antagonist)
colitis   inflammation of the colon
eosinopenia   deficiency of eosinophilic leucocytes in the blood. Eosinophiles respond to certain foreign antigens
hyperemia   localized accumulation of blood; often due to vasodilation
hyperplasia   enlargement of tissue due to number of cells
hypophysectomy   removal of the pituitary gland
neurotransmitter   chemical that transmits nerve impulses from one neuron to another
petechial   refers to small reddish spots caused by submucosal hemorrhage
psychogenic   mentally caused; of mental origin
psychosis   a pronounced mental disorder
subendocardium   tissue beneath the endothelial membrane of the heart
vagal   refers to the vagus nerve; parasympathetic in action

For Further Reading

Antelman, S. M., and Caggiula, A. R. 1977. Norepinephrine-dopamine interactions and behavior. *Science* 195:646.

Antelman, S. M.; Eichler, A. J.; Black, C. A.; et al. 1980. Interchangeability of stress and amphetamine in sensitization. *Science* 207:329.

Baldessarini, R. J. 1977. Schizophrenia. *N Engl J Med* 297:988.

Barchas, J. D.; Akil, H.; Elliott, G. R.; et al. 1978. Behavioral neurochemistry: Neuroregulators and behavioral states. *Science* 200:964.

Berger, P. A. 1978. Medical treatment of mental illness. *Science* 200:974.

Chinn, P. L., ed. 1979. Stress and adaptation. In *Advances in nursing science.* Germantown, Md.: Aspen Systems Corp.

Collins, A., and Frankenhaeuser, M. 1978. Stress responses in male and female engineering students. *Hum Stress* 4:43.

Ehrlich, Y. H.; Volavka, J.; Davis, L. G.; et al., eds. 1979. Modulators, mediators, and specifiers in brain function. In *Advances in experimental medicine and biology.* Vol. 116. New York: Plenum Press.

Eliot, R. S.; Clayton, F. C.; Pieper, G. M.; et al. 1977. Influence of environmental stress on pathogenesis of sudden cardiac death. *Fed Proc* 36:1719.

Eliot, R. S., and Todd, G. L. 1976. Stress-induced myocardial necrosis. *J SC Med Assoc* (Suppl) 72:33.

Friedman, M., and Rosenman, R. H. 1974. *Type A behavior and your heart.* New York: Alfred A. Knopf, Inc.

Glass, D. C. 1977. *Behavior patterns, stress, and coronary disease.* New York: Halsted Press.

Guillemin, R. 1978. Peptides in the brain: The new endocrinology of the neuron. Nobel Prize Lecture, 1977. *Science* 202:390.

Gunderson, E. K. E., and Rahe, R. H., eds. 1974. *Life stress and illness.* Springfield, Ill.: Charles C Thomas Pubs.

Gutstein, W. H.; Harrison, J.; Parl, F.; et al. 1978. Neural factors contribute to atherogenesis. *Science* 199:449.

Hendrix, G. H., ed. 1976. National conference on emotional stress and heart disease. *J SC Med Assoc* (Suppl) 72:1–95.

Henry, J. P., and Stephens, P. M. 1977. *Stress, health and the social environment: A sociobiological approach to medicine.* New York: Springer-Verlag.

Holden, C. 1978. Cancer and the mind: How are they connected? *Science* 200:1363.

Jenkins, C. D.; Rosenman, R. H.; and Zyzanski, S. J. 1974. Prediction of coronary heart disease by a test for the coronary-prone behavior pattern. *N Engl J Med* 290:1271.

Levi, L., ed. 1972. *Stress and distress in response to psychosocial stimuli.* New York: Pergamon Press.

Levi, L., and Kagan, A. 1980. Psychosocially-induced stress and disease— problems, research strategies, and results. In H. Selye, ed., *Selye's guide to stress research.* Vol. 1. New York: Van Nostrand Reinhold Co.

Lipowski, Z. J.; Lipsitt, D. R.; and Whybrow, P. C., eds. 1977. *Psychosomatic medicine—current trends and clinical applications.* New York: Oxford University Press.

Lown, B.; Verrier, R.; and Corbalan, R. 1973. Psychologic stress and threshold for repetitive ventricular response. *Science* 182:834.

Mason, J. W. 1975. Emotion as reflected in patterns of endocrine integration. In L. Levi, ed., *Emotions—their parameters and measurement.* New York: Raven Press.

Miller, N. E. 1980. Effects of learning on physical symptoms produced by psychological stress. In H. Selye, ed., *Selye's guide to stress research.* Vol. 1. New York: Van Nostrand Reinhold Co.

Pestronk, A., and Drachman, D. B. 1980. Lithium reduces the number of acetylcholine receptors in skeletal muscle. *Science* 210:342.

Rabkin, J. G., and Struening, E. L. 1976. Life events, stress, and illness. *Science* 194:1013.

Rahe, R. H. 1976. Stress and strain in coronary heart disease. *J SC Med Assoc* (Suppl) 72:7.

Rasmussen, A. F., Jr. 1969. Emotions and immunity. *Ann NY Acad Sci* 164:458.

Reynolds, R. C. 1974. Community and occupational influences in stress at Cape Kennedy: Relationships to heart disease. In *Contemporary problems in cardiology.* Vol 1. Stress and the Heart. Mount Kisco, N.Y.: Futura Publishing Co.

Riley, V. 1981. Psychoneuroendocrine influences on immunocompetence and neoplasia. *Science* 212:1100.

Rossier, J.; Bloom, F. E.; and Guillemin, R. 1980. Endorphins and stress. In H. Selye, ed., *Selye's guide to stress research.* Vol. 1. New York: Van Nostrand Reinhold Co.

Schwartz, M. 1978. *Physiological psychology.* 2d ed. Englewood Cliffs, N.J.: Prentice-Hall, Inc. Chapt. 14.

Selye, H. 1976. *Stress in health and disease.* Boston: Butterworths.

Sklar, L. S., and Anisman, H. 1979. Stress and coping factors influence tumor growth. *Science* 205:513.

Soloman, G. F.; Amdraut, A. A.; and Kasper, P. 1974. Immunity, emotions and stress. *Ann Clin Res* 6:313.

Stein, M.; Schiavi, R. C.; and Camerino, M. 1976. Influence of brain and behavior on the immune system. *Science* 191:435.

Tallman, J. F.; Paul, S. M.; Skolnick, P.; et al. 1980. Receptors for the age of anxiety: Pharmacology of the benzodiazepines. *Science* 207:274.

Vander, A. J. 1976. In Introduction to *Human physiology and the environment in health and disease.* San Francisco: W. H. Freeman and Co. Part 4, articles 13, 16.

Vernikos-Danellis, J., and Heybach, J. P. 1980. Psychophysiologic mechanisms regulating the hypothalamic-pituitary-adrenal response to stress. In H. Selye, ed., *Selye's guide to stress research.* Vol. 1. New York: Van Nostrand Reinhold Co.

Weiss, J. M. 1972. Psychological factors in stress and disease. *Sci Am* 226:104.

Wiener, H. 1977. *Psychobiology and human disease.* New York: Elsevier.

Wolf, H. G., and Goodell, H. 1968. *Stress and disease.* Springfield, Ill.: Charles C Thomas Pubs.

The Relation of Biologic Time to Stress and Disease

Developmental Stages and Disease Susceptibility
Fetal Stress Effects
Physiologic and Biochemical Bases of Aging
Aging, Stress, and Disease

|| **Objectives:** Upon completing this chapter you should:

1. Recognize that vulnerability to specific diseases depends upon the developmental stage of life that is stressed.
2. Be able to identify the risks of disease associated with childhood, adolescence, middle age, and old age.
3. Be well informed about the stress and damage that can occur during the fetal and perinatal periods.
4. Be familiar with the various theories of aging.
5. Understand the declining adaptability and increased susceptibility to stress and disease that characterize old age.
6. Be acquainted with the major pathophysiologic features of senescence.

Beginning with the moment the sperm penetrates the egg, each of us passes through a timed sequence of developmental changes culminating in death. Thus, despite the uniqueness of our species, with all its monumental achievements, we, as biologic entities, remain fixed to the cycle of birth, reproduction, and death, as do all organisms on this planet.

Obeying the human inclination to systematize, we divide life histories into discrete stages despite the fact that as far as Nature itself is concerned, human development is an uninterrupted continuum of change. Consequently, our points of demarcation separating the various stages are derived arbitrarily. A list of human developmental stages is shown in Table 18-1.

Although the time required for various developmental changes is genetically programmed and statistically predictable for the human species, the duration of later stages is less predictable and shows a wider range of individual variation than the earlier stages (Table 18-1). For example, duration of the gestation period and even the postnatal time required to attain puberty are relatively fixed when compared to the time involved in reaching old age and becoming senile. Such things as rate of aging and how long one lives vary considerably among individuals.

DEVELOPMENTAL STAGES AND DISEASE SUSCEPTIBILITY

It stands to reason that vulnerability to physiologic derangements depends in part upon the developmental stage being stressed. Thus, susceptibility to specific diseases may be strongly associated with a

TABLE 18-1

Major Stages of Human Development

STAGE		APPROXIMATE APPEARANCE AND DURATION
(Prenatal)	Embryo	2d through 8th week
	Fetus	3d through 9th month
(Postnatal)	Neonatal	Birth through 2d week
	Infancy	3d week through 1st year
	Childhood	2d year through 11th or 12th year
	Adolescence	12th or 13th year through 18th to 20th year
	Adulthood (prime)	20th year through 36th to 40th year
	Middle age	37th to 41st year through 56th to 64th year
	Old age and senescence	57th to 65th year until death
	Death	?

given period of development. For example, emphysema, osteo-arthritis, and advanced atherosclerosis would not ordinarily be ex-pected among adolescents and young adults. On the other hand, the onset of such disorders as cystic fibrosis and Reye syndrome would be unlikely in individuals past 20 years of age.

As a general rule the early and late periods of postnatal life are when the individual is most vulnerable to physiologic stress. A good example of this point is afforded by examining the variation in immunoglobulin reserve occurring throughout life (Figure 18-1). Compared to most adults, neither children nor the elderly are as capable of mustering effective immune reactions.

Since the earliest and latest portions of life are most suscepti-ble to stresses, most of the attention in this chapter is devoted to the problems encountered during fetal development and old age. First let us consider the periods of life from childhood through middle age.

Stress and Disease in Childhood and Adolescence

The most frequently encountered childhood stresses are related to infectious diseases and associated irregularities in the immune sys-tem, although nutritional imbalances also are common at this stage. Many children suffer from recurrent respiratory infections. For-tunately, the severity of those caused by bacteria can be checked with antibiotic therapy. Closely associated with recurrent respiratory infections is allergic disease. Indeed, the pediatrician must be con-

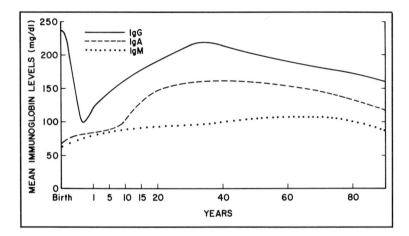

FIGURE 18-1 **Average plasma immunoglobulin levels throughout life.** Observe that the lower levels are found at the early and late periods of life, whereas the most substantial levels occur between the ages of 20 and 60, at least for IgG and IgA. (Constructed from a combination of data sources.)

stantly aware of signs and symptoms of allergic stress from both inhalants and ingestants. Of special significance in this respect is childhood asthma. Without treatment this condition can be frightening and debilitating. The offending allergens must be identified, and either they must be avoided, or the patient must be desensitized to them. Sympathomimetic agents and adrenal steroids may be necessary to alleviate attacks of bronchoconstriction. Avoidance of sudden exposure to cold air and preventing emotional disturbances also are important in controlling asthmatic distress.

For reasons that are not especially clear, the practice of pediatric allergy has lately become one of the major clinical specialties. It could be argued that childhood allergy has always existed but it simply went unrecognized in earlier times. On the other hand, it is reasonable to assume that chemical allergy is much more frequent than formerly because of the great number of new substances being released into the modern environment. Allergic disease is discussed at length in Chapter 15.

It is estimated that two of every three children in regions characterized by seasonal weather changes suffer periodic distress from infections and allergic inflammation of the ears, nose, and throat. In filtering infectious material, the lymphoid tissues in these regions become enlarged. For many years otolaryngologists routinely recommended tonsilectomy and adenoidectomy in children with recurrent problems of this nature. However, this surgery is no longer being advised, except for cases that are unusually severe. Of particular concern in these conditions is the tendency for fluid to accumulate and be retained behind the ear drum. In a procedure considered preferable to resorting to tonsilectomy and adenoidectomy, tubes are now being implanted in children's ears for periods of time in order to maintain drainage of the middle-ear region. It has been pointed out that as the individual proceeds through adolescence, the tonsils and adenoids usually shrink and cause fewer problems. Allowing these tissues to remain aids in filtering out infectious material throughout the remainder of life.

Childhood marks the time of greatest susceptibility to a number of specific infectious diseases. Contagious viral infections, such as mumps, chicken pox, and measles, occur at this time for several reasons. Foremost is the fact that children associate with other children, resulting in spread of contagion; and of course the majority of adults have already been infected with these viruses and consequently have developed immunity to them. Even when adults have escaped these infections, they are usually less likely to contract them for the same reasons that they are less susceptible than children to infectious disease in general.

Several infectious diseases of childhood can be especially serious. This is true of beta-hemolytic streptococcus infections, which in susceptible individuals incite the autoimmune inflammation that characterizes rheumatic fever. As a consequence of rheumatic fever, the heart valves and renal glomeruli can be damaged for life. Various forms of infectious meningitis and encephalitis also are dreaded childhood infections, some of which are of viral etiology, whereas others are of bacterial origin.

Reye syndrome is discussed in Chapter 15. It is a peculiar complication of childhood viral infections. The etiology of Reye syndrome is not fully understood. Processes of the disease lead to widespread damage of the liver and central nervous system, resulting in severely deranged body metabolism, convulsions, and coma. About 40% of the cases are fatal.

It is explained in Chapter 15 that several serious autoimmune diseases appear to be associated with faulty immune reactions to viral infections. Thus MS has been shown to be an aftermath of an invasion of the body by rubella virus sometime during childhood or adolescence. Furthermore, evidence is rapidly accumulating that points to a viral-autoimmune etiology of juvenile-onset diabetes. The mechanism involved is described in Chapter 15.

Accumulating data suggest that many American children are

malnourished, not because they do not eat enough but because they eat too many sugary, salty, and fatty foods. Nutritionists consider malnutritive stress to be a special problem during childhood and early adolescence. Figures from the Francis Stern Nutrition Clinic in Boston indicate that nearly 20% of children aged 6 to 11 are overweight, and nearly the same percentage have high levels of cholesterol in the blood. Furthermore, mineral imbalance in children and adolescents is not uncommon. Deficiencies in iron, magnesium, and zinc have been reported in several studies.

Adolescence is characterized by stresses related to growth processes, endocrine changes, and the need for many emotional adjustments. Puberty is frequently associated with the advent of acne, the need for orthodontic attention, intense peer pressure, changes in sexuality with consequent competition, and the experiencing of new, conflicting emotions that are strong and often labile. Psychosocial stress at this period of life in today's urban setting can be quite severe. The use of tobacco, alcohol, and illegal drugs often begins at this time, which for many individuals signals the start of a downhill course as far as health and freedom from disease is concerned. The incidence of pregnancy, accidents, and suicide continues to rise during adolescence. Fortunately in teenagers with normal constitutions, the homeostatic capacity of the body at this stage of life is strong, enabling the individual to effectively counteract the physiologic effects of emotional tensions and various other abuses. If continued into adulthood, however, these stresses eventually begin to take their toll, and homeostatic responses gradually become less effective.

There are diseases of childhood and adolescence in which little can be done so far as prevention is concerned because the conditions are genetically determined. *Cystic fibrosis* is such a form of pathology. This disorder becomes apparent early in life and is conditioned by the homozygous state of a recessive gene, meaning that the gene is carried by each of two normal parents. Each offspring from such parents has a one-fourth chance of having cystic fibrosis. In this condition there are pathologic changes involving overgrowth of fibrous tissue, accompanied by the development of cystic spaces. The exocrine gland cells are especially affected, resulting in widespread dysfunction throughout the lungs, pancreas, liver, and gastrointestinal tract (Figure 18-2). Glandular oversecretion is common, particularly from the mucous glands of the bronchial passageways. In order to prevent serious pulmonary obstruction, the bronchial secretions must be periodically loosened and mechanically aspirated. Liver cirrhosis, pancreatic deficiency, and abnormally high levels of electrolytes in the sweat are other complications

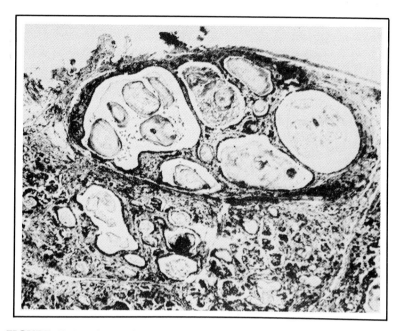

FIGURE 18-2   Cystic fibrosis of the pancreas. Note the presence of large cystic spaces. (From W. Boyd and H. Sheldon, *An introduction to the study of disease.*)

of cystic fibrosis. Although the clinical picture of the disease can be quite variable, the prognosis is poor. Death usually occurs sometime before or during young adulthood.

Hemophilia and sickle-cell anemia are two inherited blood diseases that pose serious problems for afflicted children and adolescents. A mutant, recessive, sex-linked gene determines hemophilia, in which the absence of an enzyme results in an inability of the blood to clot. The sex-linked nature of the disorder means that it is primarily males that are afflicted. Sickle-cell anemia, found primarily in blacks, is discussed in Chapter 9.

The most tragic pathologies of children and adolescents are malignancies, of which the leukemias make up the major portion. *Acute lymphocytic leukemia* is the most common form of childhood cancer. The carcinogenic transformation takes place in lymphoblasts of bone marrow. The disease is characterized by an abrupt onset with a rapid progress. Untreated cases may be fatal within 4 to 5 months of onset, and usually some of the course of the disease has already transpired before diagnosis is made. Intensive chemotherapy is the treatment of choice. Such therapy has yielded long-term

TABLE 18-2
Notable Health Problems of Childhood and Adolescence

CONDITION	CAUSE(S)
Upper respiratory infections	Pathogenic microbes, altered immunity
Asthma and other allergic diseases	Exposure to inhaled and ingested allergens
Rheumatic fever	Complication of strep infections
Chicken pox	Contagious virus
Mumps	Contagious virus
Measles	Contagious virus
Influenza	Contagious virus
Reye syndrome	Complication of virus infections
Juvenile diabetes	Autoimmune complication of virus infection
Malnutrition	Improper diet, or overindulgence in sugar, fats, and salt
Cystic fibrosis	Genetic
Hemophilia	Genetic
Sickle-cell anemia	Genetic
Acne (and scarring)	Overbalance of steroid secretions following puberty
Emotional instability and psychosomatic disorders	Psychologic conflicts of adolescence
Acute lymphocytic leukemia	Not completely understood; radiation exposures

remissions in some instances. *Acute myelogenous leukemia* and *chronic lymphocytic leukemia* are more frequently found in adults than in children. In fact, the chronic leukemias occur most commonly in persons over 35 years of age.

A partial list of major pathologies associated with childhood and adolescence is shown in Table 18-2.

Stress and Disease in the Middle-aged Adult

Much of the discussion throughout this book is probably more applicable to persons of middle age than to individuals of any other stage of life. It is during this time that progressive forms of chronic disease usually make their appearance. By the ages of 35 to 40, it is time to check for hypertension, gastrointestinal ulcers, excessive smoking and drinking, obesity, and elevated blood lipids. Also, mental disorder and autoimmune conditions usually are apparent by this time. By ages 40 to 50, emphysema, cancer, coronary artery disease, kidney disease, and diabetes may have made their appearance, and from 50 to 65 years, the risks of these same disorders become even greater.

Emotional demands are often more pronounced and unrelenting during middle age than at any other period of life. The problems created by the responsibility of teenage children on one hand, and dependent, senile parents on the other hand can make this stage of life quite stressing. In addition, this can be a time of economic strain, and the period may be characterized by depression over failing physical powers as well as boredom and resentment with numerous routine and confining responsibilities.

By the time middle age has arrived, personal habits have become well established and practiced for 20 to 30 years. Exposure to chemical hazards such as toxic substances in the occupational environment has been cumulative over the same amount of time. The middle-aged individual no longer has the adaptive powers of the young adult. After 25 years of confrontation with the various stressors outlined in previous chapters, homeostatic responses have begun to break down and disease becomes recognizable.

FETAL STRESS EFFECTS

Compared to the postnatal organism, the fetus is quite unadaptable. Even minor prenatal stress disturbances could prove to be destructive when the critical developmental changes occurring during this stage are considered. It is only because the fetus is so well protected amid uniform conditions of the intrauterine environment that it usually survives. Even so, stress-induced fetal derangements are not infrequent. What are some of the conditions that threaten fetal homeostasis?

Both the early embryo and the fetus are susceptible to disturbances brought about by most of the stressors already discussed in preceding chapters. In fact, the prenatal organism is much more vulnerable than its postnatal counterpart. One tragic piece of evidence in this regard was the unforeseen fetal effects of the drug thalidomide, sold without prescription to pregnant women as a sleeping tablet and sedative. Extensive testing of the drug in adult animals and humans had revealed no toxic effects, yet severe limb malformations developed in exposed fetuses.

TABLE 18-3
Partial List of Teratogenic Agents

PHYSICAL	INFECTIOUS	TOXIC
Hypobaric atmosphere	Rubella	Carbon monoxide
Radiation	Mumps	Nicotine
Hypothermia	Influenza	Ethanol
Hyperthermia	Syphilis	Acetaldehyde
Excessive sound intensity	Herpes	
	Gonorrhea	
	Chlamydia	
	Toxoplasmosis	
	Hepatitis	

Teratogenicity

Physical, chemical, and infective agents capable of producing embryonic or fetal damage are termed *teratogens.* Teratogenic damage may be immediate or delayed. Some deviations may not become recognizable until postnatal stages are reached. Moreover, the extent of the injury depends upon the stage of gestation during which the damage was inflicted. The first trimester of pregnancy (embryonic period) is most critical as far as risks of anatomic malformations are concerned. Such malformations could include cleft palate, spina bifida, a form of pyloric stenosis, and certain congenital heart defects. Genetic factors may play a role in the production of some of these abnormalities; yet it has been shown that without teratogenic stress, genetic predisposition alone fails in many instances to explain the abnormal development. A partial list of teratogenic agents is presented in Table 18-3.

Environmental stressors may act directly on the fetus or indirectly through the maternal organism. More often it is maternal stress being transferred to the fetus. Conditions most frequently involved in promoting fetal disorders include hypoxia, radiation exposure, hypothermia, infections, vitamin and mineral deficiencies, and drug intake.

PHARMACOLOGIC	HORMONAL
Antibiotics	Insulin deficiency
Tolbutamide	Thyroid deficiency
Amphetamines	Excessive cortisone
Barbiturates	Excessive ACTH
Thalidomide	Excessive catecholamines
LSD	Excessive estrogen
Bromides	
Morphine	
Thiazides	
Reserpine	
Antihistamines	
Anticoagulants	
Aspirin	
Benzodiazepines	
Meprobamate	

Fetal Hypoxia

Without question the foremost teratogenic agent is hypoxia. The causes of fetal hypoxia are listed in Table 18-4. Many experiments with animals strongly indicate that the major risk in fetal hypoxia is an impaired development of the central nervous system. Some of the neural effects of fetal hypoxia in humans may be subtle functional changes that could be variously manifested later as cerebral palsy, epilepsy, and mental retardation. Other effects may be in the form of organic alterations occurring early enough to produce encephalic malformations.

The developing brain of the hypoxic rat is low in total protein, DNA, and RNA, whereas studies of neonatal humans thought to have been hypoxic during fetal life have revealed a marked deficiency in nerve fiber myelination and an impairment in acetylcholinesterase activity. One of the more common causes of antepartum hypoxia is smoking during pregnancy. Carbon monoxide in the smoke promotes anemic hypoxia.

Aside from neural effects, fetal development in general can be retarded by hypoxic stress. The hypoxic fetus is usually less mature at delivery than it would have been otherwise. The birth weight is reduced, and there are greater risks of all the problems that can accompany prematurity.

TABLE 18-4
Major Causes of Fetal Hypoxia

Maternal anemia

Toxemia of pregnancy

Maternal pulmonary impairment

Cardiovascular insufficiency

Impaired placental function

Exposure to high altitude

Maternal exposure to carbon monoxide

Fetal Effects from Radiation

Exposure to radiation during pregnancy is responsible for more fetal damage than is generally acknowledged. A. C. Upton, Director of the National Cancer Institute, considers that prenatal exposure to an x-ray dose of only 1 rad is associated with a 50% increase in the risk of childhood leukemia. The leukemia can become evident within 2 to 4 years after exposure and reaches a peak within the first 10 years of life. Exposure to radiation during pregnancy has also been linked to derangements in the development of the fetal nervous system. Nerve fiber myelination and cholinergic transmission are severely altered in experimental exposures of fetal animals to x-rays. In these types of experiments the radiation doses are quite low; indeed, they are insufficient for producing any known effect on the adult organism.

Damage from Infections and Immune Reactions

Among the maternal infections having the greatest risk to the fetus during pregnancy are rubella (measles) and syphilis, both of which are capable of inflicting severe fetal damage. Cephalic malformations, cataracts, blindness, deafness, and severe mental retardation can result from these infections.

Certain immune interactions between the fetus and the maternal organism also can produce fetal injury, sometimes with surprising severity. The most noted example is *erythroblastosis fetalis*, a condition in which the red blood cells of the fetus agglutinate, resulting in an inability of the fetal blood to transport oxygen. This condition is one of the more common causes of stillbirth. In milder cases of erythroblastosis fetalis, the individual may be born alive but there can be impaired mentality. In this disorder the red blood cell agglutination is brought about by maternal Rh antibodies, developed from previous maternal exposure to Rh antigens. When there are two pregnancies, closely spaced in time, and in each pregnancy there is an Rh positive fetus developing in an Rh negative mother, then the second pregnancy stands a high risk of fetal erythroblastosis because the mother's blood was sensitized to Rh antigen during the first pregnancy.

Drug Use During Pregnancy

The use of prescribed or illegal drugs during pregnancy is contraindicated because most of these substances are potential teratogens (Table 18-3). Even use of salicylates (aspirin) is inadvisable. The fetus is vulnerable to any molecule capable of crossing the placental barrier. This includes all materials with molecular weights of 1000 or less.

Neurotropic drugs, so frequently prescribed today, have been shown to produce various adverse effects in experiments with fetal animals. Barbiturates, benzodiazepines, and amphetamines unquestionably provoke biochemical disturbances in the developing nervous system of the fetal animal. For example, the characteristic potentiation of rat locomotor responses and acoustic reflexes that normally appear in the third postnatal week was absent in animals exposed to diazepam (Valium) during the third week of gestation.

In the past, prescriptions for amphetaminelike substances were sometimes written for pregnant women at a time when it was fashionable to gain very little weight during pregnancy. One can only speculate upon the possible relationship of such a practice to the rising incidence of hyperkinesis and mental deviations that began to become more noticeable in children during the past 20 years.

Consumption of alcoholic beverages by women during pregnancy has been widely described as a significant threat to normal fetal development, and the constellation of anomalies in infants born to women drinkers has been labeled the *fetal alcohol syndrome* (FAS). The three major postnatal signs of FAS are central nervous system dysfunction, growth deficiencies, and facial malformations.

Maternal Nutrition

The relationship of maternal nutrition to fetal stress is a somewhat controversial subject. Although adequate maternal nutrition during pregnancy is important and certainly advisable, some physiologists point out that when the maternal nutrition is marginal, or even faulty, it is the mother who suffers much more than the fetus, in view of the known fetal priority for available nutrients. Along the same line of argument, it has been mentioned that among the over-populated, semistarved masses, procreation does not suffer; indeed, it appears to flourish. It is after birth that the malnutrition becomes a problem. On the other hand, there are data from numerous experiments with animals in which it would appear that fetal maturation as well as postnatal vigor and resistance to stress can be improved with optimum maternal nutrition during pregnancy, particularly in regard to minerals, vitamins, and protein quality. Of course, over-nutrition and excessive weight during pregnancy are undesirable for both fetus and mother.

Fetal Effects from Maternal Emotions

Another controversial subject in regard to adverse fetal effects is the role played by psychologic tensions of the mother during preg-nancy. As one can surmise from the nature of the matter, it is diffi-cult to determine if a cause and effect relationship exists between the two variables. Investigations with rabbits have shown that chronic fear reactions during gestation have been associated with a much greater than average percentage of defects appearing in both the fetus and the postnatal animal. Results have not been as striking in experiments with rats and dogs. We do know that intense emotional stress, especially when prolonged, can result in serious endocrine imbalances and other biochemical disturbances within the body. In pregnancies filled with emotional upsets it is certainly conceivable that the fetus would not be totally exempt from effects that may arise from the resultant chemical imbalances.

Stress During the Perinatal Period

Commensurate with the importance of fetal effects is a consideration of the stress imposed upon the organism during the transition from prenatal to postnatal life. Despite its brevity the intrapartum period is very stressful. Psychologists have made much of the idea that the transition to the outside world from the security of the womb is a most traumatic event as far as the human nervous system is con-cerned. It is true that the intrapartum interval itself together with a perinatal period of several postpartum days is especially critical and require a multitude of physiologic adjustments on the part of the

TABLE 18-5

Conditions of Prenatal and Postnatal Life

	PRENATAL	POSTNATAL
Physical environment	Fluid	Gaseous
External temperature	Constant	Fluctuates with atmospheric changes
Sensory stimulation	Very little (tactile, hearing)	Various senses stimulated by variety of stimuli
Nutrition	Hematotropic source (maternal circulation)	Depends upon food availability, ingestion, and gastrointestinal function
Oxygen supply	Maternal circulation to fetal blood stream	Atmosphere to lung to blood
Metabolic elimination	Discharged to maternal circulation	Eliminated by lung, skin, kidneys, and GI tract

neonatal organism. Some of the major adjustments are summarized in Table 18-5.

The premature infant is especially vulnerable to perinatal stresses. The normal period of human gestation is about 38 weeks. Infants delivered before the 35th week are considered premature. The major problems associated with prematurity are related to insufficient development of the respiratory, thermoregulatory, and gastrointestinal functions. Immune responses also may be underdeveloped, subjecting the newborn to a greater susceptibility to infection. Because of this the infant must be kept in a relatively aseptic environment.

Establishing a normal pattern of respiration is of particular importance in the premature infant. Oxygen may be administered in cases of cyanosis. However, this procedure is performed less frequently than formerly. When oxygen is necessary, caution must be exercised in preventing delivery of excessive amounts. A severe form of respiratory failure in newborns, *hyaline membrane disease* (also known as *respiratory distress syndrome*), results in thousands of deaths each year. Most of these casualties are premature infants. In hyaline membrane disease there is insufficient formation of surfactant in the fluid lining the alveoli. Surfactant, a lipoprotein, counteracts the surface tension of the fluid as the alveoli retract during exhalation; otherwise the alveoli collapse.

About 50% of newborns become jaundiced during the first few days of the perinatal period when the hepatic enzyme systems are immature and therefore less effective in metabolizing bilirubin.

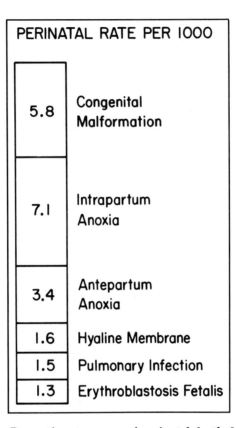

FIGURE 18-3 **Proportionate causes of perinatal death.** Insufficient oxygen during delivery is the major cause. Observe that the last four causes all relate in some way to inadequate lung ventilation or deranged blood gas transport. (Modified from P. S. Timeras, *Developmental physiology and aging*, New York: The Macmillan Co., 1972.)

Thermoregulation also may be a problem in newborns. The premature infant can neither shiver nor sweat. Because of the danger a chill represents, premature infants are usually kept under controlled temperature and humidity conditions in an incubator.

Perinatal mortality has decreased significantly in the last half century, although practically all the improvement came about prior to 1965. Since that time decreases have been minimal. The relative distribution of causes of death during the perinatal period is shown in Figure 18-3.

The period of gestation is stressing to the maternal organism as well as to the fetus. Maternal kidney mechanisms are strained, and there is perpetual risk of depleted nutrients in the expectant mother. Maternal predisposition to diabetes is usually revealed during pregnancy.

PHYSIOLOGIC AND BIOCHEMICAL BASES OF AGING

At present a great deal of attention is being focused upon the many problems associated with aging. Psychologists, sociologists, economists, government agencies, physiologists, nurses, and other health professionals are becoming increasingly concerned with the special needs of our burgeoning number of senior citizens. With each passing year the elderly constitute a progressively greater proportion of the populace. It is estimated that one of every three hospital patients exceeds the age of 55.

Growing old and dying is an evitable part of any organism's life history. Strictly speaking, the aging process begins when the individual's life begins. However, use of the term *aging* is usually reserved in reference to the later years of life when functional abilities typically begin to fail. How do physiologic stress and susceptibility to disease fit into this period of life? Before addressing ourselves more directly to this important question, let us investigate what is known of aging in terms of the underlying physiologic and biochemical changes and their causes.

Voluminous material has been written about the histology, physiology, biochemistry, and genetics of aging. Though aging is inevitable, the indomitable spirit of scientific inquiry demands that only by probing and understanding the biologic changes manifested in the process can there ever be hope of arresting, or at least delaying, the physical and mental deterioration that so often accompanies growing old.

A number of theories have been advanced as an explanation for aging. In actuality no one explanation is sufficient to account for the phenomenon. All proposed theories probably contribute to the overall picture. Indeed, there appears to be a strong interwoven relationship among the various theories (Figure 18-4).

Genetic Theory

Many evolutionary biologists and geneticists maintain that biochemical changes underlying the aging process are programmed in the DNA of cell nuclei, just as all developmental processes appear to

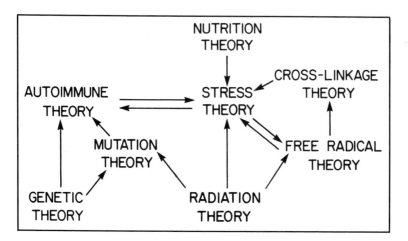

FIGURE 18-4   Theories of aging and their relationships. For an explanation of each theory and its relationship to the others, see the text.

be programmed. In support of this idea is the observation that natural selection is based upon reproduction, not prolonged survival of the individual. Hence there is no evolutionary advantage in longevity of an individual. There is no questioning the validity of the broader aspects of this concept; yet how far can one go with the idea in explaining individual variation in the rate of aging? Furthermore, what are the mechanisms by which genes bring about physiologic and biochemical changes that characterize senescence? Some biologists conceive the existence of what they term *aging genes* that are "turned on" as the later stages of life are approached, but this explanation seems an oversimplification. Others contend that as the cell ages, errors in DNA transcription to RNA and protein inevitably accumulate. According to this scheme, the more the errors in transcription, the more the aging of the cell, which in turn enhances more faulty transcription: it is an example of a typical positive feedback cycle.

On the other hand, there are developmental biologists who are wary of too much dependency upon the idea of strict gene determination of aging and cell death. They point out that though cell necrosis may appear to be a part of normal development of organs, it can be prevented by transplanting embryonic parts to other locations in the body, indicating that cellular changes leading to death are greatly influenced by environmental conditions.

Free Radical Theory

Several lines of evidence suggest that free radicals produced by lipid peroxidation progressively promote the cellular alterations that are commonly observed in aging.[1] Formation of free radicals is known to damage cell membranes by oxidizing the membrane lipids. The peroxidation of lipid can lead to a buildup of fluorescent pigments within cells. A common pigment of this type, *lipofuscin*, accumulates during senescence. Lipofuscin is especially abundant in nerve tissue of the elderly. It also appears to accumulate linearly with age in the myocardium (Figure 18-5). When lipid breakdown from free radicals occurs in the cell, the repair or removal of the damaged material is brought about by the autophagocytic action of lysosomes. When lysosomal enzymes have hydrolyzed peroxidated material, the lysosome complex becomes known as a *residual body*. It has been revealed that the lipofuscin pigments of aging are, in actuality, residual bodies. A possible reason for the pigment being so common in nerve tissue is that neurons have no cell turnover. Therefore, such cells must depend upon excellent mechanisms for repair in order to remain functional.

It has been debated whether lipid peroxidation from free radicals is a cause of aging or merely an associated phenomenon. Likewise, the accumulation of lipofuscin is looked upon by some investigators as more a result of the aging process than a cause of it. This uncertainty aside, it has been clearly demonstrated that the accumulation of lipofuscin in senescence seriously aggravates the course of pathologic changes brought about by other agents.

The acknowledged role of free radicals in aging offers support for the idea that environmental stress is instrumental in determining the rate of the aging process. As pointed out in earlier chapters, exposure to radiation, hyperoxia, drugs, and other environmental chemicals promotes the formation of damaging free radicals. Some degree of protection from peroxidation is afforded by lipid-soluble antioxidants such as alpha-tocopherol (vitamin E), which is known to bind free radicals, thereby reducing the oxidation of unsaturated fatty acids in the cell (see Chapter 11). The result of such protection is a stabilization of membrane function. Experiments with animals have indicated that an inclusion of antioxidants in the diet can increase the mean life span by 15% to 30%. Incorporation of

---

1Free radicals are discussed in Chapters 2, 6, and 9.

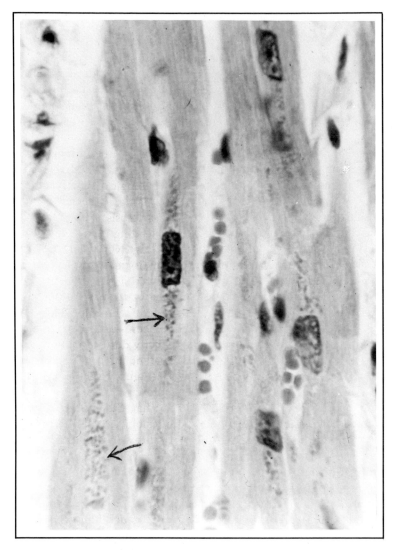

FIGURE 18-5 **Lipofuscin granules in cardiac muscle.** Arrows point to clusters of granules along the muscle fibers of an elderly subject. (Photograph by Dr. R. R. Kohn, Institute of Pathology, Case Western University School of Medicine, Cleveland, Ohio.)

these substances in animal food also can significantly reduce the incidence of tumorigenesis. Despite these interesting results, the effect of increasing dietary antioxidants in humans is uncertain at present.

Cross-Linkage—Connective Tissue Theory

Many studies have revealed that as cells age, smaller molecules have been shown to react with two macromolecules so as to effect a chemical cross-link between the larger moieties, thereby reducing their mobility and promoting formation of aggregates, which assume entirely different diffusion, permeability, and solvation properties than formerly.[2] For example, cross-linkage of DNA strands may result in mutation or even cell death.

Cross-linkage has received the most attention in respect to the proteins of connective tissue, especially collagen. As the organism ages, some of the most prominent histological and histochemical changes are to be found in connective tissue, in which a process of hardening and loss of elasticity leads to sclerosis. The process may be especially pronounced in the arteries, leading to arteriosclerosis, and in the skin dermis, leading to wrinkling. Not only is there an increased fibrous content of the connective tissue cells, but there is a highly significant increase in the cross-linking of collagen molecules. The consequence is a loss of elasticity and an increase in collagen fiber stability which is quite apparent when the material is subjected to physicochemical tests. It has been shown that these altered properties of aging collagen are directly due to the total number and chemical nature of the covalent intramolecular and intermolecular cross-links of the collagen (Figure 18-6).

A number of biochemists favor the cross-linkage theory of aging. They contend that the consequent hardening of connective tissue, particularly in key structures such as blood vessels, underlies much of the progressive physiologic failure characterizing senescence.

Mutation Theory

Mutation theory is somewhat related to the genetic theory, already discussed. Cell mutations accumulate during the life span, many of which are known to adversely affect the organism through two mechanisms. For one, there are alterations in enzyme production and action. There are numerous accounts describing a reduction of enzymatic activity of cells as they age. The repair capability for mutagenic alterations is especially critical. Indeed, there is a strong cor-

---

2When polar or ionizable atomic groups of a small molecule are adjacent to polar or ionizable atomic groups of macromolecules on either side of the small molecule, weak bonding may link the three moieties.

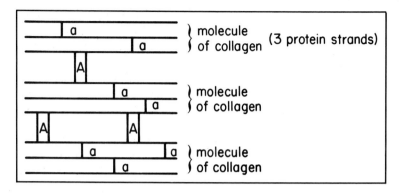

FIGURE 18-6   Simplified model of cross-linkage of collagen. A= the three molecules of collagen, which are cross-linked together by intermolecular linkages. a= protein strands within each molecule, which are intramolecularly cross-linked.

relation between the repair capability of UV-induced thymine dimers and the life span of the organism.[3]

A second possible aging effect of mutagenesis is related to impairment of immune function. The role of the immune system in aging is discussed later.

Radiation Theory

In certain respects exposure to radiation can be seen as a common denominator in some of the other theories of aging. Ionizing radiation significantly enhances the cellular production of both free radicals and mutations. Moreover, cross-linkage of macromolecules can be mediated by free radicals. Irradiated animals do exhibit a significantly decreased life expectancy due to an acceleration of aging (Figure 18-7). Japanese who were exposed to the atomic blasts at Hiroshima and Nagasaki are dying at ages significantly younger than would ordinarily be expected. It is thought that even the natural radiation present throughout a life span is of consequence in promoting changes that characterize aging.

Recent experimental evidence indicates that exposure to irradiation in some manner causes fat deposition and increased body weight, conditions that are known to promote premature onset of various degenerative diseases. Radiation is discussed in Chapter 6.

3One of the more common mutagenic alterations in DNA is the formation of bonds between two thymine nucleotides. Thymine is a pyrimidine in DNA. The DNA usually has some capability in reversing this change, however.

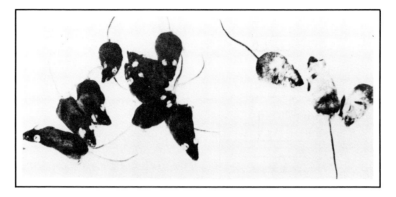

FIGURE 18-7   Effect of radiation exposure on aging. Nine young mice were given sublethal doses of ionizing radiation, and nine others (controls) were unexposed. *Left,* the controls are healthy and vigorous at 14 months of age. By 14 months, six of the exposed animals had died of old-age complications, and the remaining three, *at right,* are feeble and gray, exhibiting numerous signs of extreme aging. (Research photograph of Dr. Howard J. Curtis.)

Autoimmune Theory

The production of autoantibodies has been shown to increase with age, leading to greater risks of autoimmune damage in geriatric patients. As one grows older, thymic involution occurs, and there is a gradual decline in the production of T lymphocytes. With progressive age one also begins to lose some of the specific immunity offered by IgG and therefore must rely to a greater extent on IgM response, which is usually associated more with autoimmune phenomena. Not only do these changes subject the individual to a greater likelihood of autoimmune damage, but there are increased risks of tumorigenesis and susceptibility to microbial infections as well. Autoimmunity is thoroughly discussed in Chapter 15.

It has been demonstrated that older mice routinely produce lymphocytes that attack self. Moreover, when tumor cells are injected into a young mouse along with lymphocytes from old animals, the tumor development is enhanced, indicating that old lymphocytes in combination with tumor cells may cause the normal immunity to fail. These data confirm the concept that aging is associated with misfiring of the immune system. However, in associations of this kind we are again faced with the question of cause and effect. Do changes in immunity cause aging, or does aging bring about changes in immune competence?

Stress Theory

Stress theory emphasizes that the changes characterizing senescence are primarily a result of the constant but losing battle that engages the body in its effort to resist a more stable state, thermodynamically. In aging, stresses progressively overcome homeostatic forces, just as occurs in chronic disease. The second law of thermodynamics is not to be denied!

The stress theory is supported by most physiologists and especially by Hans Selye and his school. According to this view, accumulated wear and tear eventually exceeds the organism's capacity to repair. Connective tissue, nerve and muscle, in which there is little or no turnover of cells, are the tissues most affected by environmental stressors, and it is these tissues that show the most prominent changes in later life. Of special interest is the evidence that accumulation of the old-age pigment, lipofuscin, can result from stress, such as endocrine imbalances following cortisone injections, from chronic hypoxia, or from the administration of acetanilide, an analgesic prescribed for rheumatism.

There are volumes of data indicating that the rate of aging can be strongly influenced by exposure to stressors. It has been shown without question that chronic exposure to radiation, psychosocial stress, cold temperature, altitude hypoxia, physical fatigue, tobacco smoke, excessive food intake, infectious disease, and/or numerous drugs significantly accelerate the rate of aging in most individuals (animals or human).

Closely allied with the stress theory is the role of endocrine changes in senescence. Diseases of aging that have been linked to endocrine causes are osteoporosis, diabetes, hypertension, and some cancers. The synthesis and release of certain hormones does diminish with age. Moreover, with advancing years, membrane receptors of target cells do not bind hormones as effectively. Women experience a rather abrupt hormonal decline associated with menopause. Although men may suffer various physical and psychologic complaints during middle age, testosterone concentrations do not appear to be significantly diminished at this time.

Many older persons progressively accumulate fat due to shifts in metabolic regulation and sedentary habits. Along this line it may be recalled that middle-age stress enhances pituitary secretion of beta-endorphin and ACTH, which, along with excessive insulin, is thought to be associated with patterns of obesity that sometimes characterize older individuals. However, in regard to fat accumulation it must also be pointed out that thyroid responses characteristically decrease in later years. Even though insulin may be adequate or even excessive in quantity, responsiveness to its action is dulled in older persons, possibly because their cells have fewer receptors for binding insulin. Likewise, responsiveness to adrenal and pituitary hormones often declines with age, despite what may appear to be normal hormonal levels in the blood. Interestingly, in *progeria*, a syndrome characterized by what appears to be extremely accelerated aging, there is a pronounced reduction in tissue response to all hormones.

Nutrition Theory

A number of investigations with animals have demonstrated that the rate of the aging process and the length of life can be varied by manipulating the diet. Experiments with rats have clearly indicated that restricted caloric intake in weanlings increases the maximum life span to approximately twice that of the control animals. Restricting calories to 40% of the normal intake has the greatest effect, especially when the diet is relatively low in protein and fat. Of course, the delayed senescence observed in these experiments could be related to the absence of obesity, which protects lean animals from cardiovascular, renal, and malignant pathology, diseases ordinarily associated with advancing age. Investigations of tumorigenesis in rats are especially revealing in respect to hypercaloric intake and obesity. It has been shown that early caloric restriction inhibits tumorigenic cells. Furthermore, a positive correlation of obesity with the development of malignant disease is clearly apparent. Calorie-restricted rats do not develop tumors as often as those that are generously fed; indeed, the incidence of certain kinds of malignant growths can be predicted from knowing an animal's weight at 10 weeks of age.

In our later years the BMR progressively decreases, and the body constituent that tends to undergo a major increase is fat, given circumstances of unhampered access to food. Measurements of skin folds and body density reveal that as one surpasses the age of 40, the muscle to fat ratio begins to decrease rather sharply.

Recommended dietary allowances for individuals past 50 years of age are listed in Table 18-6.

Cell Replacement in Aging

Not only are manifestations of aging related to failing homeostatic responses of cells, but there is also a decrease in the number of functioning cells. The number of cells is determined by the balance be-

TABLE 18-6

Recommended Dietary Allowances for Persons over 50 Years

	MEN	WOMEN
Calories (kcal)	2,200	1,600
Protein (g)	50	45
Vitamin A (IU)	5,000	4,000
Vitamin E (IU)	30	30
Ascorbic acid (mg)	60	60
Niacin (mg)	16	13
Riboflavin (mg)	1.5	1.4
Thiamine (mg)	1.2	1.0
Calcium (mg)	800	800
Iron (mg)	10	10

Source: Recommended Dietary Allowances, National Academy of Science, Washington, D.C., 1980.

tween new cell production and the death of old cells. This balance shifts as age progresses. Frequency of cell division becomes limited. Some biologists consider diminished mitotic activity to be a normal, genetically programmed event. However, manipulation of the chemical environment can influence the rate of cell production. Adding large quantities of alpha-tocopherol (vitamin E) has been shown to double the number of times cultured cells divide.

Chronologic Versus Biologic Age

All of us know persons who do not look their age. And there are others who look and act much older than the calendar indicates. Obviously biologic aging does not precisely match the passing of time as measured chronologically. Merely knowing that a person is 45 years of age will not tell us the degree of aging going on in the cells and body fluids of that individual. In one such person the arteries may be loaded with atherosclerotic plaques, whereas in another the arteries may be relatively free of this sign of aging.

Premature aging characterized by such changes as cataracts and atherosclerosis can occur in individuals with metabolic disturbances, such as uncontrolled diabetes mellitus. Moreover, there are rare disorders in which certain changes usually associated with aging occur with extreme rapidity. The aforementioned progeria is an example. When present in juveniles, this condition is termed *Hutchinson-Gilford syndrome.* It is characterized by deceleration of growth, severe atherosclerosis, hyperlipidemia, lipofuscin accumulation, connective tissue fibrosis, and much cross-linking of collagen.

A form of progeria developing somewhat later in life is known as *Werner syndrome*. Each form of progeria is quite rare and appears to be genetically determined. Both forms lead to early demise of the individual. An affliction somewhat similar in appearance to progeria is *Cockayne syndrome,* diagnosed only 50 times since its discovery 43 years ago. In this genetic disorder the body appears to age at a fantastic rate of about 18 years of aging for every year of life. The cells of victims of Cockayne syndrome cannot adequately replace or repair themselves, resulting in rapid degenerative changes. Children with the affliction suffer from arthritis, cataracts, glaucoma, hearing loss, hypertension, receding gums, and arteriosclerosis. A 5-year-old victim of Cockayne syndrome, who has since died, is depicted in Figure 18-8.

Both progeria and Cockayne syndrome have been looked upon by some pathologists as a disease model for aging. Others doubt that these disorders serve as genuine examples of accelerated aging.

AGING, STRESS, AND DISEASE

There are parallels, as well as interactions, between disease and aging. Disease can promote premature aging. In turn, old age invites disease. In some of the broader aspects, disease and aging may appear to be indistinguishable. Of the two, aging is usually considered to be the more inevitable; however, disease of some form and degree is also eventual. Disturbances that we attribute to aging in the elderly are looked upon as disease in younger individuals.

In both disease and aging, homeostasis is progressively jeopardized. Steady-state balances are much more precarious in older persons than in younger ones. In advanced age a minor disturbance such as body chill, emotional upset, or a viral infection can initiate a loss of homeostatic control that the older body is slow in restoring. Before homeostasis can be reestablished, a chain of positive feedbacks may be launched. Under the circumstances a new, less effective steady state may be the utmost that the body can manage; and a compromised steady state is always more precarious than the original point of balance.

It stands to reason, then, that persons in the later stages of life are much more vulnerable to physiologic stress and much more susceptible to chronic degenerative diseases than are younger persons. Data clearly bear this out. The two major forms of pathology in in-

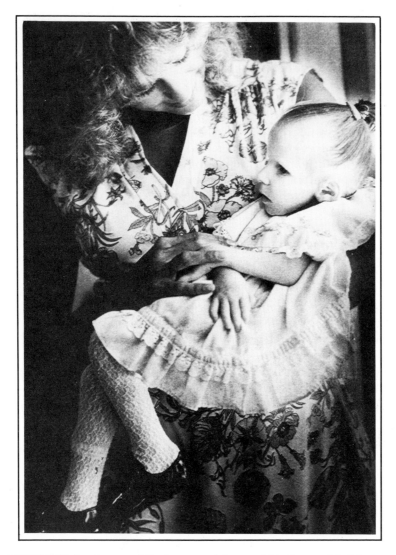

FIGURE 18-8   A case of Cockayne syndrome. This 5-year-old girl
suffered from a disorder that greatly accelerates aging processes. She
showed many degenerative changes that ordinarily are found in persons
85 to 90 years of age. (Courtesy World Wide Photos.)

dustrialized regions, cardiovascular disease and cancer, are prepon-
derant among individuals exceeding 50 years of age. Both forms of
pathology usually develop rather slowly, suggesting that it takes a
while for the counteracting resistances of the body to progressively

weaken. In this light we must consider that chronic physiologic stresses are not only important in promoting disease, but they also appear to have much to do with the rate of physiologic and biochemical changes that characterize aging.

Some Pathophysiologic Features of Senescence

Most prominent among diseases accounting for death in aging humans are arteriosclerosis, cancer, diabetes, hypertension, and renal disease. Four of these involve the blood vessels and therefore are interrelated, cancer being excepted. From this information one would surmise that we tend to go as far in length of life as our blood vessels will take us. With a decline in blood perfusion, the tissues become less effective in exchanging materials. This situation seriously jeopardizes homeostasis.

There is a pronounced decline in adaptation, physiologic and mental, in most persons of advanced age. Many organs begin to show atrophy and involution. This is not without exception, however. The prostate gland in elderly men tends to become hypertrophic, not atrophic. Some of the more striking functional declines in older individuals are related to pulmonary reserve, glomerular filtration rate, muscular strength, cardiac output, BMR, velocity of nerve conduction, and memory (Figure 18-9). In addition, there is always some degree of compromise in acuity of the special senses, vision and hearing. Furthermore, the emotions and mental adjustment of the elderly often become a major source of difficulty, not only for the geriatric patients themselves, but also for those with the responsibility of caring for these patients. *Agitated depression* is particularly common in older age. Recently it has been demonstrated that monoamine oxidase, the enzyme involved in catecholamine degradation, is significantly elevated in many older persons, and it is believed that excessive catecholamine degradation in certain brain centers causes depression. In addition, alteration of monoamine metabolism may lower the threshold for the induction of extrapyramidal symptoms. It is these symptoms that characterize Parkinson disease.

The nervous system is invariably impaired to some degree in elderly persons. Periodic ataxia, tremor, slowed reflexes, and poor autonomic regulation are not uncommon in persons past 70 years of age. Also, the brain weight decreases and the lipid turnover within it becomes diminished (Figure 18-10). The occurrence of impaired short-term memory is practically universal in older people. Although there is speculation that cross-linkage of DNA in the brain

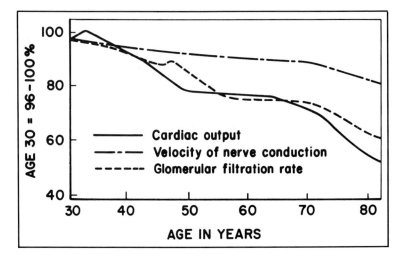

FIGURE 18-9 **Average decline in three physiologic reserves due to aging.** Prime reserve is the equivalent of 100 on the graph. Note the obvious decline in cardiac output by age 50, and the diminished glomerular filtration by age 55. After 70, all three parameters show further reduction.

occurs, memory defects are more often attributed to varied degrees of cerebral hypoxia. Indeed, one of the most dreaded complications of old age, *senile dementia*, is thought to be due to progressive cerebral ischemia from arteriosclerosis. The eventual mental deterioration in this condition is associated with gradual atrophy of the basal ganglia and portions of the cerebral cortex. Senile dementia may persist for as long as 10 years after the onset of symptoms, which initially include confusion, impaired memory, and poor judgment. A recent study of brain tissue taken at autopsy has showed that the dendritic trees of pyramidal neurons in the parahippocampalgyrus of persons with senile dementia are less extensive than in adult brains in general; whereas these dendritic trees are more extensive than average in nondemented persons of advanced age.

Psychopharmacologic, biochemical, and electrophysiologic studies suggest that cholinergic dysfunction may play a role in memory impairment of the elderly, and there is one form of dementia found in some elderly persons that appears to be associated with both a deficiency of the neurotransmitter, acetylcholine, and an accumulation of aluminum deposits among the neurons of the brain. This condition is known as *Alzheimer disease*. It is responsible for at least half the cases of senile dementia, and at present about one of every six persons over age 65 has some degree of senile dementia.

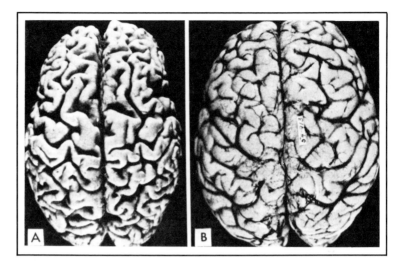

FIGURE 18-10   **Brain atrophy in old age.** A. The shrunken brain of an 82-year-old man. Note how the meninges have been stripped. B. The normal brain of a 36-year-old male. (From S. L. Robbins and R. S. Cotran, *Pathologic basis of disease.*)

Occasionally Alzheimer disease is found in persons younger than 65 to 70 years of age.

It has already been pointed out that the immune system develops deficiencies in elderly persons, leading to greater susceptibility to infections, autoimmunity, and cancer. The decline is due to selective changes in certain T lymphocyte functions, including their inability to proliferate and to promote B lymphocyte differentiation.

Some degree of COPD is often present in elderly persons. Indeed, all parameters of pulmonary function remarkably decline as one ages. The fact that maximal oxygen consumption (VO_2) decreases by over one-third from age 30 to 60 indicates a substantial reduction in exercise capacity.

The gastrointestinal system frequently becomes troublesome in old age. Gallstones, poor digestion, hiatal hernia, constipation, and diverticulosis are common complaints. Because of compromised digestion and absorption, nutritional deficiencies may develop. Elderly persons do best when eating small quantities of balanced nutrients regularly. Some seem to show a relaxing benefit from small amounts of alcoholic beverages.

Other pathologic developments of increasing incidence as one grows older include diabetes mellitus, hypothyroidism, and urogenital problems. The incidence of bladder neck obstruction, urinary tract infections, and urination frequency increase in old age. These conditions may be associated with difficulty in voiding and/or incontinence.

Degenerative changes in the skeleton, joints, and cardiovascular system are practically universal in persons past 60 years of age. Indeed, osteoporosis and osteoarthritis are considered to be normal changes associated with advancing years. *Osteoporosis* occurs much earlier in women than men. The process, in which there is a progressive demineralization of the skeleton, may begin before the age of 40 in some women. The rate of osteoporosis is increased following the advent of menopause; hence, hormonal changes are suspected.

As explained in Chapter 5, the development of cardiovascular pathology is inevitable provided one lives long enough. The aging heart muscle reveals infiltrations of fat and connective tissue, along with degeneration and atrophy of the fibers themselves. In addition, the valves undergo progressive fibrosis. Varied degrees of cardiac arrhythmia can be detected in most persons of advanced age, and by the eighth decade of life the cardiac output may decrease to half of normal. Changes in the blood vessels are even more striking. Some degree of atherosclerosis, the primary cause of arteriosclerosis, occurs in most persons by age 60 to 65. Coronary arteries, abdominal aorta, and arterial branches are the favored sites. Furthermore, blood levels of cholesterol progressively rise with age, particularly between the ages of 40 to 60 (Table 18-7).

It has been estimated that with each 5 years of aging, the peripheral resistance to blood flow increases by 5%. The consequence is a tendency for the blood pressure to rise year by year, eventually surpassing the normal limit of 140/90 torr in many individuals.

The decline in kidney function is about as striking as that shown by the heart (Figure 18-9). After age 70 the rate of glomerular filtration is only about 50% of the rate at age 40. Renal blood flow decreases from about 1100 ml/min at age 30 to only 475 ml/min at age 80, and the renal tubules are less able to concentrate the tubular fluid. The primary pathologic change in aging kidneys involves sclerosis of the glomeruli and their consequent loss of function.

Therapy in Senescence

There is no cure for old age. However, there are measures that may be effective in delaying the advent of age-related pathology. Also, there are means of relieving some of the suffering, and making the

TABLE 18-7

Increase in Average Serum Cholesterol (mg/dl) with Age

AGE IN YRS	MEN	WOMEN
0–12	194	197
13–19	197	198
20–29	227	224
30–39	242	230
40–49	246	215
50–59	254	272
60–69	259	265
70–79	258	275

Source: Combined data from several selected populations.

geriatric patient more comfortable. At present much attention is being devoted to the possibility of delaying the aging process through preventive measures. These include dietary discretion, exercise, not smoking, and a life-style that minimizes psychosocial stress. Presumably such measures would significantly increase longevity, and they certainly would improve the quality of life during later years. Research in this field is in its infancy, so it remains to be seen just how effective preventive efforts will prove to be. Preliminary data do suggest that weight control and exercise can do much to forestall age-related cardiovascular pathology.

In choosing therapeutic strategies for the elderly, basic underlying problems must be considered. Such problems stem primarily from tissue hypoxia, accumulation of free radicals, and disturbances in the macromolecular systems in the brain. Hypoxia, of course, is essentially a consequence of the vascular pathology associated with old age. Cellular hypoxia promotes degenerative damage and eventual necrosis of tissue, and cerebral hypoxia underlies senile dementia. Administration of hyperbaric oxygen is the therapy for problems stemming from tissue hypoxia. Such therapy has been successful in most instances, yet caution must be exercised in using the procedure, especially over lengthy periods. Otherwise, resulting hyperoxia may greatly increase the formation of free radicals.

Theoretically, a high intake of antioxidants such as alpha-tocopherol (vitamin E) should suppress the formation of cellular free radicals in elderly patients. Work with animals and test-tube preparations clearly show that antioxidants do significantly reduce cellular peroxidation, thereby protecting cell membranes from degenerative damage. Furthermore, the use of high dosages of antioxidants in the diet of mice delays aging and increases the life span of these animals. Whether such a procedure is effective in humans is not yet known. Controlled experimentation with humans is difficult to perform rigorously; and the usual length of human life means that many years are required to obtain results and evaluate the findings.

In view of the concept that adequate synthesis of RNA and protein in the cerebrum is necessary for normal long-term memory, it is deduced that memory impairment in old age may be related to disturbances in macromolecular systems of the brain. Accordingly, drugs such as procaine, known to prevent polyribosome instability, have been used to improve the memory of geriatric patients. At present, a procaine derivative, Gerovital H_3, is undergoing testing for potential use as a memory restorer.

The agitated depression in elderly persons often responds to use of monoamine oxidase inhibitors and the tricyclic antidepressants imipramine and amitriptyline. Such treatment brightens the patient's mental outlook and restores restful sleep at night. Persons of advanced age are especially fragile as far as mental stress is concerned. The elderly do not adapt well to change, and they frequently must be reassured.

Other therapeutic measures frequently employed in the care of aged individuals include hormonal preparations, large dosages of vitamins, and drugs that enhance vasodilation. The overall effectiveness of these measures may be questionable, although some benefit has been claimed. Long-term administration of steroid hormones is not advisable, and sustained use of estrogens and glucocorticoids may do more harm than good (see Chapter 14).

| | SUMMARY

The particular developmental stage of an organism is an essential variable in determining susceptibility to stress and disease. Because of their immature immune systems, children are especially vulnerable to infectious disease and allergic sensitivity.

Social adjustments required during adolescent years make this period one of marked vulnerability to psychosocial stress. There is a special risk of teenage pregnancy, alcohol and drug abuse, and suicide. The bodies of adolescents and young adults, however, have stronger homeostatic capability than do those of individuals of any other age.

Compared to the postnatal organism, the fetus is very unadaptable to environmental change. Physical, chemical, and infective agents capable of stressing the developing fetus are termed teratogens.

Important teratogenic stressors include hypoxia, radiation, hypothermia, infections, nutritional deficiencies and drug intake. The most significant among these is hypoxia, which results in various degrees of injury to the developing nervous system.

Adaptive requirements during the intrapartum period and the following postpartum days make this brief stage especially stressing, particularly in infants delivered prematurely.

In basic respects the physiologic and biochemical changes in old age are akin to chronic disease processes, both of which are characterized by a progressive weakening and eventual failure of homeostatic mechanisms. As such, the geriatric patient has limited adaptability and is extremely vulnerable to physiologic stress.

There appears to be an interdependent relationship among the various theories of aging. In the autoimmune theory, cross-linkage theory, and free radical theory, it is not clear whether the respective effects are causes or results of aging. The stress theory and radiation theory offer concepts that may be considered more causative, at least from the standpoint of initiating characteristic aging processes.

Universal physiologic changes in aging include various degrees of cardiovascular degeneration, osteoarthritis, osteoporosis, immune insufficiency, compromised gastrointestinal function, diminished pulmonary and renal reserves, and an impairment of vision, hearing, and memory. In addition, there often is fat accumulation, muscle-wasting, and emotional depression.

An especially dreaded complication of aging is senile dementia, primarily brought on by cerebral hypoxia, which in turn is caused by arteriosclerotic ischemia.

The use of hyperbaric oxygen, vitamins, antioxidants, antidepressants, vasodilators, and hormonal preparations has shown varied success in alleviating poor health associated with aging. Preventive measures earlier in life may prove to be more effective in preserving health in old age.

Chapter Glossary

antepartum   preceding childbirth

autophagocytic   refers to enzymes released by a cell that digests some of its own materials

basal ganglia   cerebral nuclei that relay information associated with fine muscular control

cerebral palsy   persisting motor disorder appearing in infancy; due to fetal brain damage from hypoxia

chemotherapy   the use of strong chemicals (drugs) in treating disease. The term is especially used in reference to the use of drugs in treating cancer.

diverticulosis   the development of pouches or sacs created by herniation of the intestinal mucous membrane

encephalic   pertaining to the brain

hiatal hernia   protrusion of any structure through the esophageal opening of the diaphragm

intrapartum   the period of childbirth

lymphoblasts   the developing, germinative stage of lymphocytes

macromolecules   materials of huge molecular weight such as nucleic acids and proteins

meningitis   inflammation of the three membranes that envelope the spinal cord and brain

neonatal   newborn

perinatal   pertains to the period of childbirth and the week following

spina bifida   an anomaly occurring during embryonic development in which the bony encasement of the spinal cord fails to close

For Further Reading

Bergsma, D. 1973. *Birth defects, atlas and compendium.* Baltimore: Williams and Wilkins Co.

Buell, S. J., and Coleman, P. D. 1979. Dendritic growth in the aged human brain and failure of growth in senile dementia. *Science* 206:854.

Exton-Smith, A. N., and Overstall, P. W. 1979. Geriatrics. In *Guidelines in medicine.* Vol. 1. Baltimore: University Park Press.

Finch, C. E., and Hayflick, L., eds. 1977. *Handbook of the biology of aging.* New York: Van Nostrand Reinhold Co.

Gershon, S., and Raskin, A., eds. 1975. Genesis and treatment of psychologic disorders in the elderly. In *Aging.* Vol. 2. New York: Raven Press.

Groer, M. E., and Shekleton, M. E. 1979. *Basic pathophysiology, a conceptual approach.* St. Louis: C. V. Mosby Co. Chapt. 18.

Gropp, A., and Benirschke, K., eds. 1976. *Developmental biology and pathology.* New York: Springer-Verlag.

Kalter, H. 1968. *Teratology of the central nervous system.* Chicago: University of Chicago Press.

Kanungo, M. S. 1980. *Biochemistry of aging.* New York: Academic Press.

Kellogg, C.; Tervo, D.; Ison, J.; et al. 1980. Prenatal exposure to diazepam alters behavioral development in rats. *Science* 207:205.

Mangos, J. A., and Talamo, R. C., eds. 1979. *Fundamental problems of cystic fibrosis and related diseases.* Chicago: Year Book Medical Publishers. Times Mirror.

Marx, J. L. 1979. Hormones and their effects in the aging body. *Science* 206: 805.

Moore, K. L. 1974. *Before we are born.* Philadelphia: W. B. Saunders Co.

Nandy, K., and Sherwin, I., eds. 1977. *The aging brain and senile dementia.* New York: Plenum Press.

Nelson, W. E.; Vaughan, V. C.; and McKay, R. J. 1979. *Textbook of pediatrics.* 11th ed. Philadelphia: W. B. Saunders Co.

Perl, D. P., and Brody, A. R. 1980. Alzheimer's disease: X-ray spectrometric evidence of aluminum accumulation in neurofibrillary tangle-bearing neurons. *Science* 208:297.

Persaud, T. V. N., ed. 1979. Advances in the study of birth defects. In *Teratogenic mechanisms.* Vol. 1. Baltimore: University Park Press.

Rockstein, M., and Chesky, J. 1974. *Theoretical aspects of aging.* New York: Academic Press.

Rockstein, M., and Sussman, M. 1979. *Biology of aging.* Belmont, Calif: Wadsworth, Inc.

Shephard, R. J. 1979. *Physical activity and aging.* Chicago: Year Book Medical Publishers. Times Mirror.

Smith, D., and Berwin, E., eds. 1973. *The biologic ages of man.* Philadelphia: W. B. Saunders Co.

Thorbecke, J., ed. 1975. *Biology of aging and development.* New York: Plenum Press.

Timeras, P. S. 1972. *Developmental physiology and aging.* New York: Macmillan Publishing Co.

Wilson, J., and Clarke-Fraser, F., eds. 1977. *Handbook of teratology.* New York: Plenum Publishing Co.

Appendix A
Disease Finder

    In this book discussions of various diseases are scattered about in accordance with the stressors that contribute to their development, rather than grouped in respect to the system or part of the body affected. The following diseases or groups of disorders (50) are listed in approximate order of their importance, and the chapter(s) in which information on the condition can be found is (are) designated. When more than one chapter is cited, the first number in bold print identifies the chapter giving primary attention to the topic.

Disorder	Chapter(s)
Heart disease	5, 17
Atherosclerosis	5, 17
Hypertension	5, 8, 17
Cancer (all forms)	5, 6, 13, 14, 17
Diabetes mellitus (general)	4
Diabetes (adult-onset)	12
Diabetes (juvenile-onset)	15
Infectious diseases	15
Emphysema	9, 13, 14
Allergies (except food)	15, 17
Food allergies	12
Kidney disease	11
Malnutrition	11
Anemias	9
Asthma	9, 7, 17, 18
Arthritis	15
Obesity	12
Alcoholism	14
Hearing loss	8
Mental illness	17
Autoimmune diseases	15
Multiple sclerosis	15
Neuroses	16
Depression	17
Hyperlipidemia	5, 11

Appendix B

Normal Adult Ranges for Clinical Laboratory Determinations

Cardiovascular (at rest)

Heart rate (beats/min)	48–90
Cardiac output (l/min)	3.5–6.0
Heart stroke volume (ml)	60–90
Vascular resistance (torr/l/min)	12–22
Systolic blood pressure (torr)	90–140
Diastolic blood pressure (torr)	50–90

Pulmonary

Vital capacity (l.)	3–6
Forced expiratory volume—1 sec (l.)	2.1–4.9
Maximum expiratory flow rate (l./sec)	5–11
Maximal midexpiratory flow (l./sec)	3–6
Oxygen consumption (l./min) (at rest)	0.1–0.4
Arterial-venous oxygen difference (vol %) (at rest)	3–5

Hematology

Red blood cell count (millions/mm^3)	4.0–6.0
White blood cell count (thousands/mm^3)	4.8–10.8
Platelet count (thousands/mm^3)	200–300
Hemoglobin content (g/dl)	12–18
Hematocrit (%)	36–52
Mean red cell volume (μ^3)	80–100
Mean cell hemoglobin ($\mu\mu$g)	27–31
Mean cell hemoglobin concentration (%)	32–36
Segmented leukocytes (%)	45–75
Lymphocytes (%)	25–45
Monocytes (%)	2–8
Eosinophils (%)	0–6
Basophils (%)	0–1
Reticulocytes (%)	0.6–2.5
Sedimentation rate (mm/hr)	0–10
Haptoglobin (mg/dl)	100–300

Urine

Glomerular filtration rate (ml/min)	110–140
pH	5.0–7.5
Specific gravity	1.01–1.03
Aldosterone (mcg/day)	2–23
Ammonia (mg/day)	500–1200
Calcium (mg/day)	100–300
Creatinine (mg/day)	1000–1800
Lactic acid (mg/day)	100–300
Magnesium (mg/day)	50–200
Nicotinamide (mg/day)	0.1–1.0
Total nitrogen (g/day)	12–18
Phosphorus (g/day)	1.0–1.2
Potassium (g/day)	1–3
Sodium (g/day)	3–5
Urea (g/day)	20–35
Uric acid (mg/day)	580–1000
17-ketosterioids (mg/day)	6–20

Blood Chemistry

Androgens (men) (μg/dl)	60–140
Ascorbic acid (mg/dl)	0.1–2.5
Bilirubin (total) (mg/dl)	0.2–1.2
Calcium (mg/dl)	8.6–11.0
Total cholesterol (mg/dl)	120–300
HDL cholesterol (mg/dl)	35–80
LDL cholesterol (mg/dl)	60–190
Corticosteroids (μg/dl)	6–25
Creatinine (mg/dl)	0.7–1.5
Total fatty acids (mg/dl)	250–390
Fibrinogen (g/dl, plasma)	0.3–0.6
Glucose (fasting) (mg/dl)	70–110
Iron (μg/dl)	70–105
Lactic acid (mmole/l)	0.3–1.3
Oxygen content, arterial (vol %)	16–22
Oxygen content, venous (vol %)	12–16
PO_2, arterial (torr)	80–98
PO_2, venous (torr)	30–45
pH, arterial	7.36–7.44

Blood Chemistry, cont.

pH, venous	7.28–7.35
Potassium (mg/dl)	14–22
Albumin (g/dl)	3.5–5.0
Pyruvic acid (mg/dl)	0.5–1.0
Sodium (mg/dl)	300–355
Triglycerides (mg/dl)	10–150
Urea nitrogen (mg/dl)	7–24
Uric acid (mg/dl)	3–8
Nicotinamide (mg/dl)	0.03–0.15
Tocopherols (vitamin E) (mg/dl)	0.5–1.9
Zinc (μg/dl)	175–900
T_3 (%)	25–35
Thyroxin (T_4) (μg/dl)	4–11
Phosphorus (mg/dl)	2.5–4.5
Total protein (g/dl)	6–8
Enzymes: Alkaline phosphatase (mμ/ml)	30–85
Glutamic oxalacetic transaminase (SGOT) (mμ/ml)	7–40
Lactic dehydrogenase (mμ/ml)	100–220

Color Plates

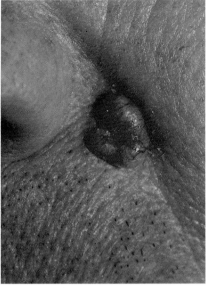

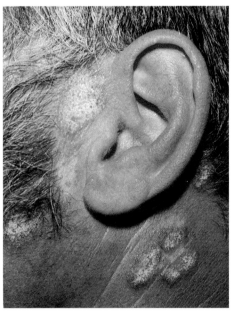

Plate 1 Basal cell carcinoma (see page 120)

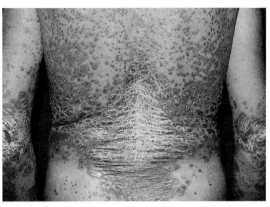

Plate 2 Psoriasis (see page 124)

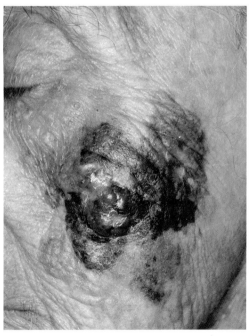

Plate 3 Discoid lupus erythematosus (see page 127)

Plate 4 Lentigo maligna melanoma (see page 133)

Plate 6 Allergic contact dermatitis (to neosporin-impregnated gauze) (see page 394)

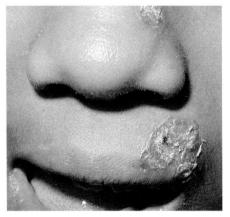

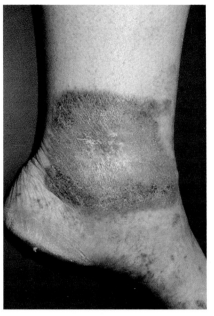

Plate 5 Impetigo (see page 385)

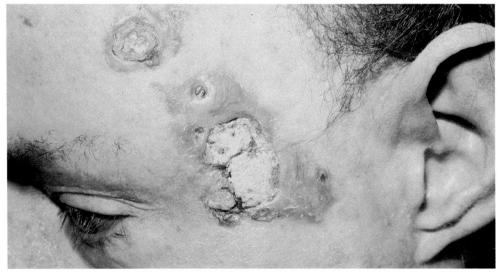

Plate 7 Scleroderma—calcinosis cutis; a collagen disease (see page 403)

Glossary

abscess—severe inflammation localized within solid tissue, characterized by purulent discharge

acclimation—process of becoming adapted or adjusted to environmental conditions or changes

acetate—organic molecule derived from oxidation of nutrient; in this form it enters the Krebs cycle

acetylcholine—a major neurotransmitter, particularly active in transmitting parasympathetic impulses

acidosis—elevated hydrogen ion concentration in the blood, may be derived from respiratory or metabolic disorders

acromegaly—thickening and overgrowth of tissue of the face and hands due to oversecretion of growth hormone in adulthood

ACTH—adrenocorticotropin; pituitary hormone that stimulates the adrenal cortex

acute—developing rapidly and running a short course

adenohypophysis—the anterior lobe of the pituitary

ADH—antidiuretic hormone secreted from the posterior lobe of the pituitary

adipose—fatty; relating to fat tissue

adrenalin—British term for epinephrine

adrenal steroids—hormones secreted by the adrenal cortex

adrenergic—nerve fibers that secrete norepinephrine

affective disorders—mood disturbances such as mania and depression

afferent—nerve impulses conducted inward from receptors to centers

agonist—a positive effector or promoter

aldosterone—steroid hormone from adrenal cortex that regulates electrolyte balance

allergenic—capable of initiating an allergic reaction

amino acid—structural subunit of proteins

amphetamine—drug that enhances transmission of catecholamine-mediated synapses in the brain

amygdala—almond-shaped group of neural nuclei comprising part of the limbic system of the brain

anaerobic—without oxygen

analgesic—an agent that alleviates pain

anaphylaxis—hypotensive shock reaction produced by sensitization to foreign protein

anemia—a decreased concentration of hemoglobin and red blood cells

anemic hypoxia—insufficient oxygenation due to a deficiency in functional hemoglobin

aneurysm—a weakened, bulging wall of a blood vessel

angina pectoris—chest pain caused by inadequate blood perfusion of the heart muscle

angiopathy—progressive disease of the capillaries

angiotensin I—small blood polypeptide generated by action of renin on angiotensinogen

angiotensin II—octapeptide formed from angiotensin I; it stimulates secretion of aldosterone

anorexia—abnormal loss of appetite for food

antagonist—something opposing or resisting the action of another material

antepartum—preceding childbirth

antibody—specialized plasma protein (immunoglobulin) capable of combining with specific antigen

antidiuresis—an effect resulting in decreased output of urine

antigen—foreign protein or protein-complex capable of stimulating a specific immune response

antihistamine—chemical that blocks the action of histamine

antioxidant—a substance interfering with oxygen combining with other materials

arrhythmia—distinct variation from normal heartbeat rhythm

articular—pertaining to a joint

asphyxia—suffocation from lack of oxygen

asthma—disorder in which there are paroxysms of bronchospasm and plugging of the airways with mucus

ataxia—staggering, uncontrolled locomotion

atherosclerosis—thickening of arterial walls with plaques of cholesterol, connective tissue, and abnormal smooth muscle cells

atopic allergy—hypersensitive reactions involving IgE antibodies and release of vasoactive mediators such as histamine

ATP—adenosine triphosphate, the compound that supplies energy for all cellular utilization

atrophy—a shrinkage or wasting of tissues or organs

autoimmune disease—damage from the body's immune reaction to its own tissues

baroreceptor—receptor sensitive to change in pressure; e.g. blood pressure

basal ganglia—cerebral nuclei that relay information associated with fine muscular control

basal metabolic rate (BMR)—minimum energy expenditure required to maintain life

bilirubin—yellowish bile pigment resulting from heme breakdown

blood-brain barrier—membrane-complex providing some degree of separation of brain circulation from the regular blood system

bone marrow depression—diminished production and maturation of erythrocytes and granulocytes

brain stem—brain subdivision consisting of medulla, pons, and midbrain; located between the spinal cord and cerebrum

bulk flow—movement of fluid or gas along a pressure gradient produced by force

Calorie—unit for measuring heat energy; amount of heat required to raise 1 liter of water 1 C

cancer—an uncontrolled growth of cells

cardiac output—volume of blood pumped by each ventricle per minute

catabolism—the phases of metabolism in which complex cellular substances are broken down to simpler form

cataract—opaque development of the lens of the eye

catecholamines—hormones such as epinephrine secreted by the adrenal medulla

cell-mediated immunity—a specific type of immune response mediated by T lymphocytes

cerebral cortex—the outermost cellular layer of gray matter covering the cerebrum

cerebral palsy—persisting motor disorder due to hypoxic brain damage

chelation—the combining or sequestering of a metallic ion into a ring form

cholesterol—a steroid carried in the blood; a precursor of steroid hormones and bile acids

cholinergic—nerve fibers that release acetylcholine

chronic—a slowly developing condition running a prolonged course

cobalamine—vitamin B_{12}

cochlea—the fluid-filled inner ear containing the organ of Corti

celiac—pertaining to abdominal viscera

colic—spasmotic pain in the abdomen

coliform—bacteria resembling the common intestinal inhabitant, *Escherichia coli*

colitis—inflammation of the colon

collagen—a fibrous protein abundant in connective tissue

coma—a deep state of unconsciousness from which one cannot be aroused

contraindication—a drug or administration that is not only inappropriate but may also be harmful

contusion—a bruise

coronary artery—artery branching from the aorta that supplies blood to the heart muscle; one to five vessels can be involved

coronary bypass—use of artery substitutes to bypass diseased coronary arteries

cortisol—glucocorticoid hormone from the adrenal cortex that responds to stress

creatinine—nitrogenous derivative of creatine phosphate that is excreted in the urine

cyanosis—dark, bluish coloration of skin and mucous membranes due to deficient oxygen in the blood

cyclic AMP (cAMP)—nucleotide within cells that serves as a second messenger for numerous nonsteroid hormones

cytotoxic—agent capable of deranging or damaging cellular organization

deamination—removal of amino group (NH_2) from an amino acid

degenerative—involving progressive loss of cellular organization

deoxyhemoglobin—hemoglobin not associated with oxygen

depressant—agent that lowers functional nervous activity

desensitization—frequent injection of small amount of antigen in order to reduce response of histamine

desquamation—a scaling off; e.g. a loss of squamous epithelium

diabetes insipidus—a disease caused by deficient secretion of ADH, characterized by increased thirst and urine output

diabetes mellitus—a disease characterized by imbalances of insulin and glucagon in which the utilization of glucose is impaired

diabetogenic—substance or condition capable of significantly elevating blood glucose

diastole—the period between ventricular contractions

2,3-diphosphoglycerate (DPG)—a substance in red blood cells that enhances dissociation of oxygen from hemoglobin

diuretic—any substance stimulating kidney action and urine excretion

diverticulosis—pouches or sacs created by herniation of intestinal mucous membrane

dopamine—an important brain neurotransmitter implicated in such diseases as schizophrenia and Parkinson's disease

dyspnea—difficulty in breathing

edema—accumulation of excessive amounts of fluid in cells and tissues

efferent—nerve impulses from centers conducted outward to effectors

electrical skin resistance—impedance to electrical conduction along skin surface

electrocardiogram (ECG)—a recording of electrical changes in the heart muscle during the cardiac cycle

electroencephalogram (EEG)—a recording of electrical changes in the cerebrum of the brain

electrolytes—ions in solution in the body fluids

electromyograph (EMG)—measurement of electrical change in muscle tension

embolism—obstruction or occlusion of a vessel

emphysema—a degenerative disease of the lungs in which alveoli break down and air flow is obstructed

encephalic—pertaining to the brain

end-diastolic volume—volume of cardiac blood just before ventricles contract

endorphins—a group of peptides of the brain and pituitary that act as neurotransmitters, neuromodulators, and hormones

eosinopenia—diminished numbers of eosinophiles in the blood

epinephrine—a catecholamine derived from tyrosine that is secreted by the adrenal medulla

erythema—inflammatory redness of the skin due to congested capillaries

erythropoiesis—production of new red blood cells and hemoglobin in the bone marrow

etiology—the causes, precipitating factors, and methods of introducing disease

euphoria—an exaggerated sense of well-being

exacerbation—an enhancement, such as an increase in severity of a condition

fetus—the developing organism during the second and third trimesters of pregnancy; from about the second or third month until birth

fibrillation—rapid, unsynchronized contractions of cardiac muscle

fibrinolysis—the dissolving of insoluble fiber making up blood clots

flatulence—distention of the gastrointestinal tract with gas

free radical—atom or groups of atoms having at least one unpaired electron; extremely reactive chemically

gallstone—a precipitate of cholesterol in the gall bladder or bile duct

gamma-amino butyric acid (GABA)—an inhibitory neurotransmitter

gamma globulin—immunoglobulin G (IgG), the most common antibody

gangrene—necrotic tissue undergoing microbial decomposition

gastroenteritis—inflammation of the stomach and intestines

glomerular filtration rate—the volume of fluid filtered from the kidney capillaries per minute or per 24 hours

glomerulus—specialized capillary in each Bowman's capsule of the kidney that performs filtration

glucagon—polypeptide hormone secreted by the alpha cells of the pancreatic islets; promotes elevation in blood glucose

gluconeogenesis—new formation of glucose in the liver from keto acids, pyruvate, lactate, and glycerol

glycolysis—anaerobic degradation of glucose to two molecules of lactic acid; occurs in the cell cytoplasm

goiter—chronic enlargement of the thyroid gland

growth hormone—large polypeptide secreted by the anterior pituitary; also known as somatotropic hormone (STH)

hair cells—mechanoreceptors in the organ of Corti of the inner ear

hallucinogen—a drug or agent that produces hallucinations

hapten—substance which becomes antigenic by coupling with larger molecules

heat exhaustion—collapse brought on by hypotension which results from depleted plasma volume caused by sweating and extreme vasodilation

heat stroke—when heat gain exceeds heat loss to the point that the thermoregulatory centers in the hypothalamus are incapable of preventing dangerous rises in body temperature

hematocrit—the percentage of whole blood that is cellular as opposed to plasma

hematoma—a small accumulation of blood within tissue

hematuria—the presence of red blood cells in the urine

hemoglobin—the ferroprotein of red blood cells that combines with oxygen in blood gas transport

hemostasis—the arrest of bleeding; blood-clotting

hernia—the protrusion of a structure through the wall of a cavity that normally contains it

Hertz (Hz)—the term used in measuring sound frequencies (cycles per second)

hiatal hernia—protrusion of a structure through the esophageal opening of the diaphragm

histamine—a potent mediator released from mast cells in inflammation; a vasodilator

hives—acute skin outbreak; urticaria

homeostasis—chemical and physical steady-state maintenance in living systems

humoral immunity—immune response performed by circulating antibodies

hydrophilic—substance attracted to water; water-soluble

17-hydroxycorticosteroids (17-OHCS)—hormones from the adrenal cortex

hypercapnia—excessive carbon dioxide in the blood

hyperemia—localized accumulation of blood

hyperglycemia—excessive levels of glucose in the blood

hyperinsulinemia—excessive levels of circulating insulin

hyperkinesis—abnormally increased motor activity

hyperlipidemia—excessive levels of cholesterol and triglycerides in the blood

hyperphagia—significantly increased intake of food; overeating

hyperplasia—enlargement of tissue due to number of cells

hypertension—high tension or pressure of circulating arterial blood; high blood pressure

hyperthermia—abnormally high body temperature

hypertrophy—an enlargement of organs or tissues

hyperventilation—a greater than usual rate and depth of breathing

hypervitaminosis—unfavorable reactions from high vitamin intake

hypervolemia—excessive extracellular fluid volume

hypobaric—significantly less atmospheric pressure than usual

hypoglycemia—an abnormally diminished level of blood glucose

hypokalemia—reduced levels of potassium in the body fluids

hypotension—lowered blood pressure

hypothalamus—a part of the brain responsible for regulating the internal environment through endocrine mediation and the autonomic nervous system

hypothermia—abnormally low body temperature

hypovolemia—decreased volume of extracellular fluid

hypoxia—an insufficient delivery of oxygen to tissue

iatrogenic—induced by medical treatment

idiopathic—disease of unknown, self-originated cause

immunoglobulin—plasma proteins that serve as antibodies

impotence—failure of erection of the penis

infarction—necrotic development resulting from occlusion of an artery

inflammation—tissue response to injury; characterized by vascular changes leading to redness, swelling, heat, and pain

innervation—a supply of functional nerve fibers

insulin—polypeptide hormone secreted by the beta cells of the pancreatic islets; promotes glucose utilization and the formation of fat and glycogen

interferon—a protein produced by the body that conveys nonspecific antiviral activity

internal environment—the extracellular fluid immediately surrounding cells of the body

intrapartum—the period of childbirth

intravenous (IV)—refers to solutions or drugs given through a vein

intrinsic factor—a glycoprotein secreted by the gastric mucosa that is necessary for absorption of vitamin B_{12}

in vitro—refers to investigations performed on test-tube preparations

in vivo—refers to investigations involving the intact, living organism

ischemia—insufficient blood supply

isometric contraction—muscle contraction in which tension develops but no shortening occurs because the opposing workload exceeds the tension

jaundice—a yellowish discoloration apparent in the skin and the whites of the eyes caused by an elevation of bilirubin in the blood

kallikrein—plasma enzyme that generates kinins such as bradykinin from their precursors

kernicterus—a condition in newborns caused by extreme elevation of bilirubin in the blood

keratin—a fibrous protein found in hair, nails, and skin epidermis

ketoacidosis—abnormally lowered blood pH due to an elevation of ketones in the blood; a complication of severe, uncontrolled diabetes mellitus

kilometer—a thousand meters; equivalent to about 3,300 feet or 1.6 miles

kinins—small polypeptides generated from plasma kininogen; a major kinin, bradykinin, is involved in inflammation

Krebs cycle—a very important metabolic pathway in mitochondria in which much energy is produced

labile—easily changeable; unstable

lactase—the enzyme that converts lactose to glucose and galactose

lactose—the disaccharide found in milk; milk sugar

lens—the adjustable component of the eye that permits appropriate focusing on the retina

lesion—a morbid change in the structure of cells, tissues, or organs

leucopenia—a substantial reduction in the number of white blood cells

limbic system—portion of the brain that mediates motivation and emotional expressions; includes the thalamus, amygdala, hippocampus, and hypothalamus

lipolysis—a breakdown of lipid stores

LSD—a potent hallucinogen

lung compliance—the elasticity of the lungs and chest wall

lymphoid tissue—includes the lymph nodes, thymus gland, spleen, tonsils, adenoids, and aggregates of lymphoid follicles as may be found associated with the liver and gastrointestinal tract

lysosome—a membrane-bound cell organelle containing digestive enzymes capable of breaking down bacteria, macromolecules, and damaged cell components

macrocytic—cells that are larger than usual

macromolecules—materials of huge molecular weight such as nucleic acids and proteins

macrophage—large white blood cells derived from monocytes that ingest foreign matter; phagocytes

malignant tumor—a mass of rapidly dividing cells that invade surrounding tissues, disrupting their function and eventually causing death of the organism

malnutrition—faulty nutrition; imbalanced food intake; can be deficient or excessive

mania—an emotional disorder characterized by great excitement, activity, exultation, and inability to concentrate and exercise judgment

mast cell—a connective-tissue cell that synthesizes and releases histamine

meningitis—inflammation of the three membranes (meninges) that envelope the spinal cord and brain

menopause—the cessation of menstrual cycling, usually appearing by the mid-40s

metabolism—the sum of the chemical changes throughout the body, especially those involving energy

metabolites—compounds degraded from key chemical substances in the body

metastasis—the breaking away of cancer cells from the parent tumor and their spread to other regions of the body

microthrombosis—occlusion of small blood vessels by blood clots

micturition—urination

mitochondria—cell organelles that are specialized for carrying out energy production and transformation

mitral valve—the valve between the left atrium and left ventricle of the heart

monoamine oxidase—an enzyme that degrades catecholamines into inactive substances

morbidity—the ratio of sick to well persons in a given population

mortality—the ratio of the number of deaths to a given population

mucosa—mucous membrane of epithelium lining such structures as the gastrointestinal tract, trachea, etc.

mutagen—a substance capable of inducing mutations

myasthenia gravis—a neuromuscular disease due to decreased acetylcholine reception at the motor end-plate of motor nerves; suspected of having an autoimmune basis

myelin—phospholipid sheath covering the axons of many neurons

myocardium—the muscle that forms the walls of the heart

myoglobin—a ferroprotein of skeletal muscle that binds oxygen; similar to hemoglobin

narcolepsy—a condition marked by a frequent, uncontrollable desire for sleep

necrosis—cell or tissue death resulting from irreversible damage

negative feedback—when the effect produced by a control system counteracts further action from the original stimulus

negative nitrogen balance—when protein catabolism exceeds protein anabolism

neonatal—newborn

nephrosclerosis—disease of the renal arteries in which the blood vessels harden

nervous breakdown—an ill-defined term indicating that emotional and nervous adjustments have failed temporarily

neuropathy—functional disturbance in the peripheral nerves; a complication of diabetes mellitus

neurosis—a functional nervous disorder of mental origin

neurotransmitter—a chemical that transmits nerve impulses from one neuron to another

niacin—nicotinic acid; one of the B complex vitamins

nocturia—the need to urinate during the night

norepinephrine—an important catecholamine neurotransmitter

normoglycemia—normal levels of blood sugar

noxious—harmful, injurious

obesity—an excessive accumulation of fat by the adipose tissues of the body

occlusion—a closing or blocking

oncogenic—tumor-producing

operant—refers to behavior that involves the operation of instrumentation

opiate—any substance having a sedative effect like opium

orthostatic—relating to or caused by erect posture

ossicular chain—the series of 3 tiny bones in the middle ear (malleus, incus, stapes)

oxidative phosphorylation—energy production and ATP formation in the mitochondria from the combining of oxygen with hydrogen

oxyhemoglobin—hemoglobin combined with oxygen

P wave—the point of the electrocardiogram reflecting depolarization of the atria

pain—sensation resulting from tissue injury that is accompanied and enhanced by emotional activation

pantothenic acid—one of the B complex vitamins

palpitation—perceptible awareness of the beating of the heart; often an increased cardiac rate that is annoying

parasympathetic—a division of the autonomic nervous system

parasympathomimetic—an agent that produces effects similar to those of parasympathetic nerves

parkinsonism—a disease characterized by tremor and rigidity in regard to control of motor function

partial pressure—the pressure or tension exerted by one gas present in a mixture of gases; e.g. the PO_2 (partial pressure of oxygen)

pathology—the study of disease

peptide—a short chain of amino acids

perfusion—supplying fluid such as blood through the bood vessels

perinatal—pertains to the period of childbirth and the week following

periosteal—pertains to two layers of fibrous tissue that form an elastic lining around bones

peripheral—situated at or near the outer portion of the body

peripheral thermoreceptors—warm and cold receptors in the skin

permissiveness—usually refers to a situation in which small amounts of one hormone enable another hormone to exert its full effect

pernicious anemia—a disease in which red blood cells do not multiply and mature normally because of a deficiency in vitamin B_{12}

petechial—refers to small, reddish spots caused by submucosal hemorrhage

pH—a logarithmic scale measuring the acidity or alkalinity of solutions

phagocytosis—the engulfing of particles such as bacteria by cells such as white blood cells; a form of endocytosis

photodissociation—chemical decomposition of substances due to exposure to light

pituitary—a major endocrine gland located just below the hypothalamus of the brain; sometimes known as the hypophysis

placebo—an inert substance in the form of a medicine given for the suggestive effect alone

plasma—the fluid portion of the circulating blood as opposed to the cellular content

platelet—cell fragment-like elements in the blood that play a role in blood-clotting

pneumoconiosis—a lung condition characterized by chronic fibrous reaction to dust inhalation

polycythemic—having significantly greater numbers of red blood cells than normal

polyoma—a virus that produces tumors in mice and hamsters

polyuria—frequent, excessive urination

positive feedback—a progressive increase or build-up in reactability due to the effect the action has in stimulating the system; a vicious cycle

postganglionic—the final efferent fiber of an autonomic nervous system pathway, running from a ganglion to an organ

postprandial—after a meal

precapillary arteriole—microscopic artery that introduces blood to a capillary bed

precursor—a preceding chemical stage or substrate

presynaptic—refers to the axon terminals of a nerve fiber which secrete neurotransmitters into the synapse

proprioceptive—neural stimulation originating from receptors in internal tissues

prostaglandins—a group of circulating chemical mediators derived from unsaturated fatty acids

proteinuria—protein in the urine; often in the form of albumin

pyrogen—a substance released from white blood cells in infection that induces an increase in body temperature by resetting hypothalamic thermoreceptors

pyruvic acid—a three-carbon intermediate in glycolysis

psychogenic—of mental origin

psychoneurosis—a nervous disorder of mental origin

psychosis—a severe mental disorder; mental illness

psychosocial—pertains to psychologic reactions prompted by social interactions

psychosomatic—a disorder in the body produced by the emotions

RAS—reticular activating system; pathways through the brain that arouse the cerebral cortex

reactive hypoglycemia—a significant reduction in postprandial blood glucose

reciprocal inhibition—when the function of one element of a dual system automatically inhibits the function of the other element

renal—pertaining to the kidney

renin—an enzyme secreted by the kidney that catalyzes angiotensinogen to angiotensin I; excessive amounts are implicated in the development of hypertension

respiratory chain—series of enzymes and substrates in the mitochondria that transports electrons to oxygen

respiratory distress syndrome—a disorder in premature infants in which there is insufficient alveolar surfactant

reticulocytes—newly produced red blood cells entering the circulation

reticuloendothelial—refers to connective tissue derivatives involved with blood cell production and the immune system

retinopathy—noninflammatory pathology of the retina; a complication of diabetes mellitus

rhinitis—inflammation of the nasal mucosa

riboflavin—vitamin B_2

rickets—a condition in which new bone matrix is inadequately calcified due to vitamin D deficiency; primarily restricted to children

rouleaux—plural of rouleau; a roll of cells, aggregated as if in a stack, like coins

schizophrenia—a mental disorder characterized by a progressive mental and emotional withdrawal from reality; hallucinations may be present

sedative—an agent or drug that quiets nervous excitement

senile—pertaining to old age, particularly the associated mental decline

serotonergic—nerve fibers that secrete serotonin

serotonin—(5-hydroxytryptamine), a neurotransmitter in the brain

serum—the fluid portion of the blood without the cells and the fibrin clot

shock—a rapid, pronounced decrease in the pressure of circulating blood

short-term memory—recall of recent events and experiences

sickle-cell anemia—an inherited disease in which one of the amino acids in the polypeptide chains of hemoglobin is different, resulting in distorted shapes of red blood cells

slough—the shedding of cells or tissue from the body; e.g. the shedding of dead, outer epidermal cells from the skin

slow virus—viruses that persist and replicate slowly, often becoming part of the host cell's own DNA; as such these viruses may stimulate autoimmune responses

somatic—pertains to the body, especially the solid framework of muscle, skin, skeleton, etc.

somatostatin—a hypothalamic hormone that inhibits secretions of growth hormone, thyroid-stimulating hormone, glucagon, and insulin

sound wave—a disturbance in the air resulting from variations in the density of air molecules, some regions having high density (pressure) and other regions having low density

spasm—intermittent involuntary muscle contractions; if painful they are referred to as cramps

specific dynamic action (SDA)—the increase in metabolism caused by eating

spina bifida—an anomaly occurring during embryonic development in which the bony encasement of the spinal cord fails to close

stasis—retardation or stoppage of normal flow or movement

stenosis—an abnormally restricted or narrowed opening

steroid—lipid molecules in which the carbons are arranged in four interconnected rings; hormones of the adrenal cortex and the gonads are steroids

stimulus—an environmental change that can be detected by a receptor

stress—a disturbance in steady state brought about by an environmental change; the disturbance must be counteracted to prevent further disorder in the system

stroke volume—the volume of blood pumped by a ventricle during one heart beat

subendocardium—tissue beneath the endothelial membrane of the heart

sulfhydryl group—a sulfur-hydrogen bonding, principally found in the amino acid, cysteine, essential for function in some enzymes

superinfections—rapid, uncontrolled growth of infective microbes

surfactant—a conjugated lipid produced by alveolar cells that counteracts surface tension in the lungs

sympathetic nervous system—a division of the autonomic nervous system that exerts widespread response throughout the body to sudden demands, threats, or changes in the environment

sympathoadrenomedullary—refers to the sympathetic nervous system and its stimulation of the adrenal medullae

sympathomimetic—produces same effect as (mimics) sympathetic nerve impulses

syncope—fainting; often due to a fall in blood pressure

synergistically—cooperative action from two or more agents such that the total effect exceeds the sum of the various individual effects

synovium—membrane lining a joint capsule

systemic—spread throughout the body as opposed to localized

systole—the period during which the ventricles are contracting

T cells—lymphocytes proliferating in lymphoid tissues from precursors that at one time were in the thymus gland

T wave—the point in the electrocardiogram that corresponds to repolarization of the ventricles

tachycardia—a rapid pulse exceeding 100 beats per minute

tectorial membrane—a structure associated with the receptor hairs in the organ of Corti of the inner ear

tetracycline—a broad-spectrum antibiotic

thalamus—an important part of the limbic system in which sensations, feelings, and emotional expressions are mediated

thermogenic—heat-producing

thiamine—vitamin B_1

thrombophlebitis—formation of blood clots in veins; brought about by inflammatory changes in the veins

thrombosis—occlusion of a blood vessel by a clot

thromboxanes—mediators that are chemically related to prostaglandins

thrombus—a clot or plug occurring in the bloodstream

thymus—a lymphoid structure located in the upper chest; secretes a hormone-like messenger called thymosin

thyroiditis—inflammation of thyroid tissue

thyroxin (T_4)—tetraiodothyronine, the major iodine-containing hormone secreted by the thyroid gland

topical—an application to a localized region of the body, usually the body surface

toxemia of pregnancy—a disorder occurring in pregnant women that is associated with fluid retention, hypertension, and proteinuria

toxin—a noxious or poisonous substance

trauma—injury; usually inflicted rather suddenly by some physical agent

tremor—shaking movement that is purposeless and uncontrolled; usually confined to the limbs

tricyclic antidepressants—drugs that elevate the mood by interfering with reuptake of norepinephrine at synapses; e.g. imipramine

triglycerides—neutral fats; the most common form of lipid in the body; found mostly in adipose cells, liver, and blood

triiodothyronine (T_3)—a thyroid hormone; not secreted as abundantly as T_4

ulcer—a lesion on the surface of the skin or mucous membranes caused by a superficial breakdown and loss of tissue

uremia—profound renal insufficiency characterized by pronounced azotemia and urea retention; kidney failure

uric acid—a nitrogenous waste product from the degradation of nucleic acids

vagal—refers to the vagus nerve, parasympathetic in action

varicose vein—a swollen, hyperdilated superficial vein of the lower extremities

vasoconstriction—decreased diameter of blood vessels brought about by smooth muscle contraction

vasodilator—an agent that promotes dilation of the blood vessels

vasomotor—neuromuscular regulation of the bore of blood vessels

vasopressin—antidiuretic hormone; another term for ADH

venipuncture—the withdrawing of blood from a vein, usually the antecubital vein; phlebotomy

venous return—the volume of blood entering the heart from the venous system per unit of time

ventilation—the movement of air in and out of the lungs

ventilation-perfusion ratio—ratio of volume of alveolar gas with the volume of capillary blood perfusing the lungs

vertigo—dizziness; a sensation of light-headedness

vesiculation—formation of blisters

visceral—refers to internal organs or structures suspended in the body cavity as opposed to the skeleton and skeletal muscles

virus—a nucleic acid core with a protein coat that behaves as a parasitic organism within living host cells

wavelength—the distance between two wave peaks in an oscillating medium

withdrawal—the unpleasant sensations and physical symptoms that occur following cessation of habitual drug use

Index